Nom
and C
Dia
Disease
and Gr

Nomenclature and Criteria for Diagnosis of Diseases of the Heart and Great Vessels

8th Edition

The Criteria Committee of the
New York Heart Association

M. Irené Ferrer, M.D., *Chairman*
Stanley E. Bradley, M.D.
Marcia B. Bull, M.D.
Martin Dolgin, M.D.
Kent Ellis, M.D.
Yale Enson, M.D.
Doris J. W. Escher, M.D.
Edward E. Fischel, M.D.
Arthur C. Fox, M.D.
Edward C. Franklin, M.D.
Sylvia P. Griffiths, M.D.
Réjane M. Harvey, M.D.
A. Gregory Jameson, M.D.
Arnold M. Katz, M.D.
Margaret M. Kilcoyne, M.D.
Marvin Kuschner, M.D.
Marianne J. Legato, M.D.
James R. Malm, M.D.

Little, Brown and Company
Boston

Eighth Edition

Library of Congress Catalog Card No. 78-71219

ISBN 0-316-60536-0 (C)

ISBN 0-316-60537-9 (P)

Printed in the United States of America

Sixth Edition, 1964

Diseases of the Heart and Blood Vessels:
Nomenclature and Criteria for Diagnosis

Fifth Edition, 1953

Nomenclature and Criteria for Diagnosis
of Diseases of the Heart and Blood Vessels

Fourth Edition, 1939

Nomenclature and Criteria for Diagnosis
of Diseases of the Heart

Third Edition, 1932
Second Edition, 1929
First Edition, 1928

Criteria for the Classification and Diagnosis
of Heart Disease

To

John Wyckoff, M.D.

who did much to develop
the New York Heart Association

Preface

It is now six years since the last (seventh) edition of the *Nomenclature and Criteria for Diagnosis of Diseases of the Heart and Great Vessels*, published in 1973, appeared. There has continued to be major extensive progress in the area of cardiology over this span, and the present edition has been revised and updated to conform with our continuously growing fund of knowledge. The basic structure of the work remains unchanged from the seventh edition since the success of this latter confirmed that the simplification effected in the seventh edition, as compared to previous editions, was warranted and well received.

The classification of the patient's overall Cardiac Status and Prognosis (which, in the seventh edition, replaced the old Functional and Therapeutic Classification) continues to be indicated in view of modern diagnostic techniques that have become capable of enlarging the concepts of a single diagnostic statement to include the stage of a disease as well as its name. Furthermore the interplay of the more specific medical and surgical therapies and their effects upon the basic disease picture must be part of modern cardiac appraisal. The use of this classification also recognizes the changing picture that may characterize the cardiac subject's performance and thus be a more practical and meaningful evaluation. Although it is difficult at times to relinquish an old and well-used method, a more vital and functional one, when it exists, is to be preferred.

The present Criteria Committee looks back with gratitude on the work of previous committees whose concepts, erudition, and devotion to clinical cardiology have made the *Criteria* the major reference work that it has been since its origin. Doctor Harold E. B. Pardee supervised its production for the first thirty years of its existence—a record of invaluable and devoted service. The present Committee therefore salutes his memory with this volume.

The Criteria Committee

Contents

Contents

Introduction

The **etiologic, anatomic,** and **physiologic** diagnosis of cardiovascular disease depend upon a careful analysis of the patient's history, a thorough physical examination, and, when indicated, a variety of laboratory examinations. Some of the latter are not specific for evaluation of the cardiovascular system, but represent an attempt to delineate the major problem. Others, such as electrocardiography, phonocardiography, echocardiography, cardiac catheterization, and a variety of radiologic techniques, are employed to detect the cause of heart disease or to identify specific anatomic and physiologic abnormalities.

The diagnostic categories are frequently dependent upon one another and, in the final synthesis, their compatibility should be examined.

The **etiology** of heart disease should be determined by considering both structural and functional disturbances. If two or more possible causes of heart disease are present, each should be mentioned. Chapter 1 delineates the etiologies of the known major structural and functional disorders of the heart, although the detailed mechanisms by which the various diseases ultimately affect the heart are not all completely understood.

Anatomic lesions of the heart and great vessels usually can be recognized clinically. In some instances their manifestations are so specific that the anatomic abnormality is easily identified. Frequently, however, the presence of a structural lesion is inferred from a recognition of the cause of the heart disease, the identification of a physiologic disturbance known to result from it, or both. More than one anatomic abnormality may be present in any one patient; each should be included in the anatomic diagnosis.

Different **physiologic** disturbances often have similar clinical manifestations; the identification of the cause of the disturbance may therefore rest upon knowledge of the etiologic or anatomic diagnoses. Frequently, more than one physiologic abnormality is present; all should be included in the physiologic diagnosis. If no disturbance is present, the physiologic diagnosis is simply: Normal Sinus Rhythm.

Each of the diagnostic items has been assigned a code number. The grading of **Cardiac Status** and **Prognosis** is also coded numerically.

A complete cardiac diagnosis should include one or more titles from each of the principal diagnostic categories of this nomenclature: **etiologic, anatomic, physiologic,** and **cardiac status** and **prognosis.** For example, a patient with rheumatic heart disease might have the following diagnoses:

Etiologic:	Rheumatic Fever, inactive
Anatomic:	Enlarged heart (left atrium, pulmonary artery, right ventricle), mitral valvular deformity
Physiologic:	Atrial fibrillation, mitral obstruction, pulmonary hypertension
Cardiac Status and Prognosis:	3.2

A patient with a patent ductus arteriosus might have the following diagnoses:

Etiologic:	Congenital Anomaly
Anatomic:	Patent ductus arteriosus, enlarged heart (left ventricle)
Physiologic:	Normal sinus rhythm, left to right shunt
Cardiac Status and Prognosis:	2.2

Certain patients may have symptoms, abnormal physical signs, or both which are referable to the heart, but which after detailed study cannot be ascribed with certainty to structural or functional cardiac disease. In such cases the diagnosis should be No Heart Disease, Unexplained Manifestation. Patients who have a disease such as systemic arterial hypertension, which can cause heart disease but which at the time of observation has not done so, are to be designated as having No Heart Disease, Predisposing Etiologic Factor (Systemic arterial hypertension).

Nomenclature and Criteria for Diagnosis of Diseases of the Heart and Great Vessels

The Etiologic Cardiac Diagnosis

1

NOMENCLATURE

1.1 Acromegaly
1.2 Alcoholism
1.3 Amyloidosis
1.4 Anemia
1.5 Ankylosing Spondylitis
1.6 Atherosclerosis
1.7 Carcinoid Tumor (Argentaffinoma)
1.8 Congenital Anomaly
1.9 Friedreich's Ataxia
1.10 Glycogen Storage Disease
1.11 Hemochromatosis
1.12 Hypersensitivity Reaction
1.13 Hypertension
1.14 Hyperthyroidism
1.15 Hypothyroidism
1.16 Infection
1.17 Marfan's Syndrome
1.18 Mucopolysaccharidoses
1.19 Neoplasm
1.20 Obesity
1.21 Polyarteritis Nodosa
1.22 Progressive Muscular Dystrophy
1.23 Progressive Systemic Sclerosis (Scleroderma)
1.24 Pulmonary Disease (Cor Pulmonale)
1.25 Reiter's Syndrome
1.26 Rheumatic Fever
1.27 Rheumatoid Arthritis
1.28 Sarcoidosis

1.29 Syphilis
1.30 Systemic Arteriovenous Fistula
1.31 Systemic Lupus Erythematosus
1.32 Toxic Agent
1.33 Trauma
1.34 Unknown
1.35 Uremia

CRITERIA

1.1 Acromegaly

Acromegaly is caused by the production of excess pituitary growth hormone after puberty, when significant linear growth of bones cannot occur. Overgrowth in the acral or distal parts of the body (hands, feet, head) is characteristic. The kidneys, liver, spleen, pancreas, adrenals, and tongue are usually enlarged. Associated endocrinopathies may include diabetes mellitus, persistent lactation, and increase in the production of 17-hydroxycorticosteroids. Multiple adenomas of endocrine glands are not unusual.

Cardiomegaly is common, especially in older patients. Heart weight well over a kilogram has been reported. Advanced coronary atherosclerosis and systemic hypertension frequently coexist. Hence, the cardiomegaly may be, in part, a result of associated hypertensive or atherosclerotic heart disease with ventricular failure. Dyspnea, fatigue, marked edema, and syncope are often the presenting symptoms. Electrocardiographic findings often include a diffuse intraventricular conduction defect or evidence of left ventricular hypertrophy.

THE FOLLOWING CRITERIA ARE REQUIRED FOR THE DIAGNOSIS OF HEART DISEASE DUE TO ACROMEGALY.

Enlargement of the heart with or without ventricular failure occurring in association with acromegaly and in the absence of coronary atherosclerosis and systemic hypertension.

1.2 Alcoholism

Chronic consumption of excessive amounts of ethyl alcohol can cause heart disease. In some alcoholic beverages, particularly beer, specific contaminants such as cobalt have been indicted as the cause of myocardial damage, but a direct effect of alcohol on the myocardium by unknown mechanisms is also suspected.

Among the symptoms of heart disease due to alcohol are palpitations resulting either from marked sinus tachycardia or ventricular irritability; more usually the symptoms result from ventricular failure. With the onset of ventricular failure, it is usual to find sinus tachycardia, arrhythmias, evidences of mitral regurgitation, or mural thrombi. Systemic and pulmonary embolization is common. Mild elevation of the systemic arterial diastolic blood pressure is frequent. Radiologic, electrocardiographic, or echocardiographic evidence of ventricular enlargement is almost invariably present. The syndrome must be differentiated from beriberi heart disease, which can occur in the alcoholic patient, but which is quickly improved by treatment with thiamine alone. The initial response to abstinence from alcohol and to therapy is often dramatic, but relapses occur with repeated use of alcohol.

THE FOLLOWING CRITERIA ARE REQUIRED FOR THE DIAGNOSIS OF HEART DISEASE DUE TO ALCOHOLISM.

The appearance of arrhythmias, cardiac enlargement, or ventricular failure in the course of chronic alcoholism and in the absence of other causes of heart disease, with the disappearance of these abnormalities after abstinence from alcohol.

1.3 Amyloidosis

Amyloidosis of the heart occurs as an isolated lesion, as part of systemic amyloid deposition, and in association with familial amyloidosis.

The isolated or senile variety is a common finding in elderly persons, but rarely produces clinical manifestations.

Systemic amyloidosis, known as secondary amyloidosis, may occur in association with chronic diseases such as rheumatoid arthritis and suppurative disease. Significant cardiac involvement is rare. Systemic amyloidosis also occurs in association with the dysproteinemias, and cardiac involvement is not infrequent in this form.

The cardiac amyloid deposition seen as a feature of primary familial amyloidosis becomes manifest in the fourth or fifth decade and is usually accompanied by evidence of involvement of the peripheral nerves and the kidneys.

Extensive infiltration of the heart by amyloid can lead to cardiomegaly, atrial arrhythmias, especially atrial fibrillation, conduction defects, low QRS–T voltage, and a reduction in myocardial compliance, with consequent interference with ventricular filling.

THE FOLLOWING CRITERIA ARE REQUIRED FOR THE DIAGNOSIS OF HEART DISEASE DUE TO AMYLOIDOSIS.

Evidence of amyloid in a biopsy specimen of skin, muscle, nerve, gum, rectal mucosa, or myocardium and one or more of the following: cardiac enlargement, disturbances in ventricular filling, atrial arrhythmias, conduction defects, or low QRS–T voltage.

1.4 Anemia

The concentration of oxyhemoglobin reflects the capacity of the blood to carry oxygen. With a decrease in hemoglobin, circulatory adjustments occur which may maintain adequate delivery of oxygen to the organs of the body. Although severe anemia, when prolonged, can lead to anatomic lesions in the heart, most of the circulatory changes encountered appear to stem from physiologic rather than structural alterations. In hereditary forms of chronic anemia, however, additional factors predispose to the development of heart diseases: in thalassemia major (Cooley's anemia), multiple blood transfusions result in hemosiderin deposition in the myocardium, and in sickle cell disease, pulmonary thromboses during crises promote the development of pulmonary hypertension.

Cardiovascular changes usually do not become evident until hemoglobin concentration is reduced by 40 percent or more. Cardiac output increases as peripheral resistance falls; coronary blood flow increases proportionately. Alterations in renal function can lead to retention of salt and water and an increase in plasma volume. Hence the circulating total blood volume can be within normal limits or only slightly above or below normal. Constriction of small veins can cause a shift of blood to the larger veins and the heart, with a consequent rise in their pressures and evidences of pulmonary and systemic congestion. Dilatation of the heart is a characteristic finding. Dyspnea can result from anemia alone and does not necessarily indicate the presence of pulmonary congestion. Other symptoms attributable to anemia are palpitations, weakness, and dizzy spells. Systolic and diastolic murmurs of any variety can occur.

Heart disease due to anemia is reversible; the signs and symptoms of congestion and cardiac dilatation should disappear with successful treatment of the anemia, and the cardiac output should fall.

The circulatory adjustments associated with anemia can also induce or aggravate the manifestations of ventricular failure or coronary insufficiency in patients with other forms of heart disease.

THE FOLLOWING CRITERIA ARE REQUIRED FOR THE DIAGNOSIS OF HEART DISEASE DUE TO ANEMIA.

Dilatation of the heart with or without congestion of the circulation in the presence of marked anemia.

1.5 Ankylosing Spondylitis (Marie-Strümpell Disease)

Ankylosing spondylitis, a chronic disease of the apophyseal joints of the spine, the sacroiliac joints, and the adjacent soft tissues, occurs chiefly in young males. It may progress to cause immobilization of the spine (poker spine) and involve the hips, shoulders, and costovertebral articulations. There is a high incidence of the tissue typing antigen HLA 27 in this disease. Inflammation and scarring of the ascending aorta occur with this disease and can produce aortic regurgitation.

THE FOLLOWING CRITERIA ARE REQUIRED FOR THE DIAGNOSIS OF HEART DISEASE DUE TO ANKYLOSING SPONDYLITIS.

Aortic regurgitation in the presence of ankylosing spondylitis and the absence of other causes of regurgitation.

1.6 Atherosclerosis

Structural or functional abnormalities of the myocardium can result from an inadequate blood supply due to atherosclerosis of the coronary arteries.

The specific etiology of coronary atherosclerosis is not known, but multiple contributing factors have been identified. Aberrations in lipid metabolism may influence the development of atherosclerotic lesions. The hyperlipoproteinemias associated with atherosclerosis are types II, III, and IV. Type II, or familial hypercholesterolemia, is characterized by markedly elevated serum cholesterol, normal or slightly elevated serum triglycerides, and an increased β-lipoprotein. Types III and IV are characterized by normal or moderately elevated serum cholesterol, elevated serum triglycerides, and an increased pre-β-lipoprotein; these abnormalities can be induced by dietary fat or carbohydrate. In some patients these conditions appear to be genetically determined.

Other systemic factors that may contribute to the development of atherosclerosis include endocrine disorders and disease states such as diabetes mellitus and systemic hypertension. Within the arterial wall itself, abnormalities in the metabolism of lipid, carbohydrate, protein, and mucopolysaccharide may be important. Diet, tobacco smoking, and emotional stress have also been implicated in the pathogenesis of coronary atherosclerosis.

The finding of slight to moderate coronary atherosclerosis by arteriography does not necessarily implicate atherosclerosis as the sole cause for existing heart disease. Regional ischemia can result in myocardial infarction or a variety of physiologic abnormalities: anginal syndrome, arrhythmias, conduction disturbances, papillary muscle dysfunction, ventricular asynergy, and ventricular failure. The size of the heart is usually normal or only slightly increased unless there has been coexistent systemic hypertension or ventricular failure.

The incidence of atherosclerotic heart disease is low in premenopausal females who do not have systemic hypertension or diabetes mellitus and is high in middle-aged males. The disease is not infrequent in young adult males, especially when there is a genetic or metabolic predisposition. Sudden death is frequent among patients with atherosclerotic heart disease, especially as a consequence of acute myocardial infarction or ventricular arrhythmias.

ONE OF THE FOLLOWING CRITERIA IS REQUIRED FOR THE DIAGNOSIS OF HEART DISEASE DUE TO CORONARY ATHEROSCLEROSIS.

1. **Anginal syndrome in the absence of aortic valvular disease, coronary ostial stenosis, or coronary arteritis.**
2. **Myocardial infarction in the absence of other obvious cause.**
3. **Ventricular failure, or arrhythmias, or conduction defects occurring in the absence of other cause in a patient in whom significant coronary narrowing is demonstrable by coronary arteriography.**

1.7 Carcinoid Tumor (Argentaffinoma)

Malignant carcinoid tumor, arising usually in the gastrointestinal tract, can produce a variety of symptoms once metastasis to the liver has occurred. These symptoms include flushing, palpitations, abdominal pain, diarrhea, and wheezing. Cardiac involvement is primarily, although not exclusively, right-sided. The manifestations of carcinoid are related to the release of serotonin (5-hydroxytryptamine) and other bioactive substances from the tumor. Serotonin is metabolized to 5-hydroxyindoleacetic acid (5 HIAA), which is excreted in the urine. Increased levels of urinary 5 HIAA are the basis of the diagnostic test for carcinoid. The proteolytic enzyme kallikrein, one of the bioactive substances released by the tumor, acts on a substrate of hepatic origin, kininogen, to produce vasodilator kinins, including bradykinin. Bradykinin and prostaglandins, which have also been found in these tumors, may be responsible for flushing, vasodilatation, and bronchoconstriction. Serotonin may be the cause of intestinal hypermobility.

Serotonin secreted by the liver metastases into the hepatic vein is the source of high blood levels of the tumor substances in the circulating blood. Endocardial lesions involving the tricuspid and pulmonic valves and the inner surfaces of the right heart chambers can result from the effect of these substances on endocardial fibroblasts. The resulting fibrosis of the valves and chordae tendineae can cause pulmonic obstruction and tricuspid regurgitation or obstruction. Endocardial fibrosis can limit ventricular filling. Serotonin is partly inactivated in the lung by monoamine oxidase. Rarely these tumors arise in the bronchial tree or metastasize to the lung and thus produce left-sided (mitral and aortic) valvular fibrosis.

THE FOLLOWING CRITERIA ARE REQUIRED FOR THE DIAGNOSIS OF HEART DISEASE DUE TO CARCINOID TUMOR.

Structural lesions of the pulmonic or tricuspid valves and evidence of metastatic carcinoid tumor in the liver.

1.8 Congenital Anomaly

Congenital cardiovascular defects result when genetic or environmental factors (intrauterine infection, metabolic disorders, drugs, irradiation) interfere with normal development of the heart and great vessels.

The criteria for diagnosis of a specific congenital anomaly are based on characteristic physical signs associated with electrocardiographic, echocardiographic, or radiologic abnormalities. In most instances, additional data must be obtained from angiocardiography or cardiac catheterization before definitive diagnosis is possible. Congenital cardiovascular anomalies are usually first manifested in infancy.

1.9 Friedreich's Ataxia

Friedreich's ataxia is a familial and hereditary neurologic disease characterized by progressive degeneration of the posterior columns and the spinocerebellar and pyramidal tracts of the spinal cord. It is manifested by unsteadiness of gait and hyporeflexia; pes cavus and scoliosis are frequent. Cardiac involvement is not unusual.

The onset of Friedreich's ataxia is insidious. In half the cases, symptoms are present by the age of 10 years and in the remainder, by early adult life. Generally, the neurologic manifestations occur first and predominate, but occasionally the discovery of a systolic murmur along the upper left sternal border or the appearance of ventricular failure can be the first indication of disease.

Electrocardiographic abnormalities are usually the earliest sign of cardiac involvement; S–T changes and T wave inversion occur, particularly in leads II, III, aVF, and over the left precordium. Arrhythmias are not uncommon in the advanced stages of the disease. Cardiomegaly is a late development.

THE FOLLOWING CRITERIA ARE REQUIRED FOR THE DIAGNOSIS OF HEART DISEASE DUE TO FRIEDREICH'S ATAXIA.

Electrocardiographic abnormalities or cardiomegaly occurring in the presence of Friedreich's ataxia.

1.10 Glycogen Storage Disease

Although there are at least six different heritable disorders of glycogen deposition, the heart is involved to a major extent only in that form of generalized glycogenosis known as Pompe's disease. This rare recessive disease is due to a lysosomal deficiency of alpha-1,4-glucosidase (acid maltase). Progressive cardiomegaly is associated with left ventricular failure due to infiltration of the myocardium with replacement of contractile units and other organelles of the myocardial cell by glycogen, and to ventricular outflow obstruction, which usually causes death in the first year of life. The infant may show macroglossia and poor skeletal muscle tone. Murmurs, if present, are inconspicuous, although a systolic ejection murmur at the base sometimes suggests left ventricular outflow obstruction. The electrocardiogram may show a P–R interval at the lower limits of normal and evidence of left ventricular enlargement.

THE FOLLOWING CRITERIA ARE REQUIRED FOR THE DIAGNOSIS OF HEART DISEASE DUE TO GLYCOGEN STORAGE DISEASE.

Cardiac enlargement with either biochemical evidence of cellular alpha-1,4-glucosidase deficiency or histologic evidence of excessive glycogen deposition in a skeletal muscle biopsy specimen.

1.11 Hemochromatosis

The heart disease associated with hemochromatosis results from excess deposition of iron in the myocardium, with consequent fibrosis. Cardiac enlargement, disturbances in ventricular filling, and conduction disturbances may ensue. The disease may be primary or secondary in origin. The primary form is a heritable disorder of iron metabolism with a marked increase in gastrointestinal absorption of iron and subsequent deposition in many organs, including the heart, liver, bone marrow, gonads, pancreas, and adrenals. The secondary form usually occurs in chronic hemolytic anemias such as thalassemia major, in association with the administration of multiple blood transfusions.

THE FOLLOWING CRITERIA ARE REQUIRED FOR THE DIAGNOSIS OF HEART DISEASE DUE TO HEMOCHROMATOSIS.

Cardiac enlargement associated with an abnormality in iron metabolism or with an hereditary hemolytic anemia requiring frequent blood transfusions.

1.12 Hypersensitivity Reaction

The cardiovascular system can be affected directly and indirectly by hypersensitivity reactions to proteins or to nonprotein haptens such as drugs. Clinically, the reactions are of several types.

Acute, immediate hypersensitivity reactions of the anaphylactic type probably reflect the prompt liberation of tissue-reactive amines, peptides, and lipids in response to the interaction of antigens with preformed antibodies. Urticaria, facial and laryngeal edema, bronchoconstriction, hypotension, and shock occur immediately or within hours after exposure to the offending agent. The effects on the heart are largely indirect and are secondary to hypoxia and systemic hypotension, but may also reflect direct action by the tissue-reactive chemicals. Arrhythmias, cardiac arrest, acute ventricular failure, and myocardial infarction can occur.

Subacute hypersensitivity reactions of the serum sickness type usually occur from four to twenty-one days after exposure to sensitizing proteins or drug haptens which stimulate production of antibodies. The antigen-antibody reaction produces damage indirectly by the activation of complement or the liberation of tissue-reactive chemicals, and directly by the effects of soluble antigen-antibody complexes or by the interaction of antibodies with cell-fixed antigens and cellular constituents. More rapid reactions can be marked by severe acute anaphylaxis. The clinical manifestations of chronic reactions include fever, arthralgias, lymphadenopathy, urticaria, neuritis, and renal insufficiency. Cardiac arrhythmias and pericarditis can occur, and in rare instances there may be myocarditis, probably as a result of coronary arteritis.

Hypersensitivity reactions of the delayed type occur when sensitized lymphocytes react with specific antigens; circulating antibodies are not involved. Although delayed hypersensitivity, as well as antibody-mediated hypersensitivity, is often suggested as a possible etiologic factor in a variety of cardiac diseases, it has been identified only as one of the mechanisms involved in the rejection occurring against transplanted hearts.

THE FOLLOWING CRITERIA ARE REQUIRED FOR THE DIAGNOSIS OF HEART DISEASE DUE TO A HYPERSENSITIVITY REACTION.

Severe systemic hypersensitivity reaction of the acute or subacute type and one or more of the following: arrhythmias, cardiac arrest, pericarditis, myocarditis, ventricular failure, or myocardial infarction.

1.13 Hypertension

Combined systolic and diastolic systemic arterial hypertension of either the primary or secondary form, can lead to ventricular hypertrophy and, more rarely, to left ventricular failure. Associated coronary artery disease can contribute to the development of left ventricular failure and arrhythmias.

In the accelerated (malignant) form of hypertension, left ventricular hypertrophy followed by dilatation and failure can occur in the absence of coronary atherosclerosis.

THE FOLLOWING CRITERIA ARE REQUIRED FOR THE DIAGNOSIS OF HEART DISEASE DUE TO HYPERTENSION.

Sustained systemic arterial systolic and diastolic hypertension and evidence of left ventricular hypertrophy or failure.

1.14 Hyperthyroidism

Hyperthyroidism produces cardiac disturbances secondary to the metabolic effect of excessive amounts of circulating thyroid hormones. These hormones affect the heart directly by increasing irritability and contractility and indirectly, by increasing the demands for delivery of oxygen to the periphery.

Weight loss, tremor, exophthalmos, and other signs of hyperthyroidism are usually but not necessarily present. Paroxysmal or sustained atrial tachycardia, atrial flutter, and atrial fibrillation are frequent, and cardiac enlargement, ventricular failure, and anginal syndrome can appear in some patients. These findings are most frequent in patients with preexisting valvular or atherosclerotic heart disease and thus occur more often in persons over 40. However, arrhythmias, cardiac enlargement, and ventricular failure can sometimes appear in previously normal hearts. Cardiac abnormalities due to hyperthyroidism usually disappear after successful treatment of the metabolic abnormality.

THE FOLLOWING CRITERIA ARE REQUIRED FOR THE DIAGNOSIS OF HEART DISEASE DUE TO HYPERTHYROIDISM.

Atrial arrhythmias (tachycardia, flutter, or fibrillation), cardiac enlargement, or ventricular failure, with clinical or biochemical evidence of hyperthyroidism and reversal of these findings following specific therapy.

1.15 Hypothyroidism

Hypothyroidism is a result of deficient levels of circulating thyroid hormones. The disease is most often idiopathic, but can follow thyroiditis, the treatment of thyroid disease by operation or with radioiodine, or can result from pituitary insufficiency. There are reductions in total metabolic rate and in cardiac output, and changes occur in connective tissues and in cholesterol metabolism. There is an increased incidence of coronary atherosclerosis among these patients; anginal syndrome and myocardial infarction are therefore frequent.

Edema and localized effusions—pericardial, pleural, and peritoneal—occur frequently in myxedema. There is retention of water, and there may be an increase in capillary permeability. Hyponatremia in these patients is thought to be due to inappropriate secretion of antidiuretic hormone.

The cardiac output is reduced; this reduction is disproportionate to the decrease in total body oxygen consumption. Blood flow to the skin is markedly diminished.

Pericardial effusion or cardiac dilatation often produces widening of the cardiac silhouette. Cardiac tamponade is, however, rare, and right atrial pressures remain normal. The electrocardiogram often shows low voltage of all complexes. Echocardiography may be useful in ascertaining the presence of pericardial fluid.

Ventricular failure in myxedema is probably not due to the endocrinopathy alone; it is usually due to concomitant atherosclerotic heart disease.

The diagnosis of myxedema is established by demonstration of a decreased capacity of the thyroid to synthesize thyroid hormone, and by the consequent alterations in total body metabolism and cholesterol metabolism.

ONE OF THE FOLLOWING CRITERIA IS REQUIRED FOR THE DIAGNOSIS OF HEART DISEASE DUE TO HYPOTHYROIDISM.

1. **Evidence of pericardial effusion and clinical or biochemical evidence of hypothyroidism.**
2. **Enlargement of the heart, clinical or biochemical evidence of hypothyroidism, and a decrease in heart size following administration of thyroid hormone.**

1.16 Infection

Any part of the heart may be involved by infection, but the valvular endocardium is most frequently affected.

Infective endocarditis is especially common when structural abnormalities exist because of rheumatic heart disease, congenital anomalies, or insertion of prosthetic valves. The infecting organisms are most often *Streptococcus viridans* and *Streptococcus faecalis*, which may transiently enter the blood during minor infections or surgical and dental procedures. Previously normal valves may also be infected, especially when there has been sustained septicemia or when cellular and antibody defenses are lowered by lymphomas or by the administration of corticosteroids and cytotoxic agents. The infecting organisms can be of any variety and include staphylococcus, pneumococcus, β-hemolytic streptococcus, *Haemophilus influenzae,* meningococcus, gonococcus, and salmonella. In certain cases, valvular vegetations may be demonstrable by echocardiography.

Fungi also may be the cause of endocarditis. An increasing proportion of such cases is observed in narcotic addicts who introduce the fungi by direct injection into the circulation. The responsible organism is usually *Candida albicans*.

Myocarditis and pericarditis can also be caused by a variety of infectious agents; viral infection is the predominant cause. Transient electrocardiographic abnormalities reflecting myocardial involvement can occur with the exanthemata. Infection with the Coxsackie, ECHO, and influenza viruses can sometimes produce significant disease.

Parasitic infestations with agents such as *Trichinella, Trypanosoma, Plasmodium malariae,* and *Echinococcus* can directly involve the myocardium, and schistosomiasis can lead to pulmonary heart disease.

Diphtheria produces a toxin which can affect the myocardium and conduction system.

ONE OF THE FOLLOWING CRITERIA IS REQUIRED FOR THE DIAGNOSIS OF INFECTION OF THE HEART.

1. Evidence of endocarditis, myocarditis, or pericarditis and demonstration of pathogenic organisms (bacterium, virus, fungus, or parasite) by culture or smear from the blood, pericardial fluid, or tissue specimen, or by inferential demonstration of their presence by serologic methods. In suspected diphtheritic myocarditis, a positive culture from the pharynx or other site of infection is required to establish the diagnosis.
2. In the presence of heart disease with valvular involvement or congenital malformation, new or changing murmurs associated either with embolic phenomena or sustained fever, anemia, and splenomegaly.

1.17 Marfan's Syndrome

Marfan's syndrome is a generalized disorder of connective tissue which usually is inherited as an autosomal dominant. The fundamental abnormality in connective tissue metabolism has not been determined, but probably involves the ground substance and is sometimes reflected in elevated plasma and urinary levels of glycosaminoglycans (mucopolysaccharides). The fully expressed syndrome is characterized by long extremities, arachnodactyly, lax joints, kyphoscoliosis, pectus excavatum, high arched palate, and ectopia lentis. Cardiovascular lesions are frequent; the most common is aneurysmal dilatation of the ascending aorta, which may result in dissecting hematoma and aortic regurgitation or aneurysms of the sinuses of Valsalva. Other lesions may include deformities of the atrioventricular valves, leading to mitral or tricuspid regurgitation. The cardiovascular lesions are the most common cause of death in Marfan's syndrome and are not always accompanied by all of the stigmata of the fully expressed syndrome.

THE FOLLOWING CRITERIA ARE REQUIRED FOR THE DIAGNOSIS OF HEART DISEASE DUE TO MARFAN'S SYNDROME.

The association of one of the cardiovascular abnormalities known to occur in Marfan's syndrome with at least one other feature characteristic of the syndrome.

1.18 Mucopolysaccharidoses

The mucopolysaccharidoses are a group of clinical syndromes produced by inborn errors of metabolism causing the deposition of mucopolysaccharide and glycolipid in many organs. Stunted growth and mental retardation usually appear in infancy. Skeletal abnormalities include clawlike hands, large head, and kyphosis, accounting for the designation "gargoylism." The myocardium and endocardium can be involved, leading to cardiac enlargement or valvular deformity. Intimal proliferation of the coronary arteries has also been described. Ventricular failure is a frequent cause of death.

THE FOLLOWING CRITERIA ARE REQUIRED FOR THE DIAGNOSIS OF HEART DISEASE DUE TO MUCOPOLYSACCHARIDOSIS.

Cardiac enlargement, with or without a murmur, and clinical and biochemical evidence of abnormal mucopolysaccharide metabolism.

1.19 Neoplasm

Tumors of the heart, primary or metastatic, produce symptoms through bleeding into the pericardium, by interference with valve function, or by interference with ventricular filling, usually resulting from extensive pericardial infiltration. Involvement of the myocardium can cause ventricular failure, arrhythmias, or conduction defects.

ONE OF THE FOLLOWING CRITERIA IS REQUIRED FOR THE DIAGNOSIS OF HEART DISEASE DUE TO NEOPLASM.

1. **Evidence of neoplasm as demonstrated by presence of tumor cells in the heart or pericardial fluid.**
2. **Pericardial effusion or restriction, not otherwise explained, in patients with advanced metastatic disease.**
3. **A cardiac tumor demonstrated by roentgenography, coronary arteriography, angiocardiography including radionuclide imaging, or echocardiography.**

1.20 Obesity

Extreme generalized obesity can cause heart disease by two mechanisms. The generalized increase in body fat and the increased circulating blood volume lead to an increase in cardiac output. Myocardial hypertrophy, reduction in ventricular compliance, or ventricular failure may ensue. In addition, gross obesity may lead to a reduction in alveolar ventilation, with resulting disturbances in respiratory gas exchange and pulmonary hypertension. Adipose infiltration may occur in these hearts, but probably is of little significance.

Since systemic hypertension and coronary atherosclerosis are associated with obesity, these etiologic factors should be carefully excluded before a diagnosis is made of heart disease due to obesity alone.

THE FOLLOWING CRITERIA ARE REQUIRED FOR THE DIAGNOSIS OF HEART DISEASE DUE TO OBESITY.

Evidence of cardiac enlargement or ventricular failure in the presence of severe obesity and in the absence of other specific causes of heart disease.

1.21 Polyarteritis Nodosa

The clinical manifestations of polyarteritis nodosa are protean and vary with the patterns of tissue damage produced by the focal inflammatory damage to small and medium arteries. Arterial obstruction or rupture may occur. The disease is most frequent in middle-aged males, but can occur at any age; a particularly accelerated form occurs in infants. Systemic effects include fever, weight loss, arthralgias, polymorphonuclear and eosinophilic leukocytosis, anemia, rapid erythrocyte sedimentation rate, and increased levels of gamma globulin. Among the local manifestations are nodular and purpuric skin lesions, muscular atrophy, pulmonary infiltrations, bronchial asthma, retinitis, uveitis, abdominal pain, hepatomegaly, splenomegaly, peripheral neuritis, paralysis of cranial nerves, and cerebrovascular occlusion. Involvement of the kidneys is frequent, with resultant hematuria, albuminuria, and secondary systemic hypertension. By involving the coronary arteries, the disease may produce arrhythmias, conduction disturbances, pericarditis, sudden hemorrhagic pericardial effusions, and myocardial infarction. Hypertension secondary to associated renal involvement may be the cause of left ventricular enlargement and failure.

Although hypersensitivity reactions and hepatitis virus have sometimes been incriminated as a cause of polyarteritis, the syndrome occurs most frequently in the absence of obvious etiology. The diagnosis depends on the demonstration of the characteristic arterial lesions in a biopsy specimen from an affected tissue.

THE FOLLOWING CRITERIA ARE REQUIRED FOR THE DIAGNOSIS OF HEART DISEASE DUE TO POLYARTERITIS NODOSA.

Demonstration of the characteristic lesion in any involved tissue and the presence of one or more of the following: arrhythmias, conduction disturbances, myocarditis, pericarditis, sudden hemorrhagic pericardial effusion, or acute myocardial infarction.

1.22 Progressive Muscular Dystrophy

The Duchenne form (pseudohypertrophic muscular dystrophy) is the commonest and most severe of all the muscular dystrophies and occurs predominantly in males through a sex-linked recessive inheritance. The skeletal muscles involved undergo severe degenerative changes, and similar lesions commonly appear in cardiac muscle. The heart can also be affected indirectly by disturbances in gas exchange due to involvement of the muscles of respiration, leading to pulmonary heart disease.

Difficulty in ambulation, the first symptom of skeletal muscle disease, usually begins between the first and sixth years of life. Rising from the prone or seated positions requires a striking and complex series of movements. The early pseudohypertrophy of the muscles below the knees, with later wasting of the upper limbs, differentiates this condition from other muscular dystrophies. The diagnosis is established on the basis of a typical clinical picture accompanied by electromyographic abnormalities, by changes in serum levels of enzymes derived from muscle, and by characteristic alterations in muscle biopsy specimens.

Cardiac symptoms are seldom prominent because physical activity is severely restricted by the skeletal muscle disease. Therefore the earliest manifestation of cardiac involvement is usually tachycardia or the incidental discovery of cardiac enlargement. Electrocardiographic abnormalities are common, with deep Q waves in the limb and left precordial leads and tall R waves in the right precordial leads. Disturbances in intraventricular conduction are frequent. Ventricular failure occasionally occurs, although most patients succumb from respiratory infection.

THE FOLLOWING CRITERIA ARE REQUIRED FOR THE DIAGNOSIS OF HEART DISEASE DUE TO PROGRESSIVE MUSCULAR DYSTROPHY.

Electrocardiographic abnormalities or cardiomegaly in the presence of progressive muscular dystrophy.

1.23 Progressive Systemic Sclerosis (Scleroderma)

In progressive systemic sclerosis there is induration and fibrosis of the gastrointestinal tract, lungs, and myocardium which resemble the lesions found in the skin (scleroderma). Raynaud's syndrome is a common and early manifestation. Occasionally, visceral involvement occurs in the absence of skin lesions.

The heart can be involved directly in the disease process; extensive myocardial fibrosis leads to disturbances in impulse conduction or ventricular filling. Systemic hypertension can develop secondary to renal involvement; pulmonary hypertension can result from diffuse fibrosis of the lung. Hypertensive and pulmonary heart disease resulting from renal or pulmonary involvement are secondary manifestations of the process, and such patients should not be designated as having heart disease due to progressive systemic sclerosis.

THE FOLLOWING CRITERIA ARE REQUIRED FOR THE DIAGNOSIS OF HEART DISEASE DUE TO PROGRESSIVE SYSTEMIC SCLEROSIS.

Disturbances in conduction or ventricular filling and evidence of progressive systemic sclerosis.

1.24 Pulmonary Disease (Cor Pulmonale)

Certain disorders of pulmonary function or structure can produce right ventricular enlargement or failure. Pulmonary arterial hypertension is the underlying process which ultimately compromises right heart function.

A variety of diseases can produce pulmonary hypertension by fundamentally different mechanisms. The pulmonary parenchyma need not be involved directly by the pathologic process. Hence the disease process responsible should always be identified when a diagnosis of pulmonary heart disease is made; for example, Pulmonary Heart Disease due to Chronic Obstructive Pulmonary Disease.

Pulmonary hypertension can stem from disturbances of respiratory gas exchange, which lead to pulmonary arterial vasoconstriction, polycythemia, and an increased cardiac output. The principal diseases that produce pulmonary hypertension by these mechanisms include obstructive diseases of the lung, structural deformities of the chest, and neuromuscular diseases.

Pulmonary hypertension can also result from anatomic curtailment of the capacity of the pulmonary vascular bed produced by massive embolization, recurrent multiple emboli, thrombosis, or occlusive vascular lesions associated with the pulmonary arteritides, sickle cell disease, or schistosomiasis. The capacity of the pulmonary vascular bed can also be reduced by fibrosing, granulomatous, or metastatic lesions. In certain diseases, such as the pneumoconioses and, more rarely, the massive fibrosis of treated tuberculosis, disturbed gas exchange can contribute to pulmonary hypertension induced by the reduction in the vascular bed.

The presence of pulmonary arterial hypertension does not of itself constitute evidence of pulmonary heart disease. Many conditions which are not primarily disturbances of pulmonary structure or function may produce pulmonary hypertension; for example, congenital heart disease with left-to-right shunt, mitral obstruction, or left ventricular failure. These disease states are not included under the heading of pulmonary heart disease, nor is this term applied to primary pulmonary disease in which pulmonary hypertension, either transient or fixed, is present, but in which there is no evidence of right ventricular disease.

THE FOLLOWING CRITERIA ARE REQUIRED FOR THE DIAGNOSIS OF HEART DISEASE DUE TO PULMONARY DISEASE.

The occurrence of right ventricular enlargement or failure in the presence of a disease process which primarily involves the lungs, pulmonary vasculature, or respiratory gas exchange and results in pulmonary hypertension.

1.25 Reiter's Syndrome

Reiter's syndrome is an inflammatory disease thought to be transmitted by the venereal route. A variety of infectious agents have been implicated but none clearly identified. Instances of the syndrome have been reported after dysentery outbreaks and in association with *Mycoplasma*. The classic syndrome is the occurrence of urethritis in a young man followed by conjunctivitis and arthritis over a period of several weeks or months. Mucocutaneous lesions and rashes of the soles and palms (keratoderma blennorrhagica) may erupt early in the disease. Single manifestations and recurrent cycles of any or all manifestations occur. The disease occurs most often in subjects with the antigen HLA B27.

Cardiac lesions due to Reiter's syndrome are rare, but may be manifested by conduction defects or aortic regurgitation. The underlying lesion is focal medial necrosis at the base of the aorta, with dilatation of the aortic ring. The similarity of the aortic lesion and certain clinical features to those of ankylosing spondylitis suggests that the two conditions may be closely related.

THE FOLLOWING CRITERIA ARE REQUIRED FOR THE DIAGNOSIS OF HEART DISEASE DUE TO REITER'S SYNDROME.

Aortic regurgitation in the presence of Reiter's syndrome and the absence of other demonstrable cause.

1.26 Rheumatic Fever

Rheumatic fever is a generalized disease characterized by inflammatory lesions in the heart, blood vessels, and joints. It follows infection with a β-hemolytic streptococcus of group A. A small percentage of patients so infected will develop clinically apparent rheumatic fever as a nonsuppurative and apparently sterile sequel. The course and manifestations of rheumatic fever are extremely variable. Permanent heart disease does not necessarily develop in patients with evidence of active carditis during an attack of acute rheumatic fever.

Certain manifestations are considered indicative of the disease and are therefore classified as *major criteria*: carditis, polyarthritis, chorea, subcutaneous nodules, and erythema marginatum. Carditis, polyarthritis, and chorea may occur independently of one another.

Other manifestations suggestive of rheumatic fever are less specific for the disease and are therefore classified as *minor criteria*: fever, arthralgia, prolongation of the atrioventricular conduction time, and an increased erythrocyte sedimentation rate or other evidence of inflammatory reaction, such as leukocytosis or an elevated C-reactive protein. Since rheumatic fever tends to recur, a previous history of the disease is also considered to contribute to the probability of the diagnosis of active rheumatic fever. Evidence of a preceding hemolytic streptococcal infection by culture or by antibody response (antistreptolysin O or other antibody titer) is an important confirmatory finding.

Rheumatic fever may also be accompanied by less specific symptoms and signs such as loss of weight, malaise, fatigability, tachycardia, precordial or abdominal pain, and erythema nodosum.

Whenever the diagnosis of rheumatic heart disease is made, the rheumatic process should be designated as active or inactive. Patients with the major or minor manifestations that have been noted should be classified as active, provided there is no other discoverable cause for these findings. If these manifestations are not present, the patient is considered as having an inactive rheumatic process. It should be noted, however, that histologic evidence of active rheumatic carditis, in the form of Aschoff's bodies, may occur without any clinical evidence of rheumatic activity.

Rheumatic heart disease can be encountered in patients who have no history of any of the manifestations of acute rheumatic fever that have been mentioned.

ONE OF THE FOLLOWING CRITERIA IS REQUIRED FOR THE DIAGNOSIS OF HEART DISEASE DUE TO RHEUMATIC FEVER.

1. Evidence of endocarditis, myocarditis, or pericarditis during an acute attack of rheumatic fever.
2. A characteristic structural lesion of the heart in a patient with a history of rheumatic fever.
3. Evidence of mitral obstruction in the absence of a history of rheumatic fever and in the absence of any other demonstrable cause.

1.27 Rheumatoid Arthritis

Fibrinous pericarditis may occur in patients with active rheumatoid arthritis. The pericardial involvement can lead to fibrosis or, rarely, to pericardial restriction.

In exceptional cases, granulomas identical with the subcutaneous rheumatoid nodule may occur in the pericardium, myocardium, or valves. These lesions infrequently produce clinical signs of cardiac involvement.

ONE OF THE FOLLOWING CRITERIA IS REQUIRED FOR THE DIAGNOSIS OF HEART DISEASE DUE TO RHEUMATOID ARTHRITIS.

1. **Evidence of pericarditis or myocarditis in the presence of active rheumatoid arthritis.**
2. **Pericardial restriction in the presence of well-established rheumatoid arthritis.**

1.28 Sarcoidosis

Sarcoidosis is a systemic granulomatous disease which can compromise cardiac function by two mechanisms. Epithelioid and giant cell granulomas with associated fibrosis but without necrosis can extensively replace myofibers. Myocardial function can also be altered if there is diffuse involvement of the lungs by the disease process, which may lead to pulmonary hypertension and right ventricular enlargement or failure.

Clinical manifestations of myocardial sarcoidosis occur infrequently and usually late in the course of the systemic disease. The abnormalities include various forms of conduction defects, including complete atrioventricular block and idioventricular rhythm, paroxysmal arrhythmias, and ventricular failure.

THE FOLLOWING CRITERIA ARE REQUIRED FOR THE DIAGNOSIS OF HEART DISEASE DUE TO SARCOIDOSIS.

Systemic sarcoidosis and one or more of the following: conduction disturbances, paroxysmal arrhythmias, S–T and T wave abnormalities, or ventricular failure.

1.29 Syphilis

Syphilitic involvement of the vascular system is usually localized to the ascending aorta, and most of the associated cardiac abnormalities are secondary to the aortitis. Dilatation of the ascending aorta, often accompanied by calcification, is apparent on the chest roentgenogram, and a systolic murmur, followed by a tambour-like second sound, can be heard at the aortic area. Involvement of the aorta usually becomes clinically overt many years after the primary infection. Aortitis can ultimately lead to fusiform or saccular aneurysms of the ascending aorta. Compression of neighboring structures by the aneurysm can produce hoarseness, cough, chest pain, and a tracheal tug. Aneurysm of the sinus of Valsalva is a less frequent occurrence.

Aortic regurgitation is a more common consequence of syphilitic aortitis than is aneurysm and is due to widening of the aortic ring. Coronary ostial stenosis is an infrequent complication which can produce the anginal syndrome by interfering with coronary blood flow. Gummata of the heart are a rare complication of late syphilis and can involve any area, including the conduction system.

Patients with syphilitic involvement of the aorta and heart often have no history of clinically apparent primary or secondary syphilis. However, modern serologic tests, which depend upon the presence of antibodies directed against the spirochete, such as the *Treponema pallidum* immobilization test or the fluorescein-tagged antibody test, are positive in almost all patients with cardiovascular syphilis.

ONE OF THE FOLLOWING CRITERIA IS REQUIRED FOR THE DIAGNOSIS OF HEART DISEASE OR AORTITIS DUE TO SYPHILIS.

1. **Widening or aneurysm of the ascending aorta in the presence of serologic evidence of syphilis.**
2. **Clinical or angiographic evidence of aortic regurgitation in the presence of serologic evidence of syphilis.**
3. **Angiographic evidence of coronary ostial stenosis in the presence of serologic evidence of syphilis.**

1.30 Systemic Arteriovenous Fistula

Systemic arteriovenous fistulae can cause a decrease in vascular resistance and an increase in circulating blood volume sufficient to cause a rise in cardiac output, stroke volume, and heart rate. These hemodynamic changes can lead to left ventricular enlargement and ultimately to left ventricular failure.

The commonest cause of significant systemic arteriovenous fistulae is a trauma, such as stab or gunshot wound, to an artery and vein. Multiple abnormal arteriovenous connections can be congenital in origin. Cerebral arteriovenous fistulae in the neonatal period may lead to unremitting ventricular failure and death. Fistulae may also arise in such acquired diseases as Paget's disease or Kaposi's sarcoma.

THE FOLLOWING CRITERIA ARE REQUIRED FOR THE DIAGNOSIS OF HEART DISEASE DUE TO SYSTEMIC ARTERIOVENOUS FISTULA.

Left ventricular enlargement in the presence of a systemic arteriovenous fistula.

1.31 Systemic Lupus Erythematosus

Systemic lupus erythematosus is a disease with multiple manifestations due to the involvement of many organ systems. The pericardium, endocardium, and myocardium can be involved in the disease process. Severe cardiac involvement is usually associated with signs of activity in other areas (cutaneous, joint, renal, or hematologic disturbances). However, pericarditis, with or without effusion, which is the most frequent cardiac manifestation of systemic lupus erythematosus, can occur episodically over several years without substantial associated signs of disease activity. Lupus valvulitis rarely causes significant valvular dysfunction. Myocarditis can produce ventricular failure. Certain drugs, such as procainamide, induce the syndrome.

ONE OF THE FOLLOWING CRITERIA IS REQUIRED FOR THE DIAGNOSIS OF HEART DISEASE DUE TO SYSTEMIC LUPUS ERYTHEMATOSUS.

1. **Evidence of pericarditis in a patient with other manifestations of systemic lupus erythematosus.**

2. **Ventricular failure in a patient with active systemic lupus erythematosus in the absence of other causes of heart disease.**

1.32 Toxic Agent

Drugs, exogenous chemicals, and high energy radiation can adversely affect the function or structure of the heart. The commonest offenders are drugs used in the treatment of heart disease. Digitalis, quinidine, and procainamide can cause severe disturbances in impulse initiation and conduction, or decreases in contractility. The toxic effects often correlate with high concentrations in the blood and usually disappear as the drug is eliminated. Drugs used for other purposes, such as emetine, imipramine, phenothiazine, and doxorubicin hydrochloride (Adriamycin) can also have direct effects on the heart, as can environmental contaminants such as carbon monoxide and nitroglycol. High energy radiation to the thorax can produce cardiac damage which often is not immediately apparent.

THE FOLLOWING CRITERION IS REQUIRED FOR THE DIAGNOSIS OF HEART DISEASE DUE TO A TOXIC AGENT.

Evidence that exposure to a drug, an exogenous chemical, or high energy radiation has produced or increased a significant disorder of cardiac function or structure.

1.33 Trauma

Blunt chest injury must be severe to produce contusion of the heart and is most common in high-speed deceleration accidents. Contusion usually causes hemorrhage in the epicardial fat and the right ventricular myocardium. Trauma to the myocardium may be accompanied by other intrathoracic injuries, such as rupture of the pericardium, aorta, or bronchus. Severe trauma may rupture the diaphragm and pericardium and result in herniation of the stomach and colon into the pericardial sac. Rarely, disruption of the pericardium by trauma (including surgical trauma) can result in herniation of the heart into a pleural space. Compression and crush injuries may also result in tearing of the atria, mitral and tricuspid valves, chordae tendineae, or coronary arteries, or in bursting rupture, which can involve any chamber.

Penetrating wounds of the chest, such as stab or bullet wounds, may produce complete disruption of the heart or result in perforation of the pericardium or atrial or ventricular myocardium, or in injury to a valve, chordae tendineae, coronary artery, papillary muscle, pulmonary artery, or aorta. Penetration of ingested foreign bodies may also injure the aorta, producing transection or aneurysm formation. Instrumentation of the esophagus, particularly dilatation of strictures, can lead to perforation of the pericardium. Foreign bodies may also reach the pericardial sac through the esophagus or the bronchi and give rise to pericarditis. Perforation of or injury to the heart may result from the passage of needles or catheters during cardiac catheterization or paracentesis of the pericardium. Trauma to the heart may also result from cardiotomy.

The clinical signs and symptoms of cardiac injury vary with the nature of the injury. Arrhythmias, abnormalities in conduction, and changes in ventricular repolarization (S–T and T wave abnormalities) may accompany myocardial contusion. Aneurysm formation can be a late complication. Hemopericardium is a common sequela of blunt and direct heart trauma and may lead to pericardial tamponade. A left-to-right shunting of blood may result from a penetrating wound of the heart. After an appropriate time interval, chest injury may be followed by a nonspecific pericarditis.

Regurgitation can follow injury to the valves, the chordae tendineae, or papillary muscles. Injury to a coronary artery can produce hemopericardium, myocardial infarction and, rarely, as a late development, a coronary arteriovenous or arterio-atrial fistula. Aortic trauma may lead to aneurysm formation.

ONE OF THE FOLLOWING CRITERIA IS REQUIRED FOR THE DIAGNOSIS OF HEART DISEASE DUE TO TRAUMA.

1. **The occurrence of major trauma and one or more of the following: the abrupt appearance of arrhythmias, conduction disturbances, pericarditis, hemopericar-**

dium, pneumopericardium, roentgenographic demonstration of herniation of the heart through the pericardial sac, valvular regurgitation, ventricular septal defect, or myocardial infarction.

2. **The occurrence of major trauma and one or more of the following: the appearance of ventricular aneurysm, aortic aneurysm, coronary arteriovenous or arterio-atrial fistula.**

1.34 Unknown

The cause should be stated as Unknown in those patients who present either definite structural changes in the heart or evidence of abnormal cardiac function for which no specific cause can be found.

1.35 Uremia

Uremia is a clinical syndrome which is associated with an abnormal elevation of urea and changes in other constituents of the blood resulting from acute or chronic renal disease. The heart and circulation can be involved in a number of different ways. Uremia is commonly associated with systemic hypertension, which can lead to left ventricular failure and pulmonary congestion. Severe anemia, an almost invariable component of the uremic syndrome, may also compromise ventricular function. Retention of salt and water due to renal insufficiency can lead to hypervolemia and congestion of the circulation. Retention of potassium can cause hyperkalemia, with subsequent ventricular fibrillation and ventricular arrest. Hypocalcemia, hyponatremia, and severe metabolic acidosis can also contribute to the abnormalities of cardiac rhythm. These electrolyte derangements frequently contribute to digitalis toxicity in patients with uremia. A frequent terminal manifestation is a sterile pericarditis with effusion, which is rarely restrictive.

ONE OF THE FOLLOWING CRITERIA IS REQUIRED FOR THE DIAGNOSIS OF HEART DISEASE DUE TO UREMIA.

1. **Evidence of pericarditis with uremia.**
2. **Arrhythmias induced by electrolytic abnormalities secondary to uremia.**

The Anatomic Cardiac Diagnosis

2

NOMENCLATURE

2.1 Diseases of the Aorta
- 2.1.1 Aneurysm of the Aorta
- 2.1.2 Aortitis
  - 2.1.2.1 Aortic arch syndrome (Pulseless disease, Takayasu's disease)
  - 2.1.2.2 Giant cell aortitis
  - 2.1.2.3 Spondylitic aortitis
  - 2.1.2.4 Syphilitic aortitis
- 2.1.3 Atherosclerosis of the Aorta
- 2.1.4 Cystic Medial Degeneration
  - 2.1.4.1 Idiopathic
  - 2.1.4.2 Marfan's syndrome
- 2.1.5 Dilatation of the Aorta
- 2.1.6 Dissecting Hematoma of the Aorta (Dissecting Aneurysm)
- 2.1.7 Embolism to the Aorta
- 2.1.8 Rupture of the Aorta
- 2.1.9 Thrombosis of the Aorta

2.2 Diseases of the Pulmonary Vasculature
- 2.2.1 Aneurysm of the Pulmonary Artery
- 2.2.2 Arteriosclerosis
  - 2.2.2.1 Atherosclerosis
  - 2.2.2.2 Medial hypertrophy
  - 2.2.2.3 Intimal fibrosis
- 2.2.3 Arteritis
  - 2.2.3.1 Generalized arteritis
  - 2.2.3.2 Localized arteritis
- 2.2.4 Arteriolitis

2.2.5 Dilatation of the Pulmonary Artery
2.2.6 Embolism to a Pulmonary Artery
2.2.7 Thrombosis of a Pulmonary Artery
2.2.8 Sclerosis of Pulmonary Veins
2.3 Diseases of the Coronary Arteries
2.3.1 Arteritis
2.3.1.1 Infective
2.3.1.2 Polyarteritis nodosa
2.3.2 Atherosclerosis
2.3.3 Embolism to a Coronary Artery
2.3.4 Stenosis of a Coronary Orifice
2.4 Diseases of the Endocardium and Valves
2.4.1 Subanular Sclerosis (Anular Sclerosis)
2.4.2 Endocardial Fibroelastosis
2.4.3 Endocardial Fibrosis (Endomyocardial Fibrosis)
2.4.4 Endocarditis
2.4.4.1 Infective endocarditis
2.4.4.2 Lupus valvulitis (atypical verrucous endocarditis)
2.4.4.3 Nonbacterial thrombotic endocarditis (marantic endocarditis, terminal endocarditis)
2.4.4.4 Rheumatic valvulitis and endocarditis
2.4.4.5 Rheumatoid valvulitis
2.4.5 Intracardiac Thrombosis (Endocardial Thrombosis)
2.4.6 Myxomatous Degeneration of a Valve (Mucoid Degeneration)
2.4.7 Neoplasm of the Endocardium
2.4.7.1 Myxoma
2.4.7.2 Papillary fibroma (papilloma)
2.4.8 Rupture of Chordae Tendineae
2.4.9 Valvular Deformity
2.5 Diseases of the Myocardium
2.5.1 Cardiomyopathy
2.5.1.1 Adipose infiltration of the myocardium

- 2.5.1.2 Amyloidosis
- 2.5.1.3 Friedreich's ataxia
- 2.5.1.4 Glycogen storage disease
- 2.5.1.5 Hemochromatosis
- 2.5.1.6 Hypothyroidism
- 2.5.1.7 Mucopolysaccharidoses
- 2.5.1.8 Nodular glycogen infiltration (rhabdomyoma)
- 2.5.1.9 Nonspecific
- 2.5.1.10 Progressive muscular dystrophy

2.5.2 Enlargement of the Heart
- 2.5.2.1 Left ventricular enlargement
- 2.5.2.2 Right ventricular enlargement
- 2.5.2.3 Left atrial enlargement
- 2.5.2.4 Right atrial enlargement

2.5.3 Infarction of the Myocardium

2.5.4 Myocardial Fibrosis

2.5.5 Myocarditis
- 2.5.5.1 Hypersensitivity
- 2.5.5.2 Infective myocarditis
- 2.5.5.3 Isolated myocarditis (Fiedler's myocarditis, idiopathic myocarditis)
- 2.5.5.4 Lupus myocarditis
- 2.5.5.5 Progressive systemic sclerosis (scleroderma)
- 2.5.5.6 Rheumatic myocarditis
- 2.5.5.7 Rheumatoid myocarditis
- 2.5.5.8 Sarcoidosis

2.5.6 Neoplasm

2.5.7 Rupture of the Myocardium: Free Wall, Interventricular Septum, or a Papillary Muscle

2.5.8 Ventricular Aneurysm

2.6 Diseases of the Pericardium
- 2.6.1 Cysts
- 2.6.2 Fibrosis, Calcification, or Both
- 2.6.3 Hemopericardium
- 2.6.4 Neoplasm
- 2.6.5 Pericardial Effusion (Hydropericardium)
- 2.6.6 Pericarditis

2.6.7 Pneumopericardium
2.6.8 Congenital Absence of the Left Pericardium
2.7 Anomalies of Cardiac Position
2.7.1 Dextrocardia
2.7.1.1 Dextrocardia with situs inversus
2.7.1.2 Dextrocardia with situs solitus
2.7.2 Levocardia with Situs Inversus
2.8 Anomalies of the Aorta and Aortic Arch System
2.8.1 Coarctation of the Aorta
2.8.2 Right Aortic Arch
2.8.3 Vascular Ring
2.9 Anomalies of the Pulmonary Arteries
2.9.1 Pulmonary Arteriovenous Fistula
2.9.2 Pulmonary Vascular Sling
2.9.3 Peripheral Pulmonary Arterial Stenosis
2.10 Anomalies of the Coronary Arteries
2.10.1 Anomalous Origin of the Left Coronary Artery from the Pulmonary Artery
2.10.2 Coronary Arterial Fistula to a Cardiac Chamber
2.11 Communications Between the Great Arteries
2.11.1 Aorticopulmonary Window
2.11.2 Patent Ductus Arteriosus
2.11.3 Truncus Arteriosus
2.11.4 Aortic Origin of the Right Pulmonary Artery
2.12 Transposition Complexes
2.12.1 Complete Transposition of the Great Arteries
2.12.2 Congenitally Corrected Transposition of the Great Arteries
2.12.3 Double-Outlet Right Ventricle
2.13 Defects at the Atrial Level
2.13.1 Patent Foramen Ovale
2.13.2 Atrial Septal Defect (Ostium Secundum)
2.13.3 Endocardial Cushion Defect (Ostium Primum and Atrioventricular Canal Defects)
2.13.4 Single (Common) Atrium
2.13.5 Cor Triatriatum
2.14 Defects at the Ventricular Level
2.14.1 Ventricular Septal Defect

- 2.14.2 Ventricular Septal Defect with Obstruction to Right Ventricular Outflow
  - 2.14.2.1 Mild or moderate obstruction to right ventricular outflow
  - 2.14.2.2 Severe obstruction to right ventricular outflow (tetralogy of Fallot)
- 2.14.3 Left Ventricular to Right Atrial Communication
- 2.14.4 Single (Common) Ventricle

2.15 Malformations of the Aortic Valve
- 2.15.1 Aortic Leaflet, Anular, or Commissural Deformities Causing Regurgitation
- 2.15.2 Aortic Atresia
- 2.15.3 Aortic Valvular Stenosis
- 2.15.4 Subvalvular Aortic Stenosis
- 2.15.5 Supravalvular Aortic Stenosis

2.16 Malformations of the Mitral Valve
- 2.16.1 Mitral Leaflet, Anular, or Commissural Deformities Causing Regurgitation
- 2.16.2 Mitral Atresia
- 2.16.3 Mitral Stenosis

2.17 Malformations of the Pulmonary Valve
- 2.17.1 Absent Pulmonary Valve
- 2.17.2 Pulmonary Atresia with Intact Ventricular Septum
- 2.17.3 Pulmonary Valvular Stenosis with Intact Ventricular Septum

2.18 Malformations of the Tricuspid Valve
- 2.18.1 Tricuspid Atresia
- 2.18.2 Downward Displacement of the Tricuspid Valve (Ebstein's Malformation)
- 2.18.3 Tricuspid Stenosis

2.19 Anomalies of Venous Drainage
- 2.19.1 Anomalous Pulmonary Venous Drainage
  - 2.19.1.1 Total
  - 2.19.1.2 Partial
- 2.19.2 Persistent Left Superior Vena Cava
- 2.19.3 Azygos Continuation of the Inferior Vena Cava

CRITERIA

2.1 Diseases of the Aorta

2.1.1 ANEURYSM OF THE AORTA

The term *aneurysm* is applied only to a saccular or sharply demarcated fusiform dilatation of the aorta. In the thoracic aorta, syphilis was formerly the commonest cause of aneurysms. However, atherosclerosis is now the usual etiologic factor in this location and in the vast majority of abdominal aortic aneurysms. Congenital and traumatic aneurysms are rare.

Atherosclerotic aneurysm is a consequence of medial atrophy and attenuation underlying extensive intimal plaque formation. The loss of muscle and elastic tissue, coupled with increasing lateral stress as distention proceeds, results in fusiform or globular dilatation. It is most frequently found in the abdominal aorta between the origin of the renal arteries and the bifurcation. Atherosclerotic aneurysms may be multiple. They commonly contain lamellated thrombus. Complications include leakage of blood, frank rupture, and erosion of vertebrae. Perforation of the aneurysmal wall with massive retroperitoneal or intraperitoneal hemorrhage is a frequent cause of death. The tear is found in the widest, and consequently the thinnest, portion of the area of dilatation; it rarely occurs at the ends or margins.

Syphilitic aneurysm results from aortitis, which causes destruction and loss of the musculo-elastic media with subsequent stretching and dilatation of the residual fibrous and scarred wall. The most common sites in order of frequency are the ascending, transverse, and descending thoracic aorta. Lamellated thrombus frequently lines and partially fills the aneurysmal sac. Complications include compression of adjacent structures such as the bronchus and recurrent laryngeal nerve and rupture and erosion of resistant neighboring structures such as the sternum and vertebrae.

Aortic aneurysms may exist without producing symptoms and are frequently discovered on routine examination of the abdomen or roentgenographic examination of the chest. Ultrasound may be helpful in diagnosis, but confirmation of the diagnosis often requires aortography. The symptoms and signs produced depend upon the size and location of the aneurysm. Thoracic aneurysms may produce pain, cough, hoarseness, dysphagia, a tracheal tug, inequality of the pulse and blood pressure in the arms, and localized or diffuse pulsation when there is impingement upon the chest wall. With aneurysms due to syphilis, there may be concomitant aortic regurgitation. Aortic regurgitation is also frequent with congenital or acquired aneurysms of the sinus of Valsalva. Abdominal aneurysms are most commonly discovered as pulsating masses, which produce pain as they enlarge or press on adjacent vertebrae and nerves. If rupture occurs, severe pain, signs of peritoneal irritation, or shock may ensue.

THE FOLLOWING CRITERION IS REQUIRED FOR THE DIAGNOSIS OF ANEURYSM OF THE AORTA.

Roentgenographic evidence of a saccular or sharply demarcated fusiform dilatation of the aorta.

2.1.2 AORTITIS

2.1.2.1 Aortic Arch Syndrome (Pulseless Disease, Takayasu's Disease)

Aortic arch syndrome is primarily a disease of young women and is seen most often in Orientals. The lesions involve the aortic arch and the origins of the great vessels from the arch. There is adventitial sclerosis, scarring of the media with disruption of the musculoelastic coats, and marked obliterative intimal fibrous thickening. Lymphocytes and plasma cells infiltrate the wall. Although rare giant cells are seen, this is not a usual feature. Thrombosis may be superimposed.

Clinically, the aortic arch syndrome is characterized by loss of pulses in the arms and a variety of manifestations of ischemia of those areas supplied by the major branches of the aortic arch. Similar findings may also be produced by syphilis, atherosclerosis, and giant cell aortitis.

THE FOLLOWING CRITERIA ARE REQUIRED FOR THE DIAGNOSIS OF AORTIC ARCH SYNDROME.

Angiographic demonstration of narrowing of the lumen of the aorta or narrowing or obliteration of the brachiocephalic vessels arising from it, in the absence of other known cause.

2.1.2.2 Giant Cell Aortitis

Giant cell aortitis is an inflammatory lesion of the aorta which occurs in older age groups. It is accompanied by similar lesions in other arteries, particularly the temporal artery. Involvement of other branches of the carotid system may result in blindness and central nervous system disturbances. All major branches of the aorta can be involved. The media, particularly its inner portion, is disrupted by an infiltration of lymphocytes, with accompanying macrophages and plasma cells. Fragmentation of the internal elastic membrane evokes a foreign body giant cell reaction. The overlying intimal fibrosis in smaller muscular arteries such as the temporal artery can produce striking luminal narrowing. Biopsy of the temporal artery may demonstrate these characteristic lesions. These lesions are frequently, but not necessarily, associated with a clinical syndrome of older persons called polymyalgia rheumatica. It is characterized by diffuse muscle aches and tenderness, a strikingly rapid erythrocyte sedimentation rate, and a salutary response to cortisone administration.

THE FOLLOWING CRITERIA ARE REQUIRED FOR THE DIAGNOSIS OF GIANT CELL AORTITIS.

Clinical or angiographic evidence of a reduction in the lumen of the aorta or obliteration or narrowing of its major branches and histologic evidence of giant cell arteritis.

2.1.2.3 Spondylitic Aortitis

Ankylosing spondylitis may be accompanied by aortic regurgitation. This is the result of aortic medial scarring with dilatation of the ring comparable to that seen in syphilis. Adventitial sclerosis, obliterating intimal thickening of the vasa vasorum, and aortic intimal fibrosis, as well as scarring of the media, characterize this lesion. Thickening of the aortic cusps, with rolling of the edges, accompanies commissural separation and, as in syphilis, is probably not related to valvular inflammation but rather, to the effects of ring dilatation. A similar lesion is seen in Reiter's syndrome.

THE FOLLOWING CRITERION IS REQUIRED FOR THE DIAGNOSIS OF SPONDYLITIC AORTITIS.

The association of aortic regurgitation with ankylosing spondylitis.

2.1.2.4 Syphilitic Aortitis

In syphilitic aortitis, involvement is most frequent in the ascending portion and arch of the aorta, less common in the thoracic part, and rare in the abdominal segment. The vessel wall is thickened and inelastic, and the lumen may be dilated. The intima contains well-defined, pearly-white, hyaline, smooth-surfaced elevations of variable size. Longitudinal wrinkling of the intima is fairly characteristic. Atheromatous deposits in the area of involvement are exaggerated and may complicate and obscure its appearance. The intimal plaques may encroach upon the orifice of any arterial branch, including the ostium of either or both coronary arteries. This encroachment frequently causes stenosis or almost complete obliteration of the orifices.

There is an increase of connective tissue in the adventitia, thickening and endothelial proliferation in the vasa vasorum, and perivascular infiltration of lymphocytes and plasma cells. The media is penetrated in flame-shaped fashion by thin-walled vascular channels and collections of lymphocytes and plasma cells. These lesions accompany areas of scarring where the elastic lamellae are ruptured and the smooth muscle cells replaced by collagen. Occasionally, the larger cell aggregates form miliary gummata with central areas of necrosis. Rarely, a few multinucleated giant cells may appear. The intima is irregularly thickened by proliferation of connective tissue.

In one-third to one-half of all cases of syphilitic aortitis, the aortic valve is affected. As a result of inflammatory change in the underlying aortic wall and dilatation of the ring, the commissures are separated, leading to aortic regurgitation. The lateral parts of the aortic cusps may coalesce with the intima of the aorta, leading to further separation of the commissures. In advanced forms of the disease, the margins of the cusps show thickening and rolling toward the ventricular aspect; this sclerosis is mechanical. Further cicatrization may reduce the cusps to cordlike structures and increase the degree of regurgitation.

In addition to fibrous proliferation, the affected leaflets and the aorta show endothelial proliferation in the vasa vasorum and infiltration by lymphocytes and plasma cells.

Syphilitic aortitis usually becomes clinically manifest only when there are complications such as aortic dilatation, aneurysm, aortic regurgitation, or coronary ostial stenosis. Aortitis may cause systolic murmurs, heard at the base of the heart; a ringing quality to the aortic component of the second sound; and radiologic evidence of dilatation, exaggerated pulsation, or calcification of the ascending aorta.

A diagnosis of syphilitic aortitis requires serologic demonstration of prior infection by *Treponema pallidum,* especially since widening of the aortic arch is frequent with systemic hypertension and in patients over 40 years of age.

THE CRITERIA REQUIRED FOR THE DIAGNOSIS OF SYPHILITIC AORTITIS ARE GIVEN IN 1.29.

2.1.3 ATHEROSCLEROSIS OF THE AORTA

Atherosclerosis of the aorta is characterized initially by intimal change. This consists of an accumulation of intra- and extracellular lipid in this layer and an increase in subendothelial connective tissue rich in mucopolysaccharide ground substance. The plaque enlarges by lipophage accretion at its periphery, and, as it ages, the center undergoes degeneration, with liberation of lipoprotein and crystalline cholesterol, which form a central grumous mass. Reactive proliferation of fibrous tissue is seen at the margins, and varying degrees of inflammatory response, consisting of lymphocytes and mononuclear cells, accompany the lesion throughout its evolution. The lipid-rich plaque frequently undergoes calcification, giving the area of involvement of the aorta a brittle character.

As the plaque expands, the underlying musculoelastic media becomes compressed, attenuated, and scarred. The internal elastic lamella may be frayed and fragmented, and the components of the plaque may penetrate and further destroy the media.

The degree of involvement of the aorta by atherosclerosis is least in the ascending portion and increases in severity from the arch to the abdominal segment. It is most marked just proximal to the bifurcation. Elsewhere in the vessel, pronounced lesions occur about the orifices of the branches and at points of fixation to surrounding structures. In children and young adults the disease has an affinity for that segment of the aorta just distal to the aortic valve and for the posterior wall of the descending thoracic aorta, particularly about the orifices of intercostal arteries.

The degenerating plaque may rupture into the lumen. This complication is common, but usually causes no detectable difficulty unless extruded components of the plaque and an associated thrombus embolize to a vessel of importance. Thrombosis and aneurysm also may result from atherosclerosis.

Atherosclerosis of the aorta produces no clinical symptoms unless there are complications of the process such as aneurysm, embolization, thrombosis, or impingement upon the orifice of arteries, with reduction in regional blood flow. The paramount physical finding is a systolic ejection murmur at the base of the heart, resulting from aortic dilatation. The aortic silhouette is elongated, tortuous, and widened, as demonstrated by chest roentgenography, fluoroscopy, or aortography. The descending aorta becomes readily visible and often curves to the left. Calcific plaques may frequently be seen in the aortic knob and in the abdominal aorta.

ONE OF THE FOLLOWING CRITERIA IS REQUIRED FOR THE DIAGNOSIS OF ATHEROSCLEROSIS OF THE AORTA.

1. **Radiologic demonstration of calcification, irregularity of outline, or aneurysmal dilatation of the aorta in the absence of syphilis.**
2. **Evidence of occlusion of major aortic branches in the absence of any other demonstrable cause.**

2.1.4 CYSTIC MEDIAL DEGENERATION

2.1.4.1 IDIOPATHIC

The changes of idiopathic cystic medial degeneration involve the aorta with moderate frequency, but rarely involve the pulmonary artery.

Slitlike spaces between the lamellae of the media of the aorta are filled with a homogenous, basophilic, mucoid material. An increase in and coalescence of these spaces produce cysts or cavities, which replace and compress muscle and elastic tissue. The abnormal mucoid substance is metachromatic and stains as acid mucopolysaccharide; its origin is unknown, but it may be a consequence of degeneration induced by intimal hyperplasia and medial hypertrophy of the vasa vasorum. Marked dilatation of the ascending aorta and dissecting hematoma are the most significant complications of this disorder. The dilatation of the ascending aorta often assumes a characteristic triangular shape.

ONE OF THE FOLLOWING CRITERIA IS REQUIRED FOR THE DIAGNOSIS OF IDIOPATHIC CYSTIC MEDIAL DEGENERATION OF THE AORTA.

1. **Dissecting hematoma of the aorta occurring in the absence of any other cause.**
2. **Marked dilatation of the ascending aorta in the absence of other cause.**

2.1.4.2 MARFAN'S SYNDROME

In Marfan's syndrome, an hereditary disease, the degeneration in the aorta is similar to that seen in the idiopathic form, but the primary lesion may be a degeneration of elastic tissue similar to that seen in other diseases. Moreover, the other features of the syndrome are present, and involvement of other vessels, including the pulmonary artery, can be seen. Dilatation of the aorta and aneurysm of the sinus of Valsalva are consequences of the medial cystic degeneration; secondary aortic regurgitation may result. As in the idiopathic form of cystic medial degeneration, the most frequent complication is dissecting hematoma.

THE FOLLOWING CRITERIA ARE REQUIRED FOR THE DIAGNOSIS OF CYSTIC MEDIAL DEGENERATION DUE TO MARFAN'S SYNDROME.

Evidence of Marfan's syndrome and any one of the following: dilatation of the aorta, aneurysm of the sinus of Valsalva, or dissecting hematoma.

2.1.5 DILATATION OF THE AORTA

The thoracic aorta can become dilated as a consequence of hemodynamic factors such as systemic hypertension, aortic valvular disease, or increased aortic blood flow. Dilatation of the thoracic and abdominal aorta may result from structural alterations due to atherosclerosis, syphilis, Marfan's syndrome, or idiopathic cystic medial degeneration.

Dilatation of the ascending aorta may produce systolic murmurs at the base of the heart, which may radiate into the neck. If the aortic ring is widened, the murmur of aortic regurgitation may be present. Radiologic examination reveals an increase in the transverse diameter of the aorta.

THE FOLLOWING CRITERION IS REQUIRED FOR THE DIAGNOSIS OF DILATATION OF THE AORTA.

Demonstration of an increase in the transverse diameter of the aorta by chest roentgenography or aortography.

2.1.6 DISSECTING HEMATOMA OF THE AORTA (DISSECTING ANEURYSM)

Dissection of the aorta is caused by a forceful penetration of blood between the layers of the vessel. The column of blood characteristically separates the outer third from the inner two-thirds of the media. The initial injury may be caused by hemorrhage from the vasa vasorum into an area of preexisting cystic medial degeneration. Subsequent expansion of the intramural hematoma leads to its rupture through the aortic intima. While areas of cystic change may be demonstrable about the primary site and in parts of the aorta not involved in the dissection, in many instances such changes are not observed.

Alternatively, the initial medial lesion may result from ischemia due to hypertensive arteriosclerosis of the vasa vasorum. The intimal tear provides an opening for extension of the lesion, with the systemic blood pressure as a driving force. The intimal tear is located most frequently in the proximal 3 cm of the aorta. It is usually transverse or circumferential and measures from 1 to 4 cm in length. The second most common site is close to the insertion of the ligamentum arteriosum.

Dissection may progress for short distances proximally or distally, or it may continue throughout the entire length of the aorta. Rupture through adventitia may produce massive hemorrhage into the pericardial sac, pleural space, peritoneal cavity, mediastinum, or retroperitoneal area. Infrequently, the hematoma reenters the main aortic lumen to form a so-called double-barreled aorta. This artificially created channel may remain functional and become endothelialized, or it may be closed by thrombus formation and fibrosis. In most instances in which the dissection continues throughout the entire length of the aorta, the smaller branches of the artery, such as the intercostals, may be severed; the coronary arteries and larger branches, such as the renal, mesenteric, and iliac vessels, may be restricted by a continuation of the pathologic process within their walls. Aortic regurgitation can result from the dissection.

Dissecting hematoma occurs predominantly in males in the middle or older age groups, particularly in the presence of systemic hypertension. Persons with Marfan's syndrome or aortic coarctation are particularly prone to this process.

The cardinal symptom of dissecting hematoma is the sudden onset of severe, continuous tearing or crushing pain in the chest which radiates to the back. The other manifestations of dissecting hematoma depend largely upon involvement of aortic branches. Thus signs and symptoms of myocardial, cerebral, renal, mesenteric, or iliac arterial insufficiency can appear.

Physical findings include agitation, the murmur of aortic regurgitation, asymmetric diminution of arterial pulses, and systolic bruits over the areas where the aortic lumen is narrowed. Systemic blood pressure is usually well maintained at the onset.

A chest roentgenogram may show widening of the aorta. Ultrasound may show aortic widening and double echoes from the aortic walls. Aortography can demonstrate a false channel, narrowing of the aortic lumen, or obstruction of aortic branches.

ONE OF THE FOLLOWING CRITERIA IS REQUIRED FOR THE DIAGNOSIS OF DISSECTING HEMATOMA OF THE AORTA.

1. **The characteristic pain associated with one or more of the following: aortic regurgitation, widening of the thoracic aorta, or asymmetric decreases in arterial pulses.**
2. **Evidence on aortography of a false channel or of the dissected membrane dividing the aortic lumen into compartments.**

2.1.7 EMBOLISM TO THE AORTA

Emboli to the aorta may originate from thrombi in the left atrium, left atrial appendage, or left ventricle. Thrombi developing over an ulcerated atherosclerotic plaque can also give rise to more distal emboli. Emboli usually lodge at the bifurcation of the aorta and can occlude the iliac arteries.

The sudden onset of pain, numbness, weakness, or paresthesias in the lower extremities, accompanied by coldness, pallor, mottled cyanosis, and absent pulsations in the same areas, is clinical evidence of an embolus lodged at the aortic bifurcation. However, sudden massive thrombosis of the terminal aorta can give rise to the same clinical picture. Aortography may delineate the site of obstruction.

THE FOLLOWING CRITERIA ARE REQUIRED FOR THE DIAGNOSIS OF EMBOLISM TO THE AORTA.

The sudden onset of the symptoms and signs of acute obstruction of the lower aorta and demonstration of a site of obstruction and/or a filling defect by aortography.

2.1.8 RUPTURE OF THE AORTA

Rupture of the aorta may result from trauma or may be associated with dissecting hematoma or aneurysm formation. Coarctation of the aorta more rarely leads to rupture. Complete rupture may be rapidly fatal, but with slow bleeding into the esophagus, pericardial sac, pleural spaces, mediastinum, or abdomen, death may be postponed for hours or days. Evidence of blood loss and shock are the major clinical manifestations.

THE FOLLOWING CRITERIA ARE REQUIRED FOR THE DIAGNOSIS OF RUPTURE OF THE AORTA.

The presence of aortic aneurysm, or dissecting hematoma, or coarctation of the aorta and evidence of bleeding into one or more of the following: pericardial sac, pleural spaces, bronchial tree, mediastinum, peritoneum, or esophagus.

2.1.9 THROMBOSIS OF THE AORTA

Thrombosis of the aorta most commonly results from atherosclerosis. When an adherent mural thrombus forms high in the aorta, it rarely increases in size sufficiently to obstruct the lumen. Complications occur if a thrombus forms at the aortic bifurcation and obstructs the lumina of the common iliac arteries. Mural thrombi at any level are potential sources of more peripheral emboli. Disengaged fragments can obstruct vessels supplying the gastrointestinal tract, kidneys, or lower extremities.

Gradual occlusion of the lumen of the terminal aorta can result in the development of collateral circulation to the lower extremities, so that their blood supply is fairly well maintained and they remain warm and their color normal. However, symptoms may include impotence and intermittent claudication, with pain appearing in the hips, thighs, and gluteal areas (Leriche syndrome).

Clinically, rapid occlusion of the lower portion of the aorta by thrombosis may be indistinguishable from occlusion due to embolism.

Aortography may delineate irregular areas of narrowing.

THE FOLLOWING CRITERIA ARE REQUIRED FOR THE DIAGNOSIS OF THROMBOSIS OF THE AORTA.

The gradual onset of the symptoms and signs of obstruction of the lower aorta and the demonstration of a site of obstruction by aortography.

2.2 Diseases of the Pulmonary Vasculature

2.2.1 ANEURYSM OF THE PULMONARY ARTERY

True aneurysms of the pulmonary artery should be distinguished from the general dilatation that may complicate chronic pulmonary hypertension. While degenerative and inflammatory vascular diseases that commonly involve the aorta are seen rarely in the pulmonary artery, syphilis, infective endocarditis, and trauma are encountered in association with pulmonary arterial aneurysms. An increased incidence of aneurysm of the pulmonary trunk or its branches, and of dissecting hematoma of the pulmonary artery, is also found in the presence of severe pulmonary hypertension, particularly when associated with congenital anomalies of the heart and great vessels. Patent ductus arteriosus, large ventricular or atrial septal defects, mitral obstruction, and recurrent pulmonary thromboembolism are therefore common predisposing conditions. Aneurysms of the main trunk are usually present when the pulmonary valve is congenitally absent or incompetent. Pulmonary arterial aneurysms may rupture either into the pericardial sac, resulting in tamponade, or into the lung, following which massive hemoptysis occurs.

THE FOLLOWING CRITERION IS REQUIRED FOR THE DIAGNOSIS OF ANEURYSM OF THE PULMONARY ARTERY.

Angiographic demonstration of aneurysm of the pulmonary artery.

2.2.2 ARTERIOSCLEROSIS

Sustained pulmonary arterial hypertension, regardless of the cause, may give rise to one or more of the following arteriosclerotic lesions: atherosclerosis, medial hypertrophy, or intimal fibrosis. These pathologic changes are encountered in the presence of: left-to-right intracardiac shunts with large pulmonary blood flow; pulmonary parenchymal disease such as the pneumoconioses; pulmonary thromboemboli; alveolar hypoxia due to chronic bronchitis, hypoventilation, or exposure to high altitude; and protracted pulmonary venous hypertension such as that encountered in mitral obstruction or protracted or recurrent left ventricular failure. In mitral obstruction and left ventricular failure the distribution of lesions is greatest in the dependent portions of the lung.

Although these arteriosclerotic lesions represent a response to increased intravascular pressure, they may themselves contribute to the levels of pressure encountered.

2.2.2.1 Atherosclerosis

Atherosclerosis of the major pulmonary arteries increases in incidence and extent with advancing years and is almost universally present, although in minor form, after the age of 40. The severity of this process appears to be independent of systemic atherosclerosis. Marked deposition of lipids and fibrous intimal plaques in the major pulmonary arteries are rare in the absence of chronic pulmonary hypertension, but in its presence, these changes become considerably more severe and widespread, especially at points of vessel division, and appear at an earlier age. Even in marked pulmonary hypertension these lesions do not rival the corresponding disease in the aorta. They rarely ulcerate, thrombose, or lead to medial hypertrophy. They rarely produce clinical manifestations and are not detected prior to death.

2.2.2.2 Medial Hypertrophy

The earliest characteristic finding in pulmonary hypertension, whether primary or secondary to pulmonary parenchymal disease, excessive pulmonary blood flow, or pulmonary venous hypertension, is muscular hyperplasia in the media of muscular arteries and arterioles. The vessels come to resemble the thick-walled pulmonary arteries and arterioles of the fetal lung. It is assumed that smooth muscle hyperplasia is stimulated by chronic spasm in response to persistent pressure evaluation, but the exact nature of the stimulus causing the cells to multiply is unknown. There is evidence that this lesion is reversible if pulmonary arterial pressure falls.

THE FOLLOWING CRITERION IS REQUIRED FOR THE DIAGNOSIS OF MEDIAL HYPERTROPHY OF THE PULMONARY ARTERIES AND ARTERIOLES.

Demonstration of the characteristic histopathologic lesion on lung biopsy.

2.2.2.3 Intimal Fibrosis

Intimal fibrosis with occasional formation of longitudinal smooth muscle bundles is a more advanced response to pulmonary hypertension than is medial hypertrophy. It also occurs as the result of organization of thromboemboli. Consequently, the origin of pulmonary hypertension in some patients has been attributed to repeated episodes of thromboembolism because the dominant pulmonary arterial structural reaction is intimal fibrosis. The intimal sclerosis seen with chronically excessive pulmonary blood flow at low pressure, as in atrial spetal defect or anomalous pulmonary venous connection, may also be due to the organization of small mural thrombi. Segmental intimal sclerosis in major pulmonary arteries has been described after intrauterine rubella infection, possibly in response to damage of the elastica in the media. Intimal fibrosis is believed to be reversible with subsidence of pulmonary hypertension.

THE FOLLOWING CRITERION IS REQUIRED FOR THE DIAGNOSIS OF INTIMAL FIBROSIS OF THE PULMONARY ARTERIES AND ARTERIOLES.

Demonstration of the characteristic histopathologic lesion on lung biopsy.

2.2.3 ARTERITIS

2.2.3.1 Generalized Arteritis

Inflammatory lesions of the pulmonary arteries occur as part of generalized collagen-vascular disease, including rheumatic fever, rheumatoid arthritis, dermatomyositis, polyarteritis nodosa, and Wegener's and sarcoid granulomatosis. There are differences in the intensity of necrosis, inflammation, and thrombosis in the various diseases, but the reactions are identical to those in systemic arteries in each disease.

Hypersensitivity angiitis, which also may be generalized, has a predilection for pulmonary arteries. There may be a necrotizing panarteritis, with many eosinophilic leukocytes in the exudate, rendering the reaction indistinguishable from polyarteritis nodosa. A granulomatous arteritis with eosinophilic infiltrate is characteristically found in pulmonary schistosomiasis. The ova released by adult worms in the liver, distal colon, or urinary bladder enter the inferior vena cava, usually by portal-to-systemic venous shunts, and are carried to the lungs, where their spines apparently contribute to entrapment in muscular pulmonary arteries with a luminal diameter of 100 to 1000 μ. Here, hypersensitivity to the foreign material leads to a granulomatous response that differs strikingly from the usual bland thrombosis accompanying other forms of emboli.

These lesions may result in increased resistance to blood flow and pulmonary hypertension.

ONE OF THE FOLLOWING CRITERIA IS REQUIRED FOR THE DIAGNOSIS OF GENERALIZED PULMONARY ARTERITIS.

1. **Demonstration of the characteristic histopathologic findings on lung biopsy.**
2. **Pulmonary hypertension and histopathologic demonstration of a systemic disease known to produce pulmonary arteritis.**

2.2.3.2 Localized Arteritis

Necrotizing inflammatory diseases of the pulmonary parenchyma may involve both arteries and veins, leading to inflammation, necrosis of the vessel wall, and thrombosis. Formerly, tuberculosis had been responsible in most such cases, but necrotizing pneumonias due to other organisms, including gram-negative bacteria, are now more common.

These lesions are rarely sufficiently disseminated to produce pulmonary hypertension.

THE FOLLOWING CRITERION IS REQUIRED FOR THE DIAGNOSIS OF LOCALIZED ARTERITIS.

Demonstration of the characteristic histopathologic finding on lung biopsy or in material obtained at lung resection.

2.2.4 ARTERIOLITIS

Necrotizing arteriolitis is the characteristic pathologic finding in the presence of severe pulmonary hypertension from any cause. It is always superimposed on arteriolosclerosis. It consists of focal fibrinoid necrosis of the media, with an acute inflammatory response in all layers of the vessel wall. Details of cells and fibers are lost in the homogeneous eosinophilic transformation of the media. A similar reaction may occur in the muscular pulmonary arteries. Thrombi form in these areas, and the necrotic vessels may rupture. Healing of such lesions is unusual, because they occur in the terminal stage of disease. There is speculation, however, that the complex plexiform and angiomatoid lesions seen in association with this arteriolitis, which occur predominantly at or near points of branching of small muscular arteries or arterioles, may develop when necrotic vessels are organized.

Arteriolitis is encountered in the presence of pulmonary hypertension so severe that the levels of pressure approach, or occasionally exceed, their counterparts in the systemic arterial circulation. These lesions in turn contribute to the level of pulmonary arterial pressure encountered. The usual disorders associated with this process are certain cases of mitral obstruction, multiple pulmonary thromboemboli, primary (idiopathic) pulmonary hypertension, and congenital lesions of the heart and great vessels associated with large pulmonary blood flow. In congenital heart disease the direction of intracardiac shunt is from right to left at this stage.

Arteriolitis does not appear to be reversible, and the level of pulmonary arterial pressure does not fall in response to either surgical correction of the underlying lesion or pulmonary vasodilating agents.

ONE OF THE FOLLOWING CRITERIA IS REQUIRED FOR THE DIAGNOSIS OF ARTERIOLITIS.

1. **Demonstration of the characteristic histopathologic findings on lung biopsy.**

2. **The presence of pulmonary arterial pressure which approaches or exceeds systemic arterial pressure and which is unresponsive to known pulmonary vasodilators.**

2.2.5 DILATATION OF THE PULMONARY ARTERY

The main pulmonary artery and its major branches may be congenitally dilated or become dilated following an increase in pulmonary arterial pressure or flow. Dilatation distal to areas of stenosis is often present. In some instances the cause of dilatation is unknown.

Dilatation of the pulmonary artery may produce systolic murmurs at the upper left sternal border. Radiographic study reveals an increase in the transverse diameter of the artery.

THE FOLLOWING CRITERION IS REQUIRED FOR THE DIAGNOSIS OF DILATATION OF THE PULMONARY ARTERY.

Demonstration of an increase in the transverse diameter of the pulmonary artery by chest roentgenography or angiography.

2.2.6 EMBOLISM TO A PULMONARY ARTERY

The pulmonary circulation filters materials exceeding 10 to 15 μ in diameter. Emboli consisting of bland or infected thrombi, bone marrow, tumor cells, amniotic fluid, fat, parasites, injected foreign materials, and air may lodge in the pulmonary arterioles or arteries, depending on their size. Embolization is closely associated with circulatory stasis, carcinoma, inflammatory diseases of the pelvic organs and lower extremities, mural thrombosis of right heart cavities, and infective endocarditis. Emboli of bland thrombi may occlude the main pulmonary artery or one of its major branches and cause sudden death or infarction or be undetected clinically. Multiple showers of small emboli can lead insidiously to a reduction in the pulmonary arterial bed and produce pulmonary hypertension. The plexiform and angiomatoid lesions of pulmonary arteries and arterioles found in patients with severe pulmonary hypertension have been attributed to organization of a vessel following thromboemboli.

The clinical picture in pulmonary arterial embolism is variable, ranging from syncope, vascular collapse, and sudden death following massive occlusion to the insidious development of severe pulmonary hypertension and refractory right ventricular failure following repeated showers of small emboli without identifiable clinical episodes of vascular occlusion.

The sudden onset of unexplained dyspnea or tachypnea is the most frequent symptom of pulmonary emboli, while pleuritic chest pain, hemoptysis, pleural effusion, and pleural friction rub are present only when infarction has occurred. Within hours after embolization, the electrocardiogram can show one or more of the following abnormalities: deviation of the electrical axis to the right; a deep S wave and depression of the S–T segment in lead I; depression of the S–T segment and inversion of the T wave in lead II; a prominent Q wave and inversion of the T wave in lead III; inversion of the T waves in the right precordial leads; or the appearance of right bundle branch block. Most of these findings are transitory. Atrial arrhythmias can also appear with embolization.

Chest radiographs may be normal or show evidence suggesting infarction, local reduced vascular filling, central pulmonary arterial distention, or right ventricular enlargement. Changes in the distribution of blood and air in the lungs can occur and result in evidence of increased dead space ventilation at rest or with exercise, associated with a decreased single-breath diffusing capacity and a partially compensated respiratory alkalosis.

ONE OF THE FOLLOWING CRITERIA IS REQUIRED FOR THE DIAGNOSIS OF EMBOLISM TO A PULMONARY ARTERY.

1. **The demonstration of filling defects causing complete or partial occlusion of some portion of the pulmonary artery tree, preferably by selective pulmonary angiography.**

2. The demonstration of regional pulmonary ischemia on lung scan following intravenous injection of radioactive macroaggregated albumin, in the absence of other diseases known to be capable of producing such local ischemic changes. Accuracy may be helped by an associated ventilation lung scan.
3. Unexplained dyspnea or tachypnea and the presence of one or more of the following: clinical or radiographic evidence of pulmonary infarction or the transient electrocardiographic abnormalities described above.

2.2.7 THROMBOSIS OF A PULMONARY ARTERY

Primary thrombosis in the pulmonary arteries is rare and may indicate defects in the intrinsic clotting mechanism or a tendency of the red blood cells to agglutinate (as occurs in sickle cell anemia or polycythemia). It can also result from chest trauma. It is not unusual as a secondary phenomenon in areas of pneumonitis that impinge on the vessel wall. Thrombi are found frequently in cases of cyanotic congenital heart disease, such as tetralogy of Fallot, because pulmonary blood flow is reduced, and the polycythemic response to hypoxemia leads to increased blood viscosity.

Thrombosis of the major pulmonary arteries is manifested by partial occlusion of the vessels by a smooth, polypoid mass of thrombus which projects into the main divisions and is attached to the endothelial surface of the intrapulmonary vessels. Organized thrombi in the muscular arteries may appear as an eccentric plaque or a polypoid mass of fibroelastic tissue attached to the wall, or the lumen may be divided into channels by bridging strands of fibroelastic tissue. Because the conditions under which thrombosis is likely to occur also predispose to embolism, and since the clinical features of both processes may be indistinguishable, it is often difficult, if not impossible, to ascertain on clinical grounds whether intravascular thrombi are local or embolic in origin.

2.2.8 SCLEROSIS OF PULMONARY VEINS

Obliterative sclerosis of small intrapulmonary veins can occur without evidence of antecedent inflammation or other pulmonary parenchymal lesions. The walls of the veins are the site of fibrosis, and the lumina are severely narrowed or occluded. Secondary changes in the lung are indistinguishable either from those due to extrinsic compression of pulmonary veins by scarring or tumor or from those due to mitral obstruction.

The clinical picture is a nonspecific one of progressive pulmonary congestion in the absence of other abnormalities known to be capable of producing pulmonary venous hypertension. Diagnosis prior to death is difficult and unusual.

THE FOLLOWING CRITERION IS REQUIRED FOR THE DIAGNOSIS OF SCLEROSIS OF PULMONARY VEINS.

Lung biopsy which demonstrates characteristic lesions of the intrapulmonary veins.

2.3 Diseases of the Coronary Arteries

2.3.1 ARTERITIS

2.3.1.1 Infective

Infective arteritis results most commonly from septic emboli in infective endocarditis and more rarely by direct extension from contiguous suppurative processes such as tuberculous pericarditis. The inflammation can spread to all coats of the artery and lead to myocardial infarction, mycotic aneurysms, or myocardial abscesses. The diagnosis is rarely made before death, since the primary disease usually dominates the clinical picture.

2.3.1.2 Polyarteritis Nodosa

The outstanding features of arteritis due to polyarteritis nodosa are inflammation of all layers of the coronary arteries, with conspicuous medial and adventitial involvement and perivascular infiltration. Necrosis of the wall may result in the formation of aneurysms or rupture of a vessel. Thrombosis or obliteration of the lumen by scar formation can result in small areas of myocardial infarction. It is not clear whether ventricular enlargement and failure seen in conjunction with coronary arteritis result from these vascular lesions or from systemic arterial hypertension, which is a frequent manifestation of vascular involvement elsewhere in the body, especially in the kidney.

THE FOLLOWING CRITERIA ARE REQUIRED FOR THE DIAGNOSIS OF POLYARTERITIS NODOSA OF THE CORONARY ARTERIES.

Evidence of a myocardial infarction occurring in the presence of established systemic polyarteritis nodosa.

2.3.2 ATHEROSCLEROSIS

Atherosclerosis of the coronary arteries primarily involves their intima; changes in the media and adventitia occur secondarily. The intimal lesions may include thickening by connective tissue rich in ground substance, aggregation of lipid-laden macrophages, and accumulation of extracellular lipid deposits, including cholesterol crystals. These deposits are associated with proliferation of collagenized connective tissue. Calcification and, rarely, ossification may develop in the intimal lesion. Fraying, fragmentation, and rupture of the internal elastic lamina may also occur. Thinning of the media results from atrophy and destruction of medial muscle, together with fibrous replacement. The extent of the medial lesion appears to be proportional to the thickness of the adjacent intimal plaque. Adventitial collagenous sclerosis and varying degrees of lymphocytic infiltration involving the outer coats may be seen.

Consequent to the alterations in the intima, there is often a rich capillary formation that usually originates from the vasa vasorum.

The surface of the intimal lesion may become necrotic and ulcerate, or may be the site of hemorrhage or thrombus formation.

Occlusion of a coronary artery may be gradual or rapid. Gradual occlusion is produced by eccentric or concentric thickening of the intima, to which any or all of the foregoing processes, except intraluminal thrombosis, may have contributed. Gradual occlusion is not commonly total, but may be very nearly so. Rapid occlusion may be caused either by rupture of intramural capillaries in a necrotic plaque, by hemorrhage into an ulcerated plaque, or by intraluminal thrombosis. The site of thrombosis is most commonly over an ulcerated plaque into which there has been hemorrhage. Intraluminal thrombosis may also occur over a nonhemorrhagic plaque which has narrowed the lumen of the vessel.

The lesions which impinge on the lumen of the vessel can vary in length from a few hundred micra to a centimeter or more in length.

Clinically significant atherosclerosis leading to anginal syndrome or myocardial infarction may vary from a small segmental lesion in one vessel to widespread lesions in all of the arteries and their major branches.

Selective coronary arteriography can reveal the presence of atherosclerosis by demonstrating partial or complete occlusion of the larger vessels or occasionally by showing aneurysms of the coronary arteries. If collateral circulation is present, the occluded vessel can fill by retrograde flow.

ONE OF THE FOLLOWING CRITERIA IS REQUIRED FOR THE DIAGNOSIS OF ATHEROSCLEROSIS OF THE CORONARY ARTERIES.

1. Anginal syndrome in the absence of aortic valve obstruction or coronary ostial stenosis.
2. Evidence of myocardial infarction in the absence of evidence of coronary emboli.
3. Evidence by coronary arteriography of the vascular abnormalities described.

4. **Evidence of calcification of an artery by radiographic techniques or at the time of surgery.**

2.3.3 EMBOLISM TO A CORONARY ARTERY

Embolism to a coronary artery occurs most commonly in the course of infective endocarditis. Emboli can also originate from thrombi on prosthetic valves or components of these valves. Emboli may arise from mural thrombi on the left side of the heart or from valve fragments released from mitral or aortic valves during a surgical operation.

Emboli can produce myocardial infarction or myocardial abscesses. The anterior descending branch of the left coronary is the vessel involved most frequently.

THE FOLLOWING CRITERIA ARE REQUIRED FOR THE DIAGNOSIS OF EMBOLISM TO A CORONARY ARTERY.

Evidence of recent myocardial infarction in the presence of any of the following: infective endocarditis; a recent operation on aortic or mitral valves; aortic or mitral prosthesis or homograft.

2.3.4 STENOSIS OF A CORONARY ORIFICE

Stenosis of a coronary orifice is most often the result of syphilitic aortitis, but can occasionally be found with atherosclerosis of the supravalvular aorta or following trauma during cardiac surgery. Dissecting hematoma of the aorta can also result in compression of the coronary arteries at their origin.

Anginal syndrome, myocardial fibrosis, and myocardial infarction can result from these lesions. These manifestations of coronary insufficiency are most frequently due to coronary atherosclerosis or aortic valvular lesions; hence the diagnosis of coronary ostial stenosis requires arteriographic demonstration.

THE FOLLOWING CRITERION IS REQUIRED FOR THE DIAGNOSIS OF STENOSIS OF A CORONARY ORIFICE.

Arteriographic evidence of coronary ostial stenosis.

2.4 Diseases of the Endocardium and Valves

2.4.1 SUBANULAR SCLEROSIS (ANULAR SCLEROSIS)

The zone of attachment of the mitral valve, and occasionally that of the aortic valve, marks the site of a fibrocalcific deposit in older persons. The deposits of calcium are variable in extent and mainly involve the junctional myocardium immediately below the valve anulus. These lesions usually do not produce obstruction or regurgitation and are not related to antecedent endocarditis. The valves are usually not involved, or only slightly so at their base, and valvular function usually remains undisturbed. However, the calcification occasionally may extend into the mitral leaflets and produce mitral regurgitation. In rare instances the calcific deposits may affect the conduction system and result in conduction defects.

The characteristic finding is a C-shaped band of calcium on radiologic examination.

THE FOLLOWING CRITERION IS REQUIRED FOR THE DIAGNOSIS OF SUBANULAR SCLEROSIS (MITRAL ANULUS CALCIFICATION).

Radiographic evidence of a C-shaped band of calcium between the left atrium and left ventricle.

2.4.2 ENDOCARDIAL FIBROELASTOSIS

Endocardial fibroelastosis is characterized by diffuse thickening of the endocardium, primarily of the left ventricle, giving it a milky-white appearance and relatively smooth lining. In addition to left ventricular involvement, the left atrium is frequently affected; although the endocardium of the right ventricle may show some thickening, it is always less prominent than on the left. There is a characteristic hyperplasia of fibroelastic tissue in and beneath the endocardium, with extension of fibrous bands into the myocardium.

The etiology and pathogenesis of endocardial fibroelastosis as an isolated phenomenon is unknown, although it is thought to originate in utero from environmental factors or an infectious agent. It may be present at birth and cause death from left ventricular failure in infancy. The occurrence of patchy areas of endocardial thickening in association with congenital malformations, notably those involving left-sided valves (aortic stenosis or atresia, mitral stenosis), and coarctation of the aorta is considered a "secondary" reaction to hemodynamic stress and injury.

The clinical picture of endocardial fibroelastosis is frequently that of a baby who fails to thrive and manifests signs of progressive left ventricular failure. Heart murmurs are inconspicuous, although an apical systolic murmur may occasionally reflect mitral regurgitation. The chest roentgenogram usually shows marked cardiac enlargement, and the electrocardiogram primarily reflects left ventricular enlargement.

The diagnosis is made with certainty only at necropsy. However, endocardial fibroelastosis may be considered to be present if in such clinical situations the following are excluded: active myocarditis, glycogen storage disease, and cardiovascular malformations, notably anomalous origin of the left coronary artery from the pulmonary artery.

2.4.3 ENDOCARDIAL FIBROSIS (ENDOMYOCARDIAL FIBROSIS)

This lesion is characterized by extensive endocardial and subendocardial fibrosis. The opaque, milky-white endocardium differs from that of endocardial fibroelastosis in that there is no increase in elastic tissue. The sclerosing process frequently extends to the inner myocardium. It is encountered in black people in some parts of Africa and has been described in other parts of the world in patients of African descent.

While focal degrees of endocardial thickening may be seen in other patients with hypertrophy of the heart of unknown cause, it is never so extensive as that found with endocardial fibrosis.

Patients with endocardial fibrosis may have an enlarged heart and evidence of ventricular failure. The diagnosis is rarely made prior to death.

2.4.4 ENDOCARDITIS

2.4.4.1 INFECTIVE ENDOCARDITIS

A wide variety of bacteria may cause endocarditis. The majority of cases are caused by *Streptococcus viridans* and are seen in patients with valves previously damaged by rheumatic fever or deformed by congenital defects. Infection can also occur on prosthetic valves and with congenital anomalies such as patent ductus arteriosus and ventricular septal defect. Other bacteria known to cause infection include staphylococcus, pneumococcus, β-hemolytic streptococcus, *Haemophilus influenzae,* meningococcus, and salmonella. These often cause infection of previously normal valves, especially in debilitated patients. Fungi can also be the cause of infection, particularly in heroin addicts, and the responsible organism is usually *Candida albicans*.

The valves are the site of a destructive process with superimposed vegetations. The vegetations are located principally on the contact surfaces of the valves, but may extend to contiguous mural endocardial surfaces, chordae tendineae, and papillary muscles. The left side of the heart is preponderantly involved.

The vegetations consist of masses of fibrin with enmeshed red cells. Bacteria grow on the surface and are entrapped within the friable fibrin mass. The underlying valve or mural endocardium is ulcerated, necrotic, variably invaded by polymorphonuclear leukocytes, and may be the site of frank abscess formation. An acute inflammatory reaction may be seen throughout the involved valve. As the infection is prolonged, either because of the nature of the infecting organism or because of antibiotic therapy, the lesion may contain large numbers of mononuclear cells. Evidences of repair are seen in the proliferation of connective tissue in the valve and in the growth of granulation tissue into the vegetation itself. With control of the infection, the vegetations undergo fibrosis, hyalinization, and often calcification, forming irregular nodular masses and deforming the valve.

Serious consequences of the active stages include destruction of a portion of the valve leaflet, perforation or aneurysm of a leaflet, rupture of the chordae tendineae, and embolization. If the patient survives to the healed stage, such defects may be the cause of continuing hemodynamic disability.

The clinical picture is characterized by fever, anemia, splenomegaly, new or changing murmurs, and embolic phenomena involving the skin, mucous membrane, brain, spleen, kidneys, and extremities. Right-sided endocarditis is frequently associated with septic emboli to the lungs; this can occur in narcotic addicts. Shaking chills, sweating, clubbing, and arthralgias are common. Osler's nodes, Janeway lesions, and splinter hemorrhages, although well known as associated findings, are not often seen today. With severe valvular damage, signs and symptoms of valvular regurgitation may become prominent, and ventricular failure may develop abruptly. In certain cases, valvular vegetations may be demonstrable by echocardiography.

ONE OF THE FOLLOWING CRITERIA IS REQUIRED FOR THE DIAGNOSIS OF INFECTIVE ENDOCARDITIS.

1. **Positive blood cultures associated with new or changing murmurs or with embolic phenomena.**
2. **In a patient with a congenital cardiac anomaly or with prior valvular damage, new or changing murmurs associated either with embolic phenomena or sustained fever, anemia, and splenomegaly.**

2.4.4.2 Lupus Valvulitis (Atypical Verrucous Endocarditis)

Valvulitis can occur in association with systemic lupus erythematosus. The lesions may vary in size from small verrucae to large vegetations and consist of granular fibrinous masses in which red and white blood cells are enmeshed. When present, hematoxylin bodies provide a distinctive feature of the lesion. Infiltration with macrophages and lymphocytes is present at the bases of the fibrinous masses, and occasionally there are plasma cells and evidence of organization. The masses are usually located on the ventricular aspect of the valves and extend in some cases onto the neighboring mural endocardium. The mitral and tricuspid valves are most often involved. Perforation of the valve and rupture of the chordae tendineae have not been described with the lesion.

These lesions rarely produce valvular obstruction or regurgitation and hence are not recognized clinically. However, superimposition of infective endocarditis is not unusual and may produce significant deformity of the valves.

2.4.4.3 Nonbacterial Thrombotic Endocarditis (Marantic Endocarditis, Terminal Endocarditis)

This type of endocarditis is seen most frequently in patients succumbing to chronic wasting diseases such as malignant tumors with metastases or severe malnutrition. The origin of the lesion is not clear. The lesion consists of firm, gray, yellow, or pink flat or raised nodules along the line of closure of the mitral valve and occasionally of the aortic valve. The lesions are larger than rheumatic verrucae and occasionally may be seen as large polypoid or pedunculated vegetations. The underlying valves may show some degenerative change. The mural endocardium and the chordae tendineae are usually not involved. The vegetations consist largely of agglutinated platelets and an admixture of red blood cells and fibrin, often with some evidence of organization at the periphery. Polymorphonuclear leukocytes are rarely found in these lesions, and bacteria are not present. Embolic phenomena, particularly cerebral, occasionally occur with this type of endocarditis. The lesion is rarely recognized prior to death.

2.4.4.4 Rheumatic Valvulitis and Endocarditis

During the acute phase of rheumatic heart disease, tiny, wartlike nodules (verrucae), 1 to 3 mm in size, occur along the line of closure of the valvular leaflets. These are firm and occur singly, in clusters, or in a continuous chain. Being strongly adherent, they do not easily become emboli. The mitral valve is most frequently affected, followed closely in frequency by the aortic valve. The tricuspid valve is involved less often and less severely, and the pulmonic valve is affected only rarely. Verrucae may be present along the chordae tendineae, which become swollen and fused. The affected leaflets are edematous and often adhere to each other.

The vegetations consist of small platelet and fibrin thrombi deposited on damaged proliferated endocardial cells. The underlying valvular tissue is edematous and contains a cellular infiltrate. The verrucae undergo organization, with an ingrowth of connective tissue cells, and the surface becomes covered by a smooth layer of endothelium. Within the leaflet and in the valve ring there is also a concomitant diffuse inflammatory process characterized by edema, an ingrowth of capillaries, the presence of polymorphonuclear cells, and occasionally Aschoff's bodies. Subsidence of this interstitial valvulitis is followed by an increase in connective tissue and an ingrowth of new blood vessels.

The acute insult to the valves, with or without recurrent attacks of rheumatic carditis, leads to progressive scarring and deformity. The leaflets become fused, retracted, thickened, vascularized, and calcified. The edges of the aortic valve cusps become thickened and rolled; the fusion of the cusps may be so extensive that the valve assumes a bicuspid appearance. The chordae tendineae also become fused, thickened, and shortened, thus adding to the mechanical deformity of the valve. At this stage the valves contain masses of hyaline fibrous tissue, numerous thick-walled blood vessels, irregular collections of calcium, and foci of lymphocytes and monocytes. These structural alterations in the leaflet lead to stenosis of the orifice and incompetence of the valve and to valvular obstruction or regurgitation, or both.

Some thickening and vascularization of the mitral valve, slight fusion and thickening of the chordae tendineae, and slight fusion of the commissures of the cusps of the aortic valve are not infrequent incidental necropsy findings in older patients. Whether they are all due to rheumatic inflammation or whether other disease processes are implicated is not clear at the present time.

The endocardium of the left atrium just above the posterior leaflet of the mitral valve is often the site of a zone of fibrinoid necrosis with associated Aschoff's cells. Aschoff's bodies are frequently observed in the endocardium of atrial appendages and ventricular endocardium.

Initially, there may be no clinical evidence of these structural abnormalities, although other "major" or "minor" evidences of acute rheumatic fever may be present. Systolic murmurs which appear may result from an increase in blood flow resulting from fever or anemia, or to cardiac dilatation secondary to myocardial involvement, and hence do not necessarily indicate valvular involvement. The appearance of an holosystolic murmur at the apex suggestive of mitral regurgitation usually indicates mitral valve involvement even if it subsequently disappears. Basal and apical diastolic murmurs usually suggest the presence of aortic or mitral valvulitis even if the murmurs are transient.

THE FOLLOWING CRITERIA ARE REQUIRED FOR THE DIAGNOSIS OF VALVULITIS DUE TO RHEUMATIC FEVER.

The appearance of an apical holosystolic murmur or of a diastolic murmur in association with one or more of the following: evidence of infection with β-hemolytic streptococcus of group A or one of the other major or minor criteria of rheumatic fever.

2.4.4.5 Rheumatoid Valvulitis

The unusual but specific form of rheumatoid involvement of valves is the presence of granulomas. These have central areas of fibrinoid necrosis surrounded by palisaded rows of macrophages and are identical to the subcutaneous rheumatoid nodule. They are usually accompanied by similar granulomatous involvement of pericardium and pleura.

The valvular lesions rarely produce valvular obstruction or regurgitation and hence are not recognized clinically.

2.4.5 INTRACARDIAC THROMBOSIS (ENDOCARDIAL THROMBOSIS)

Intracardiac thrombosis may result from inflammation, injury, necrosis and fibrosis, and slowing and abnormal eddying of the bloodstream. Thrombi may form on the endocardium of any of the cardiac chambers and are especially frequent in the atrial appendages. They may be the source of systemic or pulmonary emboli.

The marantic thrombus (stasis thrombus) is often found in the atrial appendages, most often associated with atrial fibrillation and ventricular failure. Ball, or globoid, thrombi occasionally lie free in the atrial chambers or may be attached to the atrioventricular orifices. They are most often found in association with obstruction of the mitral or tricuspid valves.

The majority of mural thrombi in the ventricles form as complications of myocardial infarction, particularly with ventricular failure. Although they are found predominantly in the left ventricle, they may involve both sides of the interventricular septum. In ventricular aneurysms incidental to myocardial infarction, mural thrombosis is common. The large thrombi are attached at their bases and are friable, laminated, and may be organized. Thrombosis of the ventricles is also seen in heart disease due to alcoholism or in hearts hypertrophied from an unknown cause.

Mural thrombi may be the source of systemic or pulmonary emboli.

While echocardiography may demonstrate the presence of a filling defect in a cardiac chamber, a negative study does not rule out such a lesion.

ONE OF THE FOLLOWING CRITERIA IS REQUIRED FOR THE DIAGNOSIS OF INTRACARDIAC THROMBOSIS.

1. **Angiocardiographic evidence of a filling defect in a cardiac chamber.**
2. **Evidence of intermittent valvular obstruction.**
3. **Evidence of systemic embolization in the presence of myocardial infarction, atrial fibrillation, valvular obstruction, or ventricular failure.**

2.4.6 MYXOMATOUS DEGENERATION OF A VALVE (MUCOID DEGENERATION)

Myxomatous degeneration of the mitral and aortic valves may lead to regurgitation. The central skeleton of fibrous tissue is transformed into a loose accumulation of connective-tissue ground substance, and the outer layers of the leaflets are secondarily thickened by increases in collagen and elastic fibers. Both leaflets of the mitral valve may be thickened and enlarged and balloon into the left atrium. Usually, the posterior leaflet is more seriously affected; the anterior leaflet is sometimes spared entirely. The histologic appearance is similar to that in patients with Marfan's syndrome, but other stigmata of that syndrome may be absent. The diseased valves may be the seat of superimposed infective or nonbacterial thrombotic endocarditis. The attenuated chordae tendineae contribute to valvular malfunction. They may rupture, with abrupt appearance of severe mitral regurgitation.

THE FOLLOWING CRITERION IS REQUIRED FOR THE DIAGNOSIS OF MYXOMATOUS DEGENERATION OF THE VALVES.

Histologic evidence of myxomatous change in valves removed at operation for correction of aortic or mitral regurgitation.

2.4.7 NEOPLASM OF THE ENDOCARDIUM

2.4.7.1 MYXOMA

Myxomas of the endocardium are almost invariably benign and are usually single. They occur most frequently in the atria, predominantly on the left, and their location determines their hemodynamic effects. Left atrial myxomas, particularly if they are pedunculated, can produce intermittent obstruction of the mitral orifice. Obstruction of venous flow into the left atrium may also cause pulmonary hypertension. Sudden movement of the tumor mass with atrial systole can cause an audible early diastolic sound. Myxomas in the right atrium can produce intermittent obstruction of the tricuspid orifice. Similarly, myxomas arising in the ventricles can produce intermittent obstruction to outflow from the right or left ventricle. Such intermittent obstruction can cause the sudden onset of severe hemodynamic abnormalities in patients who have no antecedent history of heart disease, and the signs and symptoms may be unique in their alterations with changes in body position.

Right-sided myxomas can produce emboli to the pulmonary arteries and left-sided myxomas, emboli to the peripheral arteries. In addition, the presence of the tumor mass itself can cause fever, weight loss, alterations in serum globulins, and an anemia which is sometimes hemolytic.

The hemodynamic effects of myxomas can be demonstrated by cardiac catheterization, but confirmation of the presence of a tumor mass requires echocardiographic or angiocardiographic examination. Occasionally, the tumors are calcified.

2.4.7.2 Papillary Fibroma (Papilloma)

Papillary fibromas of the heart valves are rare lesions which can produce murmurs and intermittent or fixed obstruction of the valve orifices. The findings, as with myxomas, depend on the anatomic location, size, and shape of the masses, which may arise from thrombus material rather than from valvular tissues.

ONE OF THE FOLLOWING CRITERIA IS REQUIRED FOR THE DIAGNOSIS OF HEART DISEASE DUE TO NEOPLASM OF THE ENDOCARDIUM.

1. **Demonstration by angiocardiography or echocardiography of an intracavity tumor mass.**

2. Histologic demonstration of myxomatous tissue in an embolus removed from a peripheral artery.
3. Demonstration of tumor tissue removed from the endocardium at operation.

2.4.8 RUPTURE OF CHORDAE TENDINEAE

Nonpenetrating, crushing injury to the chest may result in rupture of the chordae tendineae of either atrioventricular valve. Rupture of the chordae tendineae may also occur spontaneously or result from infective endocarditis, rheumatic valvulitis, or myxomatous degeneration.

The physiologic consequence of rupture of the chordae tendineae is valvular regurgitation. The abrupt onset of the disturbance can lead to the rapid development of pulmonary or systemic congestion.

While the sudden appearance of mitral or tricuspid regurgitation following trauma or occurring during the course of infective endocarditis or rheumatic valvulitis suggests rupture of the chordae tendineae, tear or perforation of a valve or detachment of a papillary muscle may be associated with the same findings.

THE FOLLOWING CRITERION IS REQUIRED FOR THE DIAGNOSIS OF RUPTURE OF CHORDAE TENDINEAE.

Demonstration at operation.

2.4.9 VALVULAR DEFORMITY

Valvular deformity, a frequent cause of valvular dysfunction (obstruction, regurgitation), is most often the sequel of rheumatic endocarditis and, less frequently, of infective endocarditis. In syphilitic aortitis, the aortic valve may become deformed on a mechanical basis. Hemodynamic trauma caused by turbulence or jet impact may contribute to the progression of abnormality in a valve previously damaged by inflammation, or induce deformity in a congenitally malformed valve. Valvular deformity may have a chemical origin, as in carcinoid heart disease. In older persons without a history of rheumatic fever, the aortic cusps may be the seat of sclerotic and calcific changes, which produce rigidity and deformity. It is not clear whether this form of aortic valvular disease (often termed *calcific aortic disease* or *calcific aortic stenosis*) stems from changes in a congenitally malformed valve (bicuspid, unicuspid) or in one damaged by undiagnosed rheumatic fever or is a primary lesion in an otherwise normal valve. Myxomatous degeneration in the aortic, mitral, or tricuspid valves may occur alone or in association with Marfan's syndrome.

Single or recurring episodes of inflammatory reaction in a valve lead to healing by proliferation of granulation tissue, which matures to produce dense collagenized scar tissue. Thick-walled small arteries extend into the valve substance from the base of the valve. Such vascularization is particularly prominent in rheumatic heart disease. The dense fibrous tissue in a scarred valve interrupts and replaces the normal collagen and elastic-tissue skeleton of the valve. Inflammation, with subsequent scarring, leads to obliteration of the commissures of the atrioventricular valves. Chordae tendineae are shortened, thickened, and fused. Scarring with or without calcification produces a relatively rigid, unyielding valve, with consequent disturbances in valve function. Calcification is not infrequently superimposed on fibrous scarring and increases the degree of rigidity and malfunction.

Infections of the valve may lead to aneurysm. Frank perforation may occur during infective endocarditis. Similarly, a defect at the free edge and line of closure of a valve in the form of irregular scalloping or extensive erosion may be seen after infection and may result in abnormalities of valve closure.

Angiocardiography can frequently demonstrate valvular deformity which results in stenosis. In patients with aortic stenosis, the valve may be seen to bulge convexly into the aorta during systole, forming a dome, and may be seen to be thickened, with decreased mobility and an eccentric orifice. A narrow jet of contrast material may be seen to enter the aorta during systole. Mitral stenosis may be revealed by a dome-shaped anterior bulging of the mitral valve into the left ventricle during diastole. A jet of contrast material may enter the left ventricle through the stenotic orifice, which is diminished in width. Valve leaflets may be shortened and thickened and have diminished mobility. Tricuspid stenosis may result in a doming of the thickened valve leaflets into the right ventricle during diastole. In pulmonic stenosis the thickened valve cusps may show decreased mobility and a dome shape as the valve bulges into the pulmonary artery during systole. A jet of contrast material may enter the pulmonary artery through a narrowed and eccentric orifice.

In patients with mitral stenosis, echocardiography may show that the anterior leaflet of the valve does not open well and does not close rapidly in early diastole and that the total amplitude of leaflet motion is decreased.

ONE OF THE FOLLOWING CRITERIA IS REQUIRED FOR THE DIAGNOSIS OF VALVULAR DEFORMITY.

1. Evidence of valvular obstruction or regurgitation in the presence of causes known to produce or result in valvular deformity.
2. Radiologic evidence of calcification of a valve.
3. Angiocardiographic evidence of thickening or abnormal motion of a valve.
4. Echocardiographic evidence of abnormal motion of a valve.

2.5 Diseases of the Myocardium

2.5.1 CARDIOMYOPATHY

2.5.1.1 ADIPOSE INFILTRATION OF THE MYOCARDIUM

Adipose infiltration of the myocardium is seen particularly in obese persons with excess epicardial fat. The right ventricle is predominantly involved. Adipose tissue extends into the myocardium, infiltrating between fibers, which may undergo atrophy and extensive replacement when the infiltration is extremely severe. The role of such adipose infiltration in the production of clinical heart disease due to obesity is not clearly established.

2.5.1.2 Amyloidosis

In the isolated or senile form associated with a plasma cell dyscrasia and in the familial form, amyloid (an altered or fibrillar protein) is deposited in the interstitium of the myocardium and conduction system. The myofibers are surrounded, compressed, rendered atrophic, and eventually replaced by amyloid. Neighboring muscle fibers may be hypertrophied, but the weight of the heart is often not increased. Multiple small subendocardial nodules may be present in the atria.

In the systemic or secondary form, amyloid is predominantly deposited in the small arteries and arterioles, although it may also be deposited in the interstices of the myocardium.

Extensive involvement can occasionally lead to cardiac enlargement and to disturbances in ventricular filling and congestive phenomena. The electrocardiogram may show left axis deviation, prolongation of the P–R interval, or complete atrioventricular block. Atrial fibrillation is a common finding. The voltage of the QRS complexes and T waves often is reduced, and there may be poor progression of R waves in the precordial leads.

THE CRITERIA REQUIRED FOR THE DIAGNOSIS OF CARDIOMYOPATHY DUE TO AMYLOIDOSIS ARE GIVEN IN 1.3.

2.5.1.3 Friedreich's Ataxia

Myocardial degeneration without pericardial or valvular disease has frequently been found in Friedreich's ataxia. There is cardiac enlargement, with focal destruction of myofibers, replacement fibrosis, and hypertrophy of intact fibers. Focal interstitial myocarditis characterized by infiltration by lymphocytes and occasionally by polymorphonuclear leukocytes may be observed. Small coronary arteries are often involved and may be occluded. The conduction system may be involved in this process.

THE CRITERIA REQUIRED FOR THE DIAGNOSIS OF CARDIOMYOPATHY DUE TO FRIEDREICH'S ATAXIA ARE GIVEN IN 1.9.

2.5.1.4 Glycogen Storage Disease

Abnormal glycogen deposition in the myocardium due to alpha-1,4-glucosidase deficiency (Pompe's disease) results in marked cardiac enlargement, particularly of the left ventricle and ventricular septum. The myofibers are infiltrated and swollen with glycogen and contain few myofibrils. Left ventricular failure may result from this lesion. In some instances, subaortic obstruction is produced by encroachment of the thickened interventricular system upon the left ventricular outflow tract.

Huge deposits of glycogen can also be found in the tongue, skeletal muscle, and other organs.

THE CRITERIA REQUIRED FOR THE DIAGNOSIS OF CARDIOMYOPATHY DUE TO GLYCOGEN STORAGE DISEASE ARE GIVEN IN 1.10.

2.5.1.5 Hemochromatosis

Involvement of the myocardium is common in hemochromatosis and consists in the accumulation of hemosiderin within the myofibers. This begins as perinuclear deposition and spreads to involve much of the fiber. It is associated with degenerative changes within the fiber, fragmentation, and focal scarring.

Cardiac enlargement and conduction disturbances commonly occur. Disturbances in ventricular filling may be terminal.

THE CRITERIA REQUIRED FOR THE DIAGNOSIS OF CARDIOMYOPATHY DUE TO HEMOCHROMATOSIS ARE GIVEN IN 1.11.

2.5.1.6 Hypothyroidism

In myxedema, the properties of collagen and mucoproteins are probably altered, and soluble complexes are converted into unstable gels. These are deposited in the interstitium of the heart and in the pericardium. Consequently, an increase in basophilic and metachromatic material can be demonstrated between muscle fibers and in the pericardium, particularly in untreated patients. The deposits in the pericardium are probably the cause of the frequently observed pericardial effusion. The functional significance of the myocardial deposits is unknown.

THE CRITERIA REQUIRED FOR THE DIAGNOSIS OF CARDIOMYOPATHY DUE TO HYPOTHYROIDISM ARE GIVEN IN 1.15.

2.5.1.7 Mucopolysaccharidoses

This group of genetic disorders is characterized by inborn errors of metabolism which result in the deposition of excess quantities of mucopolysaccharides in connective tissue. Fibroblasts are swollen and vacuolated, and there is an increase in intercellular ground substance. In the heart there is nodular thickening of the valves and shortening and thickening of the chordae tendineae. Regurgitation or obstruction of the mitral or aortic valves may result, as may pulmonic regurgitation. Deposition of mucopolysaccharide in the intima of coronary vessels, with reactive intimal fibrous proliferation, may produce striking narrowing. Enlargement of the heart is usually attributable to valvular defects, but direct involvement of myocardial connective tissue may play a role.

THE CRITERIA REQUIRED FOR THE DIAGNOSIS OF CARDIOMYOPATHY DUE TO MUCOPOLYSACCHARIDOSES ARE GIVEN IN 1.18.

2.5.1.8 Nodular Glycogen Infiltration (Rhabdomyoma)

This form of cardiac glycogen deposition is most often observed in association with tuberous sclerosis. The nodular lesions usually occur in the ventricular septum, but may be present in the wall of any of the chambers or the atrial septum. They compress surrounding normal myofibers and are made up of a lacy network of cell membranes encompassing large vacuolar spaces that contain glycogen. The masses so formed may seriously encroach upon the lumina of the chambers.

Symptoms in infancy may result from left ventricular failure or arrhythmias. In older children and adults with tuberous sclerosis (manifested by mental retardation, intracranial calcification, or adenoma sebaceum), cardiomegaly may be the only evidence of glycogen deposition in the heart.

THE FOLLOWING CRITERIA ARE REQUIRED FOR THE DIAGNOSIS OF CARDIOMYOPATHY DUE TO NODULAR GLYCOGEN INFILTRATION (RHABDOMYOMA).

Angiocardiographic evidence of local mural or septal tumor masses encroaching upon the cavities of the heart in association with tuberous sclerosis.

2.5.1.9 NONSPECIFIC

Cardiomyopathy may be caused by anemia, thiamine deficiency, or prolonged hypovolemic shock. The heart may be enlarged, dilated, and flabby, with fatty change visible through the endocardium as transverse yellow markings, or "tigering." The lesions in these conditions are similar, consisting of fatty change, hydropic degeneration, and swelling of the myofibers. In the advanced form, this damage may progress to actual necrosis.

Clinically, there may be ventricular dilatation, ventricular failure, and arrhythmias.

THE FOLLOWING CRITERIA ARE REQUIRED FOR THE DIAGNOSIS OF NONSPECIFIC CARDIOMYOPATHY.

The presence of ventricular dilatation, ventricular failure, or arrhythmias in the course of profound anemia, hypovolemic shock, or thiamine deficiency.

2.5.1.10 PROGRESSIVE MUSCULAR DYSTROPHY

The heart in progressive muscular dystrophy may show fine or gross areas of fibrosis. Residual atrophic myofibers are encompassed by the fibrous tissue. Other muscle fibers are hypertrophied.

THE CRITERIA REQUIRED FOR THE DIAGNOSIS OF CARDIOMYOPATHY DUE TO PROGRESSIVE MUSCULAR DYSTROPHY ARE GIVEN IN 1.22.

2.5.2 ENLARGEMENT OF THE HEART

Enlargement of the heart results from hypertrophy of the myocardium or dilatation of the cardiac chambers or a combination of these changes. One chamber or all four may be involved, depending upon the nature of the underlying disease and its degree of progression.

2.5.2.1 Left Ventricular Enlargement

Hypertrophy of the left ventricle usually involves both the free wall and the interventricular septum. The papillary muscles and trabeculae carneae are thickened and may reduce the luminal dimensions of the chamber. In the hypertrophied myocardium the cardiac cells increase in diameter and length, but do not increase in number. The thickening of the cells results from an increase in the number of sarcomeres and mitochondria. Depending upon the stimulus to hypertrophy, the proportion of the cell occupied by either mitochondria or contractile units becomes disturbed so that one population of organelles hypertrophies out of proportion to the rest of the cellular components. The cell, for example, that has enlarged in response to a volume overload has an increased number of mitochondria, compared to the normal; the cell that hypertrophies in response to a pressure overload responds by an increase in sarcomeric units. Connective tissue cells often increase in number. When hypertrophy exists without dilatation, it is sometimes called *concentric hypertrophy*.

Hypertrophy of the left ventricle can be caused by increases in pressure or volume load. Dilatation of the left ventricle is usually accompanied by hypertrophy and can result from left ventricular failure, sustained arrhythmias, aortic and mitral regurgitation, ventricular septal defect, and patent ductus arteriosus.

In certain persons, marked hypertrophy of the left ventricle, with or without ventricular dilatation, occurs in the absence of a generally accepted cause. Although the primary alteration in these cases may be hypertrophy of the myofibers, varying degrees of muscle necrosis and patchy fibrosis are also usually found in the myocardium. These latter alterations tend to be subendocardial in location and are frequently associated with mural thrombosis. Within the myocyte itself, accumulations of Z substance are a prominent feature; they may be involved in the generation of new sarcomeric units in the cell. These types of cardiomyopathy have been termed *idiopathic myocardial hypertrophy, idiopathic or primary myocardial disease,* and *familial cardiomegaly.*

In some instances, marked hypertrophy, particularly of the interventricular septum, may result in obstruction to blood flow from the left ventricle during systole as the septum abuts against the anterior leaflets of the mitral valve. This leaflet often shows endocardial thickening. The obstructive syndrome caused by this lesion has been termed *idiopathic hypertrophic subaortic stenosis, idiopathic hypertrophic subvalvular aortic stenosis, hypertrophic obstructive cardiomyopathy, muscular subaortic stenosis*. This type of hypertrophy can occur early in life and in some instances seems to be of familial or congenital origin. Left ventriculography shows impingement of the hypertrophied septum on the left ventricular outflow tract and variations in the contour of the left ventricular cavity. The electrocardiogram may show unusually prominent Q waves in addition to left ventricular hypertrophy. Diagnosis of this type of hypertrophy requires demonstration of obstruction to left ventricular outflow below the level of the aortic valve. Here, echocardiography has become extremely important in demonstrating increased septal thickness and systolic anterior motion (SAM) of the anterior leaflet of the mitral valve. The latter may not be present at rest, but because of the dynamic nature of the obstruction, may be brought out by provocation with the Valsalva maneuver, amyl nitrite, inotropic agents, or premature beats.

Marked hypertrophy decreases the compliance of the left ventricle and elevates the end-diastolic pressure in the chamber.

When dilatation accompanies hypertrophy, it produces what is sometimes termed *eccentric hypertrophy.* General enlargement of the ventricle occurs, and the apical portion of the chamber becomes conspicuous. The trabeculae carneae and papillary muscles are flattened and less prominent than in pure hypertrophy.

Enlargement of the left ventricle usually causes the

point of maximum impulse to be displaced to the left and downward on physical examination. In the presence of hypertrophy the apical thrust tends to be prolonged and vigorous. A fourth heart sound is commonly present.

Mild to moderate hypertrophy may not alter the electrocardiogram. However, marked hypertrophy of the left ventricle can cause changes in the electrocardiogram which are due to a change in the position of the heart in the thorax and an increase in muscle mass, with a consequent shift in orientation of the vector of depolarization. The mean electrical axis of the QRS (Table F, Appendix) may be shifted considerably to the left (left axis deviation is present when angle alpha lies between +29° and −90°), but in thin-chested persons and those with a vertical heart, this may not occur. Increased QRS voltage is often seen and is considered significant when the largest positive or negative deflection in the limb leads (at normal standardization) is greater than 20 mm (2.0 mv); or when S in V1, V2 or V3 is more than 30 mm (3.0 mv); or when R in V5 or V6 is more than 30 mm (3.0 mv); or when the sum of R in V5 or V6 and the deeper of the S waves in V1, V2 or V3 is 40 mm or more. The duration of the QRS complex is often, but not always, prolonged and may range between 0.10 and 0.12 sec. The intrinsicoid deflection, or time from the onset of the QRS complex to the peak of R, in V6 may be delayed (longer than 0.045 sec). Secondary changes in repolarization (S–T segment and T wave) may occur with marked hypertrophy and are manifested by depression of S–T segments and negative T waves in leads I, aVL, and V4–V6 (Fig. 1).

In children, the voltage of the QRS complex tends to be higher than in adults. Hence voltage criteria for left ventricular hypertrophy in children are different. Left ventricular hypertrophy can be suspected when the sum of R in lead I and S in III is more than 30 mm, the sum of R in V5 and S in V2 is greater than 60 mm, and the R/S ratio in V1 is less than the maximum normal for the age: under 1 year, 0.8; 1 to 5 years, 0.2; and 6 to 14 years, 0.1 or less. The intrinsicoid deflection in V6 may exceed 0.04 sec, but this is a late manifestation of left hypertrophy, as are depressions of S–T segments and inversions of T waves in the left ventricular leads (I, aVL, V4–V6).

The vectorcardiogram can show alterations in the presence of left ventricular hypertrophy. The mean QRS vector tends to be rotated leftward, posteriorly, and superiorly and has increased magnitude (2.0 mv or more) and counterclockwise rotation. When hypertrophy is advanced, the mean S–T and T vectors are directed away from the QRS vector (that is, to the right and anteriorly), resulting in a wide spatial QRS–T angle, which usually exceeds 120° and may reach 160° to 180°. The electrocardiogram and vectorcardiogram often reflect hypertrophy more readily than dilatation.

Radiologic examination of the heart is a more reliable indicator of dilatation than of hypertrophy. In the posteroanterior projection, concentric hypertrophy (that is, hypertrophy without dilatation) may cause increased rounding of the lower left heart (ventricular) border in the absence of an overall increase in heart size. When hypertrophy and dilatation coexist, enlargement of the ventricular region occurs, with lengthening and increased prominence of the lower left heart border. When left ventricular enlargement is minimal, the change from normal size may be revealed only by serial roentgenograms. Right ventricular enlargement or pericardial effusion can at times exactly resemble left ventricular enlargement on plain chest films.

Angiocardiography is necessary to define the sizes, shapes, and positions of the cardiac chambers in some cases. In the hypertrophied ventricle, angiocardiography will demonstrate thickening of the free wall and papillary muscles and accentuation of the trabeculae. Dilatation is readily apparent on angiocardiography. Ultrasound is also useful in measuring left ventricular free wall and septal thickness as well as left ventricular dilatation.

ONE OF THE FOLLOWING CRITERIA IS REQUIRED FOR THE DIAGNOSIS OF ENLARGEMENT OF THE LEFT VENTRICLE.

1. **A displacement of the point of maximum impulse downward and to the left on physical examination**

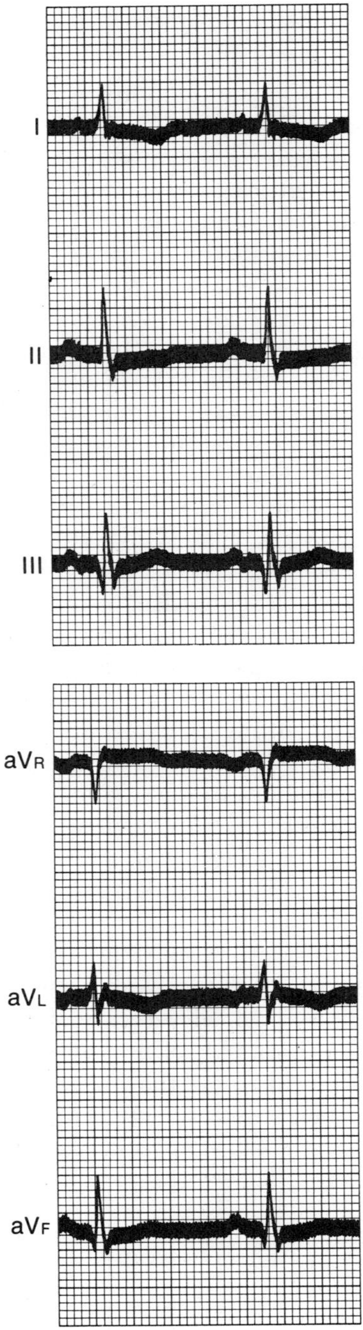

Figure 1

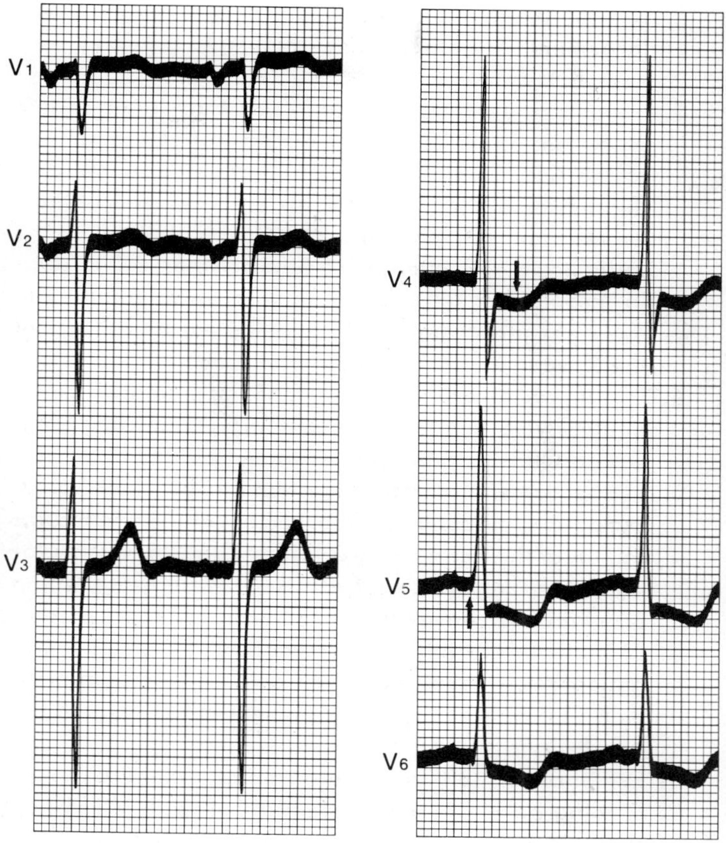

Figure 1. *Left ventricular hypertrophy.* There is a normal mean electrical axis of QRS and an increased voltage of S waves in V2 and V3 and of R waves in V4 and V5; the sum of S in V3 and R in V5 is 51 mm. The QRS duration is 0.10 sec, and the peak of the R waves (intrinsicoid deflection) in V5 and V6 is delayed (0.055 sec). A small arrow in V5 points to the Q wave and marks the onset of QRS. The arrow in V4 marks the depression of the S–T segment, which is also present in V5 and V6, where the T waves are negative. There are negative T waves also in leads I and aVL. (The leads are recorded in four sets of three simultaneous leads each: I, II, III; aVR, aVL, aVF; V1, V2, V3, V4, V5, V6. The standardization is 1 mv = 10 mm in all twelve leads.)

(unless there is accompanying right ventricular enlargement, in which case this sign becomes less specific).

2. Either a moderate degree of left axis deviation (angle alpha between +29° and −30°) or increased voltage of the QRS complexes, or both, coupled either with depression of the S–T segments and inversion of the T waves in leads I, aVL, and V4–V6 or with delay in the intrinsicoid deflection in V6 (greater than 0.045 sec.)
3. In infants, left axis deviation with an rS complex in the right precordial leads and increased voltage of the R wave in the left precordial leads.
4. In the vectorcardiogram, a QRS loop rotated counterclockwise to the left, posteriorly, and superiorly, with a QRS–T angle greater than 120°.
5. In the posteroanterior projection of the chest roentgenogram, evidence of enlargement of the ventricular region of the heart (not explained by right ventricular dilatation or pericardial effusion), with lengthening or increased convexity of the lower left heart border, or both. In the lateral projection of the chest roentgenogram, a relatively thick anteroposterior dimension of the heart should be present at the level of the diaphragm.
6. Evidence of left ventricular enlargement by ventriculography or echocardiography: with dilatation there is an increased left ventricular volume; with hypertrophy, an increase in total muscle mass of the left ventricular wall and increased thickness of the left ventricular wall at the end of diastole.

2.5.2.2 Right Ventricular Enlargement

Hypertrophy of the right ventricle results in thickening and increased prominence of the trabeculae carneae. Hypertrophy of the right ventricular infundibulum, the crista supraventricularis, and the papillary muscles also occurs. Pure hypertrophy of the right ventricle is usually caused by chronic pressure overloads. Considerable hypertrophy may be present without overall enlargement of the heart apparent on chest roentgenograms.

Marked hypertrophy may lead to a decrease in compliance of the right ventricular wall and elevation of the end-diastolic pressure in the right ventricle. Muscle hypertrophy, particularly of the right ventricular outflow tract or infundibulum, may be so marked as to cause an obstruction to right ventricular ejection.

Dilatation of the right ventricle tends to broaden and flatten the trabeculae carneae. A dilated right ventricle may secondarily displace the left ventricle toward the left and lift the cardiac apex off the diaphragm, as is typical of tetralogy of Fallot.

Dilatation is usually due to right ventricular failure or volume overload, as in left-to-right shunts at the atrial level or regurgitation across the tricuspid or pulmonary valves. Hypertrophy typically accompanies chronic dilatation. Dilatation without hypertrophy can result from the sudden appearance of pulmonary hypertension following massive pulmonary embolism.

Enlargement of the right ventricle can cause an epigastric pulsation. Considerable hypertrophy can result in a pronounced systolic pulsation along the left border of the sternum.

Marked hypertrophy of the right ventricle can lead to changes in the electrocardiogram which are in part related to a change in position of the heart in the thorax and in part to an increase in muscle mass. The mean electrical axis of the QRS (Table F, Appendix) may be shifted rightward (right axis deviation is considered present when angle alpha lies between +91° and −91°). The axis is usually at +100° to +120°, but occasionally is as far to the right as +180°. The QRS duration remains normal. If large R waves occur in the right precordial leads, especially if in V1 the R is preceded by a Q wave, and if the intrinsicoid deflection in V1 exceeds 0.025 sec, the pattern is diagnostic of right ventricular hypertrophy. Hypertrophy is likely if the R/S ratio in V1 is 1.0 or more, the R/S ratio in V5 or V6 is 1.0 or less, and the height of the R wave in V1 is 5 mm or more; or if there is an RSR′ in V1 (and a normal QRS duration), and the first or second R wave is greater than 8 mm in height. In more advanced

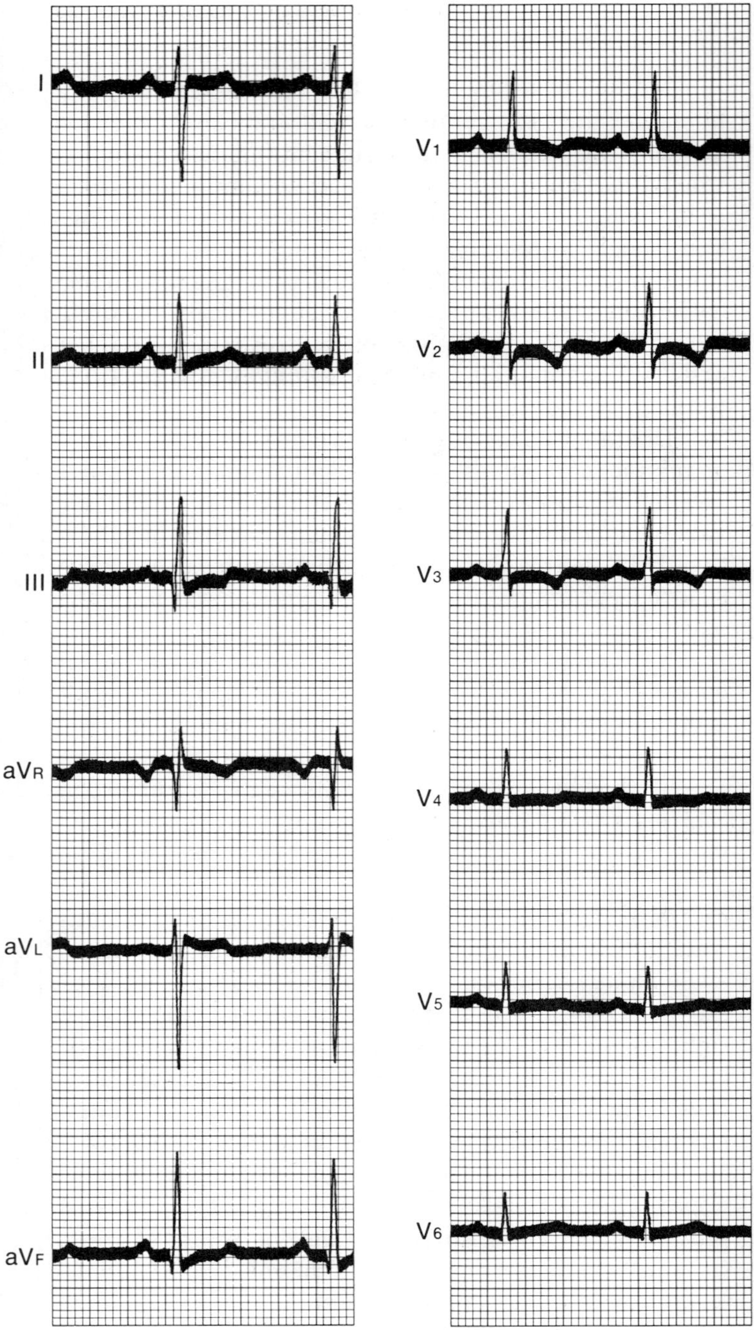

Figure 2

stages there are depression of the S–T segments and negative T waves in leads II, III, aVF, and the right precordial leads, V1–V3 (Fig. 2).

The vectorcardiogram may also show changes in the presence of right ventricular enlargement. When hypertrophy is moderate to severe, the mean QRS vector loop is displaced to the right and anteriorly, usually inferiorly, and, more rarely, to the right and posteriorly. There is usually clockwise rotation of the loop, and there are secondary changes in spatial S–T and T vectors, which are most frequently displaced leftward and posteriorly; the spatial QRS–T angle may exceed 150° to 180°.

The changes in the mean electrical axis which suggest an electrocardiographic diagnosis of right ventricular hypertrophy in adults are not applicable to infants. Infants normally may have considerable right axis deviation at birth and shortly thereafter. However, in infants, if a Q wave precedes the large R in V1 or V3R, the pattern is diagnostic of right ventricular hypertrophy unless ventricular inversion with congenitally corrected transposition of the great arteries or papillary muscle infarction is present. In infants with hypertrophy the intrinsicoid deflection in V1 may also be delayed beyond the normal of 0.025 sec. With hypertrophy the R/S ratio in V1 or V3R may exceed 6.0 up to 3 months of age, 4.0 up to 6 months, 2.0 up to 5 years, and 1.0 up to 15 years, while the R/S ratio in V6 is 1.0 or less. With hypertrophy the amplitude of R in V1 or V3R may exceed 20 mm in infants under 1 year or 16 mm in children over this age. Right hypertrophy is likely if there is an RSR′ in V1, with a normal QRS duration, and the height of one of the two R waves

---

Figure 2. *Right ventricular hypertrophy.* The mean electrical axis of QRS is +158°, and the QRS duration is normal (0.07 sec). The large R in V1 is preceded by a small Q wave, and the peak of R (intrinsicoid deflection) is delayed (0.045 sec). There are depressed S–T segments in leads III, aVF, V2, and V3 and negative T waves in V1–V3. (The leads are recorded in two sets of six simultaneous leads each: I, II, III, aVR, aVL, aVF, V1–V6. The standardization is 1 mv = 10 mm in the six limb leads and 1 mv = 5 mm in the six V leads.)

exceeds 8 mm, especially if the R/S ratio is larger than 1.0. The direction of T waves in right ventricular leads (V3R, V1–V2) is upright in the first 24 hours of life, but after a few days, and certainly after 3 weeks of age, T waves in the right precordium are normally negative and remain so up to 1 year of age. Thus between age 3 weeks and 1 year, a positive T wave may appear in right V leads due to right ventricular hypertrophy; this is usually seen only when the QRS criteria for hypertrophy previously described are also present. Depression of the S–T segment in leads II, III, and aVF are seen with advanced right hypertrophy.

The chest roentgenogram may show changes induced by hypertrophy and dilatation. In the posteroanterior projection, the apex of the heart can be rounded and elevated. Frontal, lateral, and the right oblique projections can show bulging of the left upper and ventral (anterior) cardiac borders due to increased prominence and dilatation of the right ventricular outflow tract and main pulmonary artery. Enlargement of the main pulmonary arteries and the right atrium suggests that the right ventricle is likely to be enlarged.

When right ventricular enlargement is slight and when the diaphragm is very low (for example, in obstructive pulmonary disease), right ventricular enlargement may not be appreciated unless serial roentgenograms are available to show the increase in heart size.

On other occasions, dilatation of the right ventricle may rotate the interventricular septum to the left and dorsally, so that in extreme cases the dilated right ventricle actually forms the left heart border. Under this circumstance, in the frontal projection of the chest roentgenogram a long, convex or straight left heart border continuous with the pulmonary artery segment is produced and can be confused with left ventricular enlargement or dilatation of the left atrium.

Marked enlargement of the ventricular region of the heart in the presence of exceptionally clear lungs with small pulmonary vessels suggests either pericardial effusion or right heart dilatation secondary to congenital or acquired tricuspid regurgitation. In the presence of left heart enlargement or pericardial effusion, evidences of right ventricular enlargement can be obscured. Ventriculography is useful for demonstrating both dilatation and hypertrophy. Echocardiography has limited usefulness as a measurement of right ventricular hypertrophy, but can be useful in detecting dilatation.

ONE OF THE FOLLOWING CRITERIA IS REQUIRED FOR THE DIAGNOSIS OF RIGHT VENTRICULAR ENLARGEMENT.

1. Pronounced systolic pulsation or heave along the left border of the sternum or under the xiphoid process in the epigastrium.
2. Right deviation of the electrical axis coupled either with depression of S–T segments and inversion of T waves in leads II, III, aVF, and V1–V3, or a single, tall peak or R in V1, with a delay in the intrinsicoid (greater than 0.025 sec).
3. Vectorcardiographic evidence of a QRS loop rotated clockwise, rightward, and anteriorly, with a QRS–T angle of greater than 150°.
4. In the frontal projection of the chest roentgenogram, unusual prominence of the central pulmonary arteries (indicating that pulmonary hypertension is present) and rounding and elevation of the apex of the heart. Enlargement of the main pulmonary artery and right atrium, accompanied by enlargement of the ventricular region of the heart, particularly in the absence of left atrial enlargement or evidence of pulmonary capillary hypertension.
5. In the lateral roentgenographic projection, encroachment of the heart on the retrosternal clear space, as well as dorsal displacement of the posterior margin of the intrathoracic inferior vena cava.
6. Ventriculographic or echocardiographic evidence of dilatation or hypertrophy of the right ventricle.

2.5.2.3 Left Atrial Enlargement

Hypertrophy of the left atrium produces a thickened muscular atrial wall and prominent pectinate muscles in the base of the atrial appendage. Hypertrophy of the left atrium is usually the result of chronically increased left atrial pressure, as in left ventricular failure and mitral valve dysfunction.

Left atrial dilatation of variable degree usually accompanies left atrial hypertrophy. Dilatation sometimes reaches enormous proportions, especially in rheumatic mitral regurgitation. Dilatation is often seen in both chronic pressure and chronic volume overloads (as in mitral regurgitation and, less strikingly, in large left-to-right shunts through ventricular septal defects or a patent ductus arteriosus). Atrial dilatation often occurs in the presence of chronic atrial fibrillation and tends to perpetuate the arrhythmia.

The electrocardiographic and vectorcardiographic criteria either for left or right atrial enlargement are not so reliable as the roentgenologic criteria. However, certain features may assist in this diagnosis. In left atrial enlargement there is often an intra-atrial block, as shown by an increased duration of the P wave (exceeding 0.07 sec in infants under 1 year old; 0.08 sec from 1 to 12 years; 0.09 sec from 12 to 16 years; and above 0.11 sec in adults). The mean electrical axis of the P wave is shifted to the left (usually falling between +30° and −30°). In V1 the P wave may be diphasic, with the second and negative component 0.04 sec in duration or longer and 1 mm (0.1 mv) or more in depth. There may or may not be notching of the P wave.

The mean P vector is shifted posteriorly, leftward, and inferiorly and is increased in duration. In the frontal plane it may assume a horizontal and leftward orientation, often approaching an axis of 0°, in contrast to the normal P axis of +30° to +60°. Thus P waves in leads I and aVL are more prominent than those in III and aVF.

The size of the left atrium can usually be accurately estimated on chest roentgenogram. Following opacification of the esophagus by ingestion of barium, slight left atrial enlargement may be apparent only in the lateral or right anterior oblique projections. Even the slightly enlarged left atrium will often displace the esophagus posteriorly. As seen in the frontal chest roentgenogram, this posterior bulging of the left atrium tends to increase the cardiac opacity over the region of the left atrium. On the frontal chest roentgenogram the left atrial margins can be roughly approximated by noting the right and left main bronchi, the double density on the right heart border due to the additional shadow of the left atrium, and the prominence (or lack of it) of the left atrial appendage on the left heart border in the junctional region between the pulmonary artery and the ventricular region. Enlargement of the left atrium can produce a widening of the subcarinal angle and elevation of the right or left main bronchi or of both.

Correlation has been excellent between echocardiographically and angiographically determined left atrial dimension.

ONE OF THE FOLLOWING CRITERIA IS REQUIRED FOR THE DIAGNOSIS OF LEFT ATRIAL ENLARGEMENT.

1. A wide P wave, with a leftward P axis at or near 0° and a prominent deep negative component to a diphasic P wave in V1.
2. An abnormal frontal cardiac configuration on the chest roentgenogram due to one, and preferably several, of the following features: widening of the subcarinal angle, abnormal elevation of the right or left main bronchi, or both; a prominent second contour along the mid right heart border; straightening or convexity along the left heart border in the region of left atrial appendage.
3. On lateral or right anterior oblique projections of the chest roentgenogram, abnormal displacement of the barium-filled esophagus by the enlarged left atrium.
4. Angiocardiographic or echocardiographic evidence of dilatation or hypertrophy of the left atrium.

2.5.2.4 Right Atrial Enlargement

Hypertrophy of the right atrium, which results in a thickened muscular wall and prominent pectinate muscles, is usually due to chronically increased right atrial pressure, as in right ventricular failure, tricuspid valvular disease of acquired or congenital origin, or chronic atrial fibrillation.

Dilatation of the right atrium is usually accompanied by hypertrophy, but this is variable in degree. Dilatation tends to be most marked in the presence of chronic tricuspid regurgitation, especially when caused by congenital heart disease. Both dilatation and hypertrophy may result from large left-to-right shunts due to atrial septal defects or anomalous pulmonary venous connection to the right side of the heart.

Right atrial enlargement can produce changes in the electrocardiogram, vectorcardiogram, and chest roentgenogram.

In right atrial enlargement the P wave duration is not longer than normal, but its amplitude may be large (3 mm [0.3 mv] or more in leads II, III, and aVF), and, indeed, the P wave may appear somewhat narrow as well as tall. The mean P axis is shifted rightward beyond +60°, but seldom further than +90°, and the biphasic P wave in V1 is large (3 mm or more), with a positive initial component predominating.

The mean P vector is increased in magnitude in right atrial enlargement and is rotated rightward (or occasionally slightly leftward), inferiorly, and anteriorly.

ONE OF THE FOLLOWING CRITERIA IS REQUIRED FOR THE DIAGNOSIS OF RIGHT ATRIAL ENLARGEMENT.

1. A P wave which is less than 0.12 sec in duration, associated with large P waves in II, III, and aVF, a P wave axis more than +60°, and a large positive initial component to the biphasic P wave in V1.
2. In the frontal projection of the chest roentgenogram an unusually long and prominent right heart border, whose edge extends 2 fingerbreadths beyond the right vertebral edge.
3. On the lateral projection of the chest roentgenogram an unusually posterior location of the intrathoracic inferior vena caval margin and encroachment on the retrosternal clear space from below.

4. Angiocardiographic evidence of right atrial dilatation or hypertrophy.

2.5.3 INFARCTION OF THE MYOCARDIUM

Infarction of the myocardium can result from impaired coronary blood flow secondary to a variety of underlying lesions of the coronary arteries and their ostia. Atherosclerosis is by far the most frequent cause. It can also result from an anomalous origin of the left coronary artery from the pulmonary artery.

The area of ischemic necrosis or infarction of the heart may vary from focal and minute to diffuse and massive. Infarcts do not ordinarily involve the myocardial wall uniformly throughout their extent. The same infarct may be transmural in one area and subendocardial or intramural in another. When the infarct involves the pericardium, it may be followed by fibrinous pericarditis; when it involves the endocardium, it may be followed by mural thrombosis. Generally, the process does not involve all of the muscle fibers within a circumscribed area, nor is the involvement uniform in age. Hence there is commonly a mixture of healthy and dead or dying muscle, infiltrated with leukocytes, showing condensation of reticulum, and focal hemorrhages. Shrinkage following removal of necrotic muscle begins between the first and second week, when young granulation tissue appears. In the next few weeks this is replaced by fibrous tissue. The lesion becomes a scar within two or three months.

Infarcts occur in the apical portion of the anterior wall of the left ventricle and the contiguous portion of the ventricular septum as a result of obstruction of the anterior descending branch of the left coronary artery; in the basal diaphragmatic or inferior (formerly called posterior) wall and contiguous septum as a result of obstruction of the right coronary artery; and in the lateral wall of the left ventricle as a result of obstruction of the left circumflex artery. Very rarely, there may be isolated infarction of the right ventricle or of one of the atria. Even in conjunction with left ventricular infarction, only 5 percent of hearts will show right ventricular infarction, and about 15 percent will show infarction of the atria, of the right more often than of the left atrium.

Narrowing of the right main coronary artery or of the left circumflex artery before the origin of the sinus node artery may produce pathologic changes in the sinoatrial and atrioventricular nodes, the His bundle, and the bundle branches; if the narrowing is distal to the origin of the sinus node artery, the sino-atrial node may be spared. Narrowing of the posterior descending coronary artery may produce changes in the left posterior fascicle (posterior radiation) of the left bundle branch. Narrowing of the anterior descending coronary artery before the origin of the second perforating branch may produce changes in the right bundle branch and left anterior fascicle (anterior radiation) of the left bundle branch; narrowing distal to this point may produce changes in the left anterior fascicle of the left bundle branch alone. It is possible to have narrowing of only the artery supplying the atrioventricular node and His bundle. The reduced arterial lumina may be associated with severe degeneration, necrosis, and fibrosis of any of the specialized structures, resulting in atrioventricular, bundle branch, or fascicular blocks.

The typical patient with myocardial infarction presents with severe anterior precordial chest pain or discomfort; this is usually, but not necessarily, of a pressing or squeezing character and not relieved by rest or nitroglycerin. The pain may also be felt in the neck, jaw, left shoulder or arm, or occasionally in the midback. Sweating, fainting, nausea, weakness and, occasionally, vomiting, along with a subjective sense of doom, accompany the other symptoms. The attack may be preceded by a period of days or weeks marked by anginal episodes which progressively increase in duration and severity. In some cases, pain and other symptoms may be slight, may even be absent, or may not fit the characteristics described.

The physiologic consequences of an infarct include ventricular failure, cardiogenic shock, the frequent appearance of various arrhythmias (ventricular more often than supraventricular), as well as disturbances in atrioventricular and intraventricular conduction.

The patient may appear acutely ill and agitated, frequently is sweating, and often has pallor, cyanosis, and a lower-than-normal blood pressure. The heart may be of normal size in the absence of antecedent disease. Heart sounds are often of poor quality. A fourth heart sound is frequently present, and there may be paradoxical splitting of the second sound. A pericardial friction rub, a third heart sound, pulsus alternans, evidence of pulmonary congestion, and a wide variety of arrhythmias may be present. In some cases only minimal signs, if any, of physiologic derangement may be noted.

Subsequent to the attack the patient may have a fever, commonly to 101°F, but sometimes to 103°F; an elevated white cell count (as high as 20,000 cells per cubic millimeter); and a significant rise in the serum levels of several intracellular enzymes, such as glutamic oxaloacetic transaminase (SGOT), glutamic pyruvic transaminase (SGPT), lactic dehydrogenase (LDH), and creatinine phosphokinase (CPK). Some or all of these enzymes may increase minimally or maximally following an infarction. The rise generally appears within twenty-four hours and precedes at variable rates over the subsequent days or weeks. However, occasionally there is no elevation of temperature, white cell count, or enzymes, especially if the area of necrosis is small. A rapid erythrocyte sedimentation rate (ESR) often appears after three to seven days and returns to normal only after several weeks.

Characteristic electrocardiographic changes accompany most, although not all, infarctions. Three types of changes are seen: alterations of the QRS complex, elevation of S–T segments, and serial T wave changes; in the diagnosis of myocardial infarction the most reliable of these are abnormalities of the QRS.

Changes in the QRS complex consist of either a Q wave which is larger than normal and usually wider than 0.03 sec in duration in those leads which face the area of infarction, or a loss of amplitude of R or disappearance of the R wave in one or more of the precordial V leads. The normal size and variation of the Q and the R wave in these leads can be found in Tables A, B, and E of the Appendix.

Elevation of the S–T segment will be found during the acute phase of the infarction in those leads facing the area of necrosis. This S–T elevation is usually accompanied by a reciprocal depression in the leads opposite those facing the infarction. For example, in anterior myocardial infarction the S–T is elevated in lead I and depressed in lead III, whereas in inferior myocardial infarction the S–T is elevated in standard leads II and III and depressed in standard lead I.

Serial T wave changes occur over a period of several days. The T wave at first may be diphasic, but later becomes negative in the leads facing the area of myocardial infarction. With healing, negative T waves may revert to normal or may persist indefinitely.

Estimation of the sites of myocardial infarction can be determined from the electrocardiographic findings. Since the V leads are actually anterior precordial leads, they will reflect the various forms of anterior myocardial infarction. Depending upon the site of these anterior infarcts, standard leads I and II as well as lead aVL will also be involved. Inferior myocardial infarctions are located for the most part on the diaphragmatic surface of the left ventricle. Lead aVF faces this area. Thus in inferior myocardial infarction, leads II, III, and aVF will contain the diagnostic evidence.

In anteroseptal myocardial infarctions the changes will be found in leads V1, V2, and V3 and there is no abnormality in the standard or aV leads (Fig. 3). Anterior or apical myocardial infarction will show its effects in V2, V3, or V4 (Fig. 4), whereas the anterolateral myocardial infarction will produce changes in V4 to V6 as well as leads I and II (Fig. 5). When the entire anterior wall is involved in the necrotic process, all six V leads will be affected (Fig. 6). When infarction is located high on the lateral wall near the base, the effect will be noted in lead aVL only. The precordial V leads taken in the fourth intercostal space (the usual site) will not be abnormal. When a deep Q and elevated S–T segment or serial T wave changes appear in aVL, one can confirm this diagnosis by finding these same abnormalities in the V leads taken two interspaces above the usual position, that is, in the second intercostal space. Inferior (diaphragmatic) myocardial infarction affects leads II, III, and aVF. If the inferior myocardial infarction extends laterally, as occasionally occurs, one will find the evidences of necrosis in leads II, III, and aVF and also in V5 and V6, which are laterally oriented (Figs. 7 and 8).

True posterior (posterobasal or dorsal paravertebral, not diaphragmatic) infarcts are rare, but when present, are accompanied by an increase in size in R in V1 and V3R, with large upright T waves in these leads. They are usually accompanied by an inferior or a lateral infarct.

Isolated subendocardial myocardial infarction is rare; the usual location of infarcts is epicardial or intramural. Subendocardial infarctions often almost completely encircle the interior of the left ventricle, producing a ringlike type of necrosis. The electrocardiographic evidence consists of depression in the S–T segments in all leads save aVR. The S–T segment is elevated in the latter because it faces the interior of the left ventricle and hence the necrotic surface. QRS changes do not usually appear with this infarct. The depression of the S–T segments remains fixed for several days, rather than disappearing in minutes or hours, as is the case with the transitory S–T segment abnormalities of coronary insufficiency.

Although the papillary muscles of the left ventricle may be infarcted along with subendocardial infarction, papillary muscles may be scarred or infarcted separately. Hence infarction of the posteromedial papillary muscle is associated with the depression of the S–T segment in V1 through V4 and infarction of the anterolateral papillary muscle, with these changes in V4 through V6.

Electrocardiographic changes can indicate the age of the myocardial infarction to some degree. The actual changes may not appear immediately and indeed may be delayed for several days after the onset of chest pain. Usually, they exist in some form by the fifth to seventh day, but occasionally appear as late as the second or third week of the illness. As the necrosis resolves and replacement fibrosis begins, changes in T waves occur serially (Figs. 6 and 9), and conduction defects may appear (Figs. 6 and 8). Instability of the electrocardiogram is usual for three to six weeks. The S–T segment deviations subside early in the course. An acute infarction is accompanied by serial changes in the S–T segment; an older infarct, by an unchanging or stable electrocardiogram (which usually means that the T wave abnormalities are not varying in form), this stabilization usually occurring by the second or third month. The electrocardiogram may or may not return to normal with final healing.

Vectorcardiographic changes may assist in the diagnosis of myocardial infarction in most patients; the major QRS loop configurations, described in the transverse, sagittal, and frontal planes, can be examined for this purpose.

In anteroseptal infarction, with loss of anterior septal forces, the early QRS vectors and the efferent limb of the QRS loop are displaced posteriorly and to the left (the normal early forces being directed anteriorly and rightward). This is best seen in the transverse (horizontal) plane (XZ leads of the Frank lead system). The afferent limb and terminal deflection are inscribed normally in a counterclockwise direction. In the right sagittal plane (ZY leads) the initial part of the QRS vector loop moves posteriorly and usually inferiorly. The afferent limb is inscribed in a normal clockwise direction. The QRS loop in the frontal plane (ZY leads) is normally located.

In anterior or apical infarction, with loss of anterior

Figure 3. *Anteroseptal myocardial infarction.* Leads V1–V3 have a QS deflection; there is no R wave in these leads. The S–T segment is elevated in V1–V4, and T waves are diphasic or negative in V1–V4 and low in V5, V6. The standard and aV leads are normal (the T wave in lead I is low because of the vertical electrical position of the heart). (The leads are recorded as in Figure 2.)

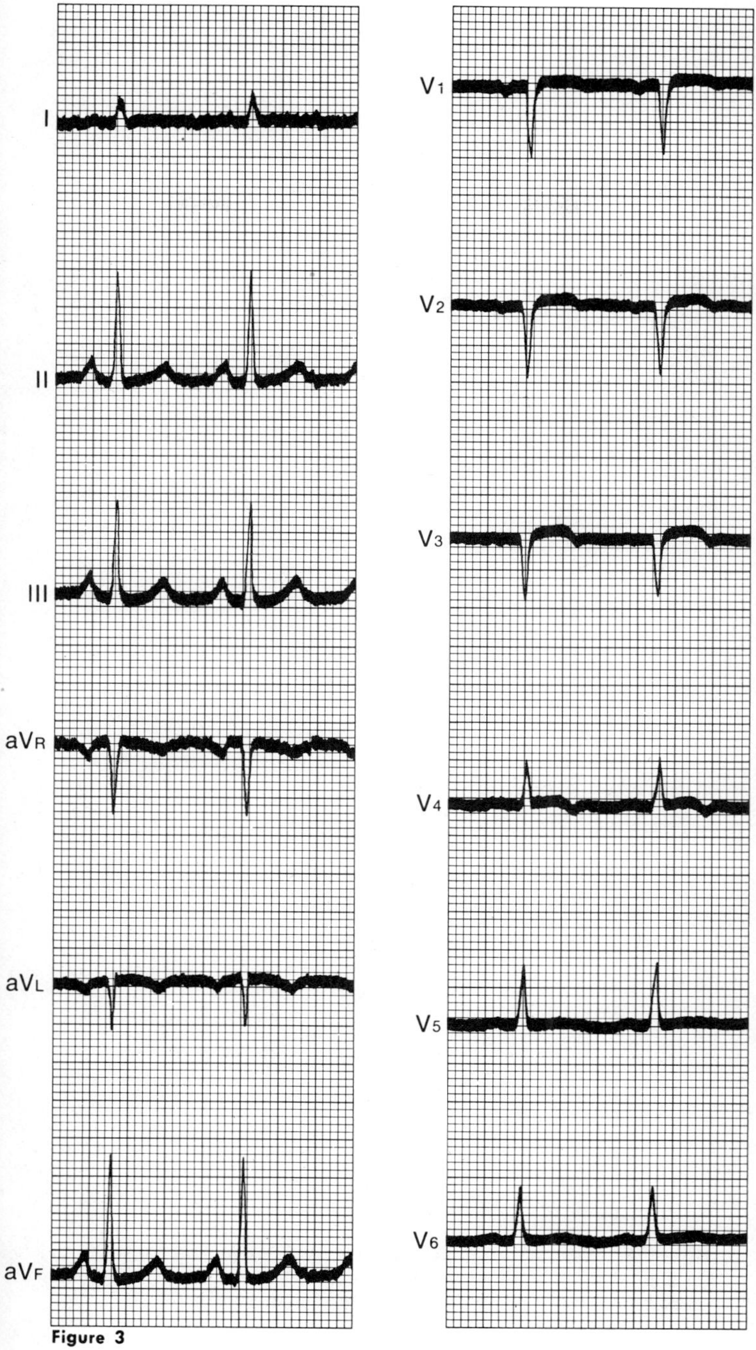

Figure 3

Figure 4. *Anterior or apical myocardial infarction.* There is a QS and no R in lead V2, with a normal R wave in V1 and V3–V6. The other leads are normal. (The leads are recorded as in Figure 1.)

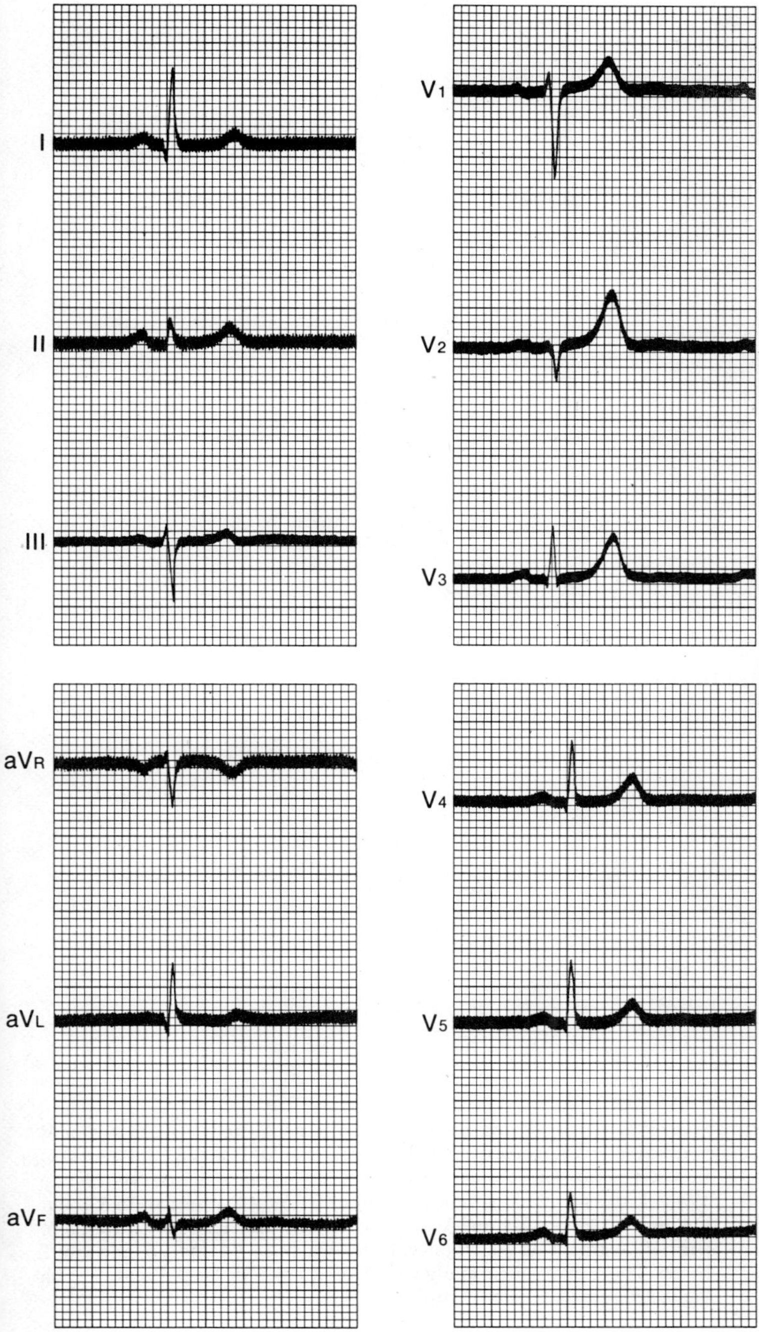

Figure 4

Figure 5. *Anterolateral myocardial infarction.* There is a QS and no R wave in lead V4, a deep and wide Q with a small R in V5, and a wide Q in V6. The normal R wave progression (an increase in size from V1 to V6) is lost, as R in V3 is smaller than in V2, and R is absent in V4 and low in V5. Only in V1 and V6 is R of normal size. There is elevation of the S–T segment in V3–V5, negative T waves in V4 and V5, and low T in V6. There is an abnormally wide Q and low T in leads I and II. (The leads are recorded as in Figure 1.)

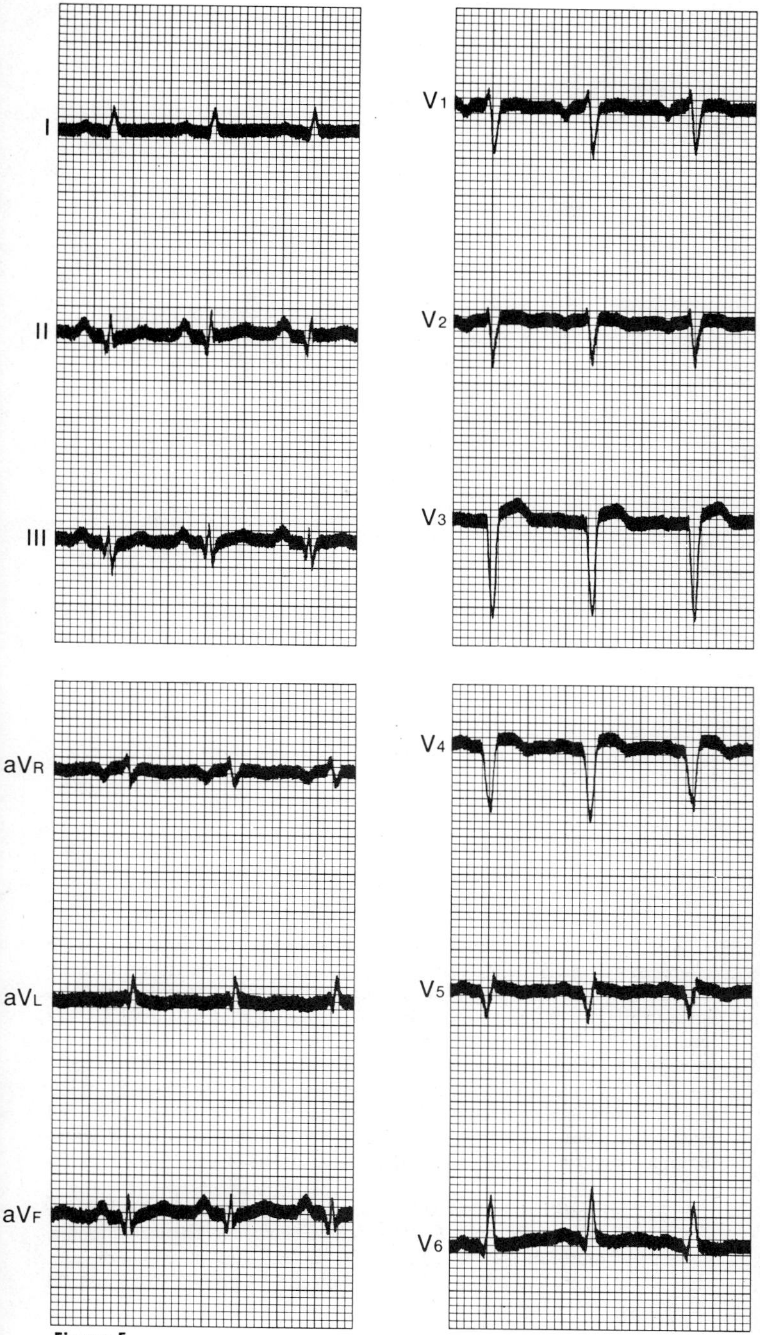

Figure 5

Figure 6 A–E. *Extensive anterior myocardial infarction: serial changes.* All six V leads are involved in the abnormalities indicating anteroseptal, apical, and anterolateral infarction. The serial changes seen in the five tracings (Figs. A–E) were recorded on the second, third, fifth, twelfth, and fourteenth days of the illness. Leads I and aVL have elevated S–T segments (at arrows), while reciprocal depressions of S–T segments are seen in III and aVF early in the illness (Fig. 6A). There are elevations of S–T segments (at arrows) and loss of R waves in V1–V4, and subsequently (Figs. 6B–E) V5 and V6 are also involved. T waves become negative in leads I, II, aVL and in most of the V leads as the changes evolve.

In Figure 6B the QRS axis has shifted from a moderate left axis deviation (–20°), as shown in Figure 6A, to a marked left axis deviation as shown in Figure 6B (–47°); in Figure 6C the axis lies at –11°, indicating that a transitory left anterior fascicular block was present in Figure 6B. (The leads are recorded as in Figure 2.)

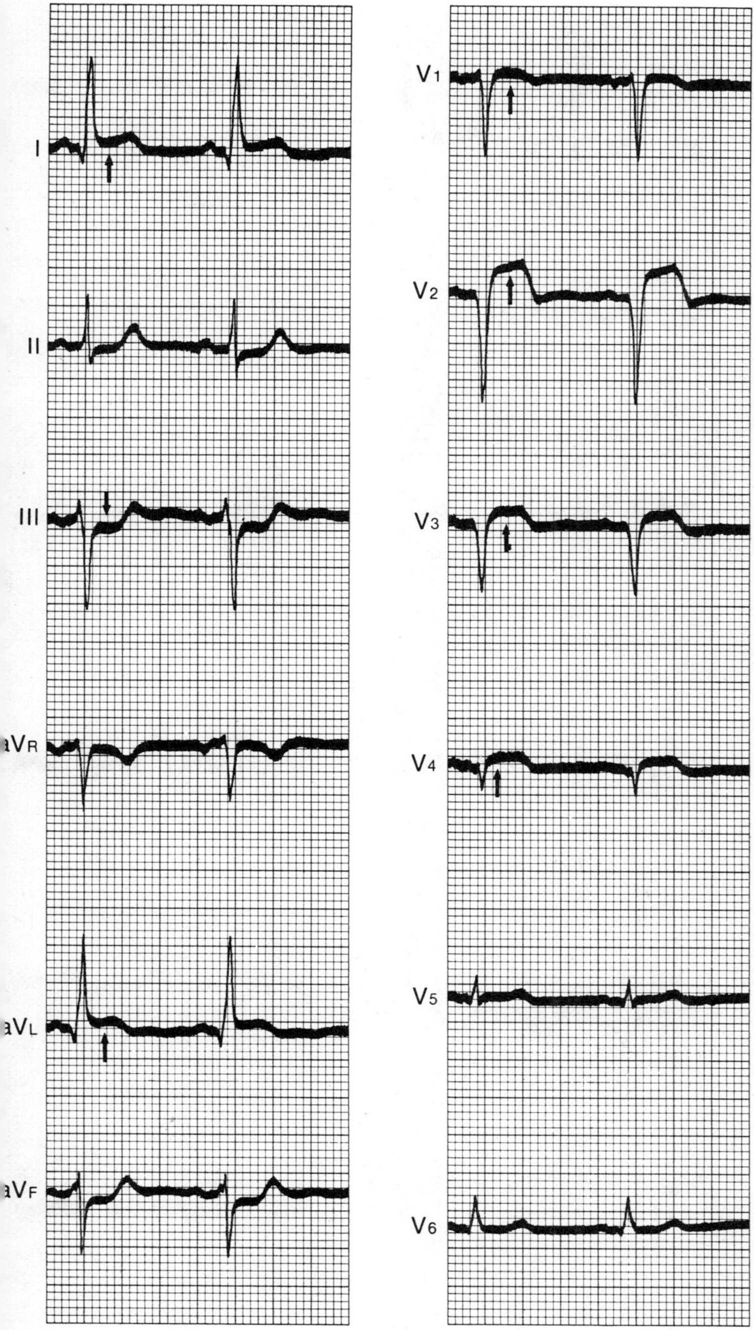

Figure 6A. *Extensive anterior myocardial infarction: serial changes.* Second day of the illness.

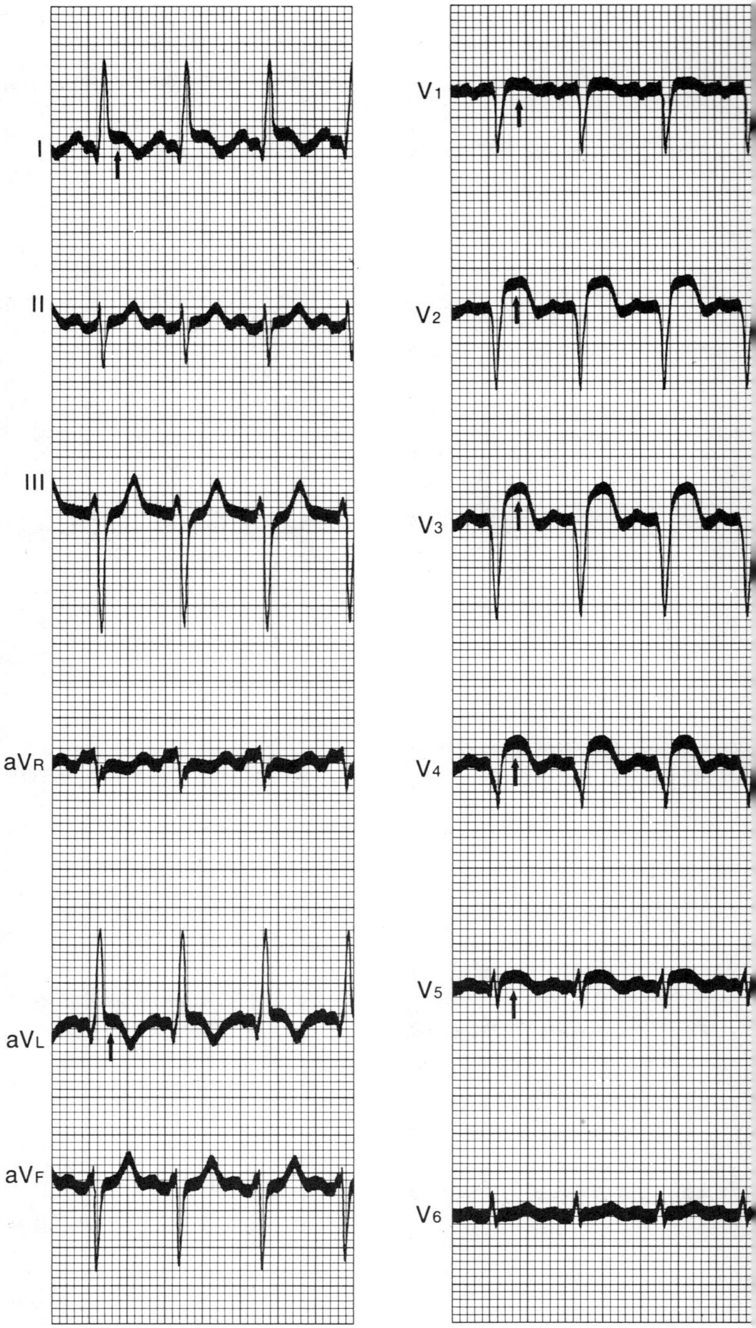

Figure 6B. *Extensive anterior myocardial infarction: serial changes.* Third day of the illness.

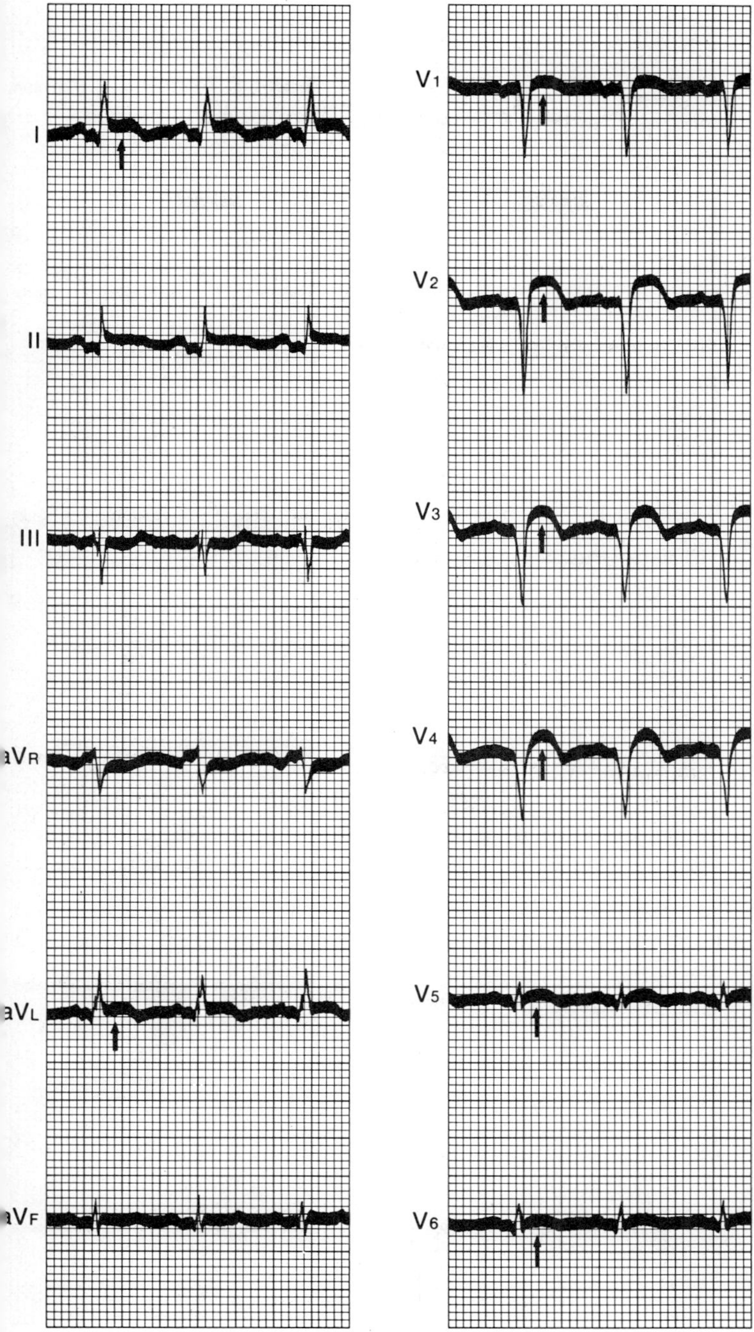

Figure 6C. *Extensive anterior myocardial infarction: serial changes.* Fifth day of the illness.

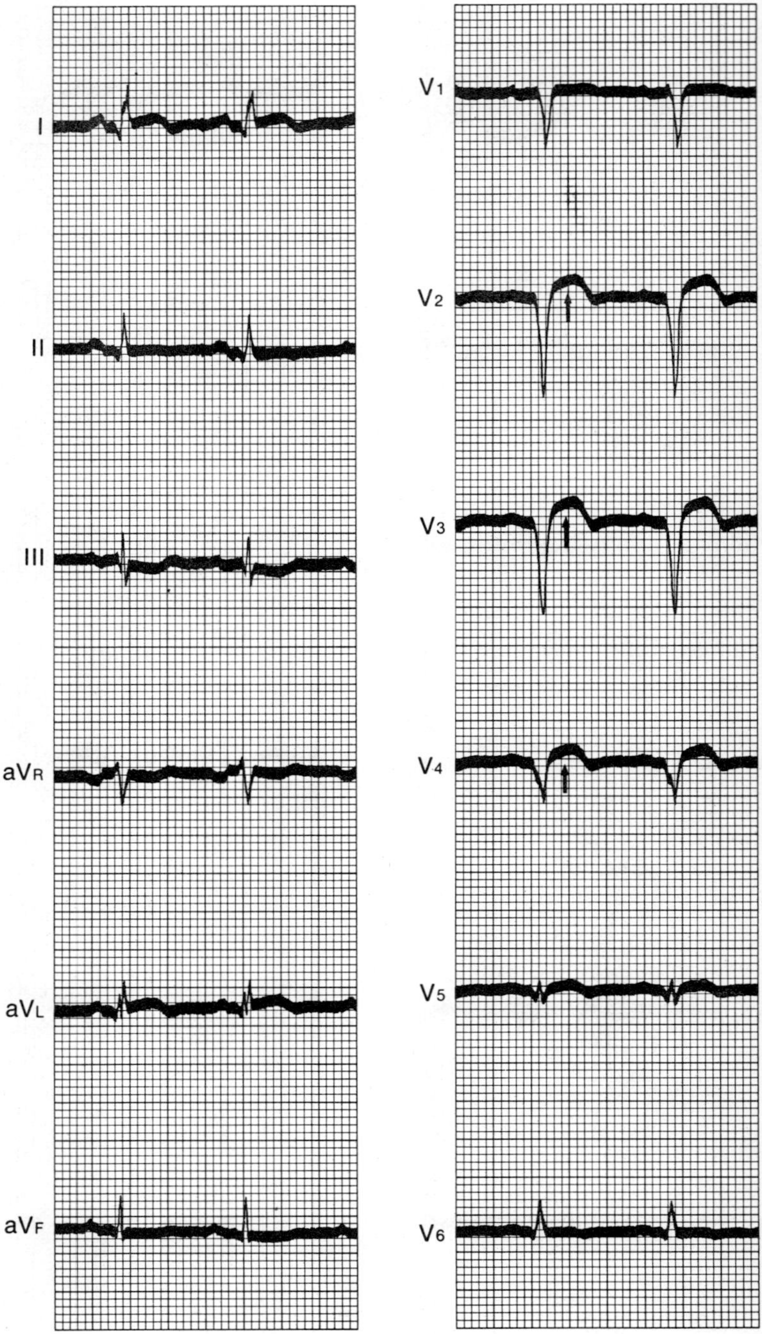

Figure 6D. *Extensive anterior myocardial infarction: serial changes.* Twelfth day of the illness.

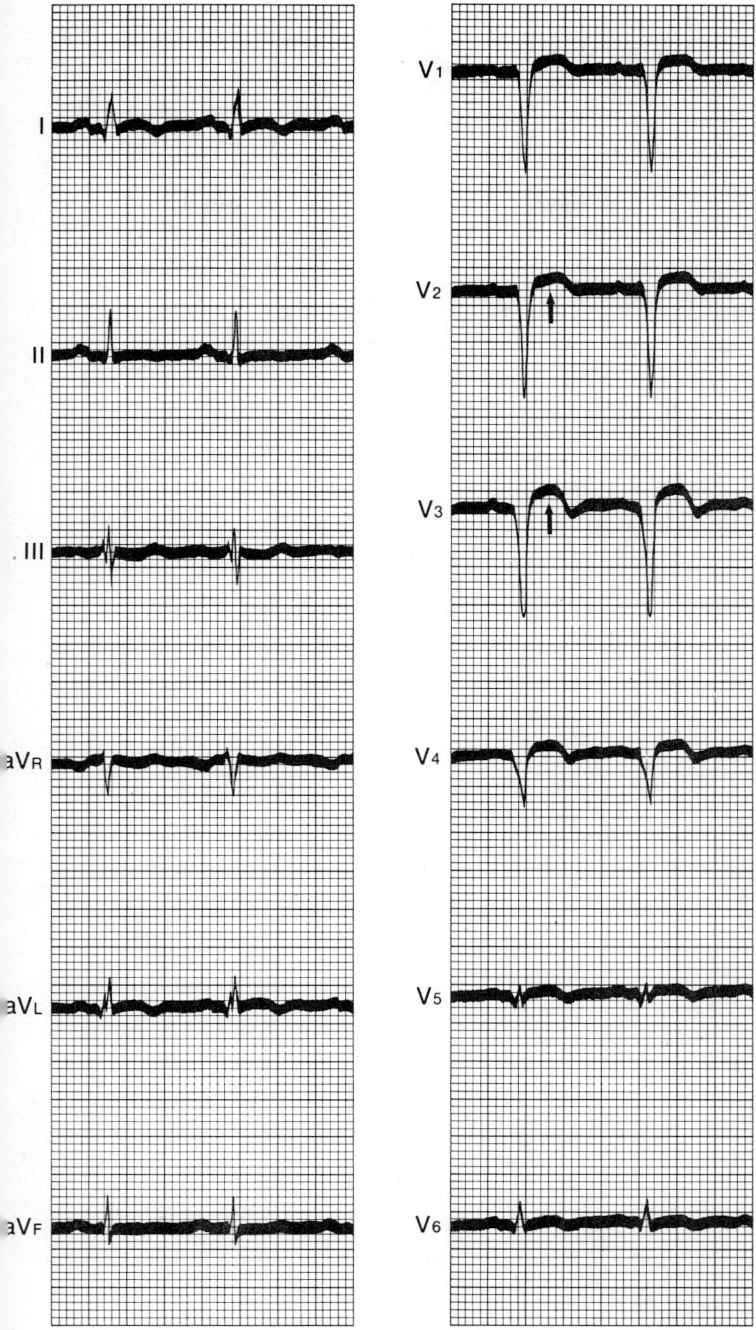

Figure 6E. *Extensive anterior myocardial infarction: serial changes.* Fourteenth day of the illness.

Figure 7. *Inferolateral myocardial infarction.* There are elevations of S–T segments and negative T waves in leads II, III, aVF, V4–V6. (The leads are recorded as in Figure 1.)

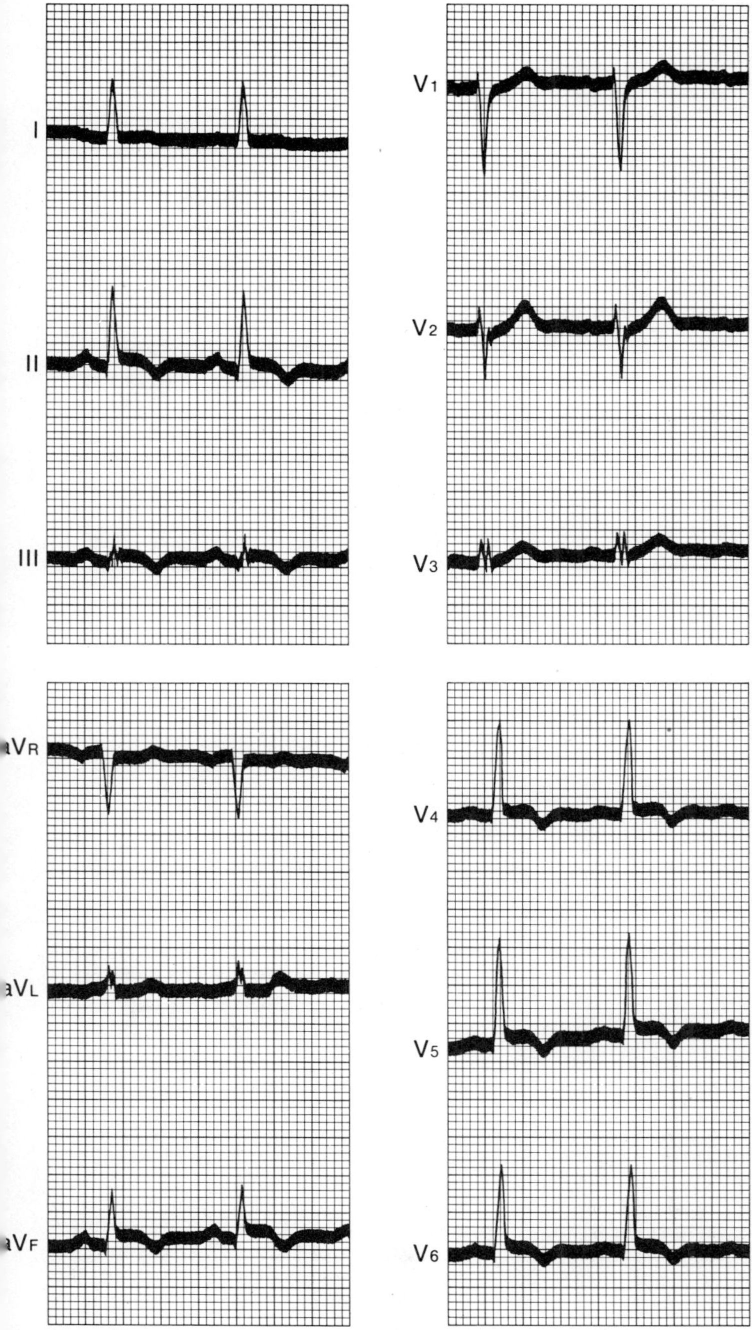

Figure 7

Figure 8 A–C. *Inferolateral myocardial infarction: serial changes.* There are abnormally wide Q waves (Figs. 8A and 8B) in leads II, III, aVF, and V4–V6, with elevated S–T segments in these same leads (indicated by arrows in leads II, III, V5, V6). Reciprocal S–T depressions are seen in I, aVL, V1, V2 (indicated by arrows in I, aVL). In Figure 8C, S–T deviations have disappeared, and negative T waves are seen in II, III, aVF, and V3–V6. The tracings A–C were recorded on the second, fifth, and fourteenth days of illness. (The leads are recorded as in Figure 1.)

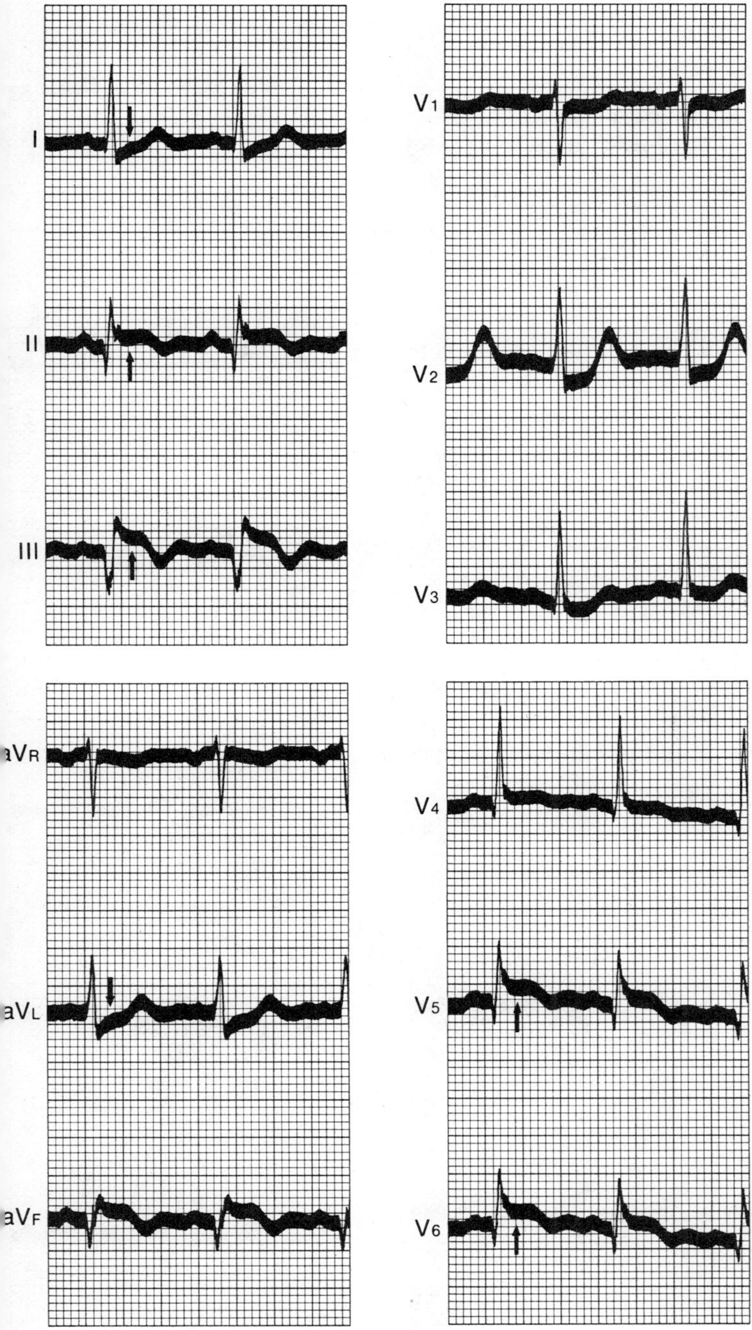

Figure 8A. *Inferolateral myocardial infarction: serial changes.* Second day of the illness.

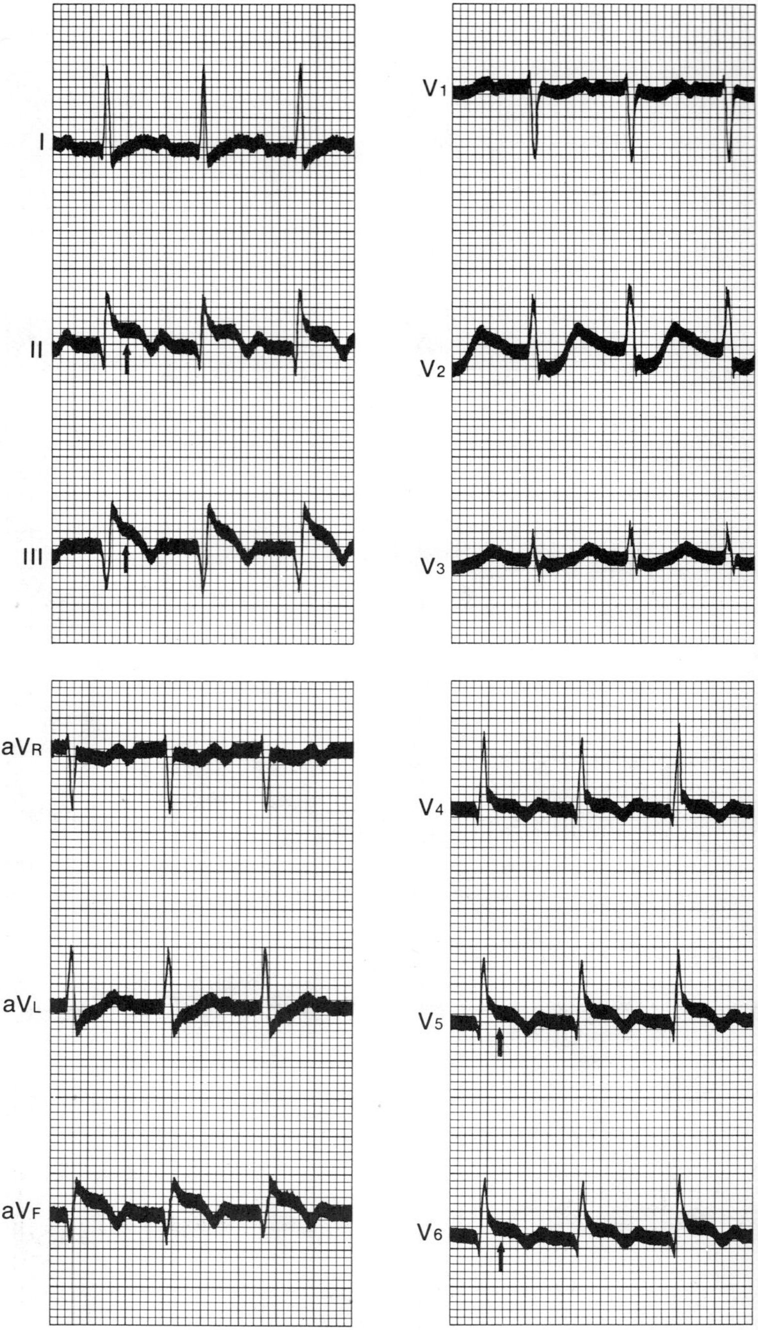

Figure 8B. *Inferolateral myocardial infarction: serial changes.* Fifth day of the illness.

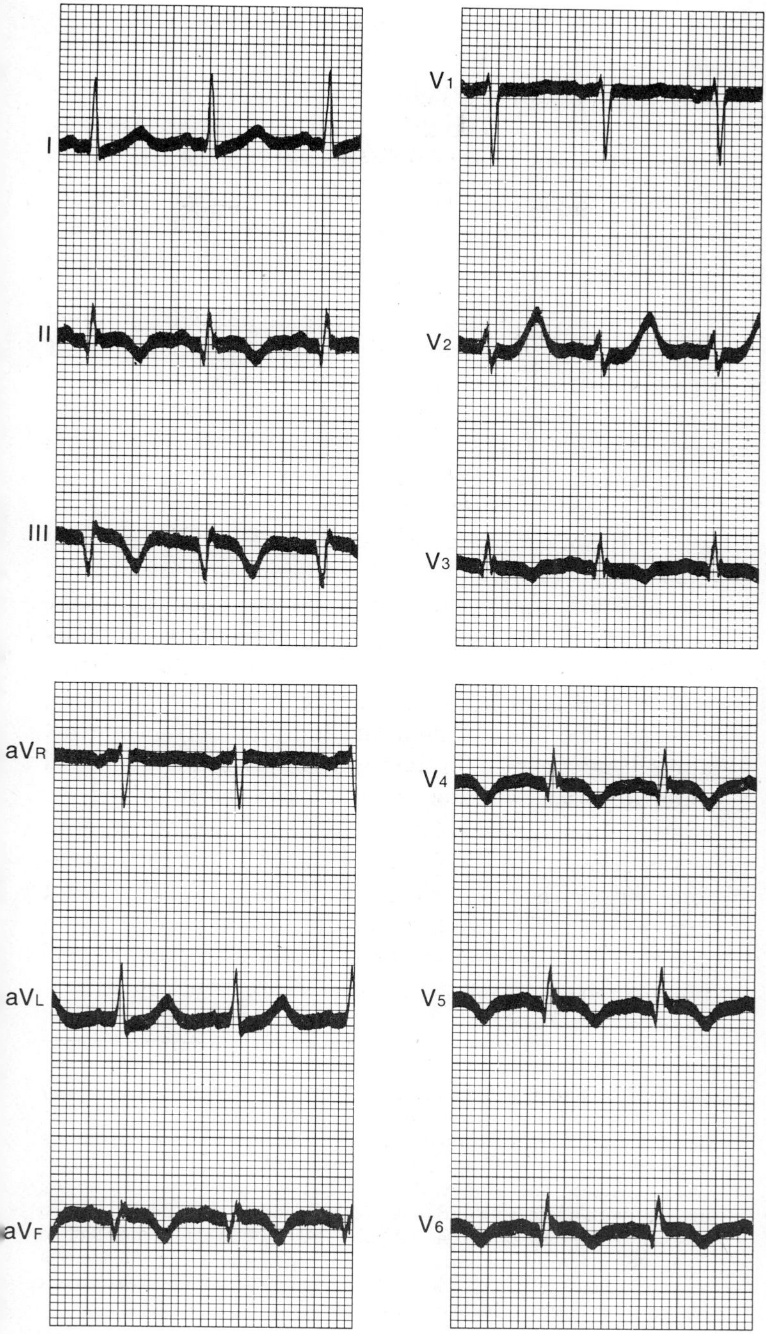

Figure 8C. *Inferolateral myocardial infarction: serial changes.* Fourteenth day of the illness.

forces only, the normal initial rightward and anterior QRS vector is preserved, and the abnormality involves the subsequent efferent limb of the QRS loop. In the transverse plane the initial deflection is anterior and rightward, the efferent limb is displaced posteriorly and leftward (instead of the normal anterior direction), and the afferent limb and terminal deflection are normally directed. In the right sagittal plane the initial deflection is normally directed superiorly and anteriorly, while the abnormal efferent limb, its normal anterior convexity lost, is displaced posteriorly; as in the transverse plane, this remains the diagnostic feature. The afferent limb and terminal deflection remain essentially unchanged. There is no abnormality demonstrated in the frontal plane.

With infarction of the anterolateral wall, the initial QRS forces are normal, but the efferent limb and part of the afferent limb of the QRS loop are affected. In the transverse plane the initial part of QRS loop is normally directed, anteriorly and to the right, but the efferent limb is displaced posteriorly and to the right in a clockwise rotation. The afferent limb and terminal portion are not altered significantly. In the right sagittal plane the initial anterosuperior deflection appears, as is normal, and the efferent limb moves posteriorly and may be either anterior or posterior to the afferent limb; the QRS loop may therefore be clockwise or counterclockwise, and a figure of eight may be seen. The frontal plane displays a normal initial vector, with the efferent limb displaced rightward and lying to the right of the afferent limb. The loop thus is

---

Figure 9 A and B. *Anteroseptal myocardial infarction with right bundle branch block (A) and later, left anterior fascicular block (B).* In both A and B there is a deep and wide Q (indicated by upward-pointing arrows in V1, V2), with elevated S–T segments in V–V5, a prolonged QRS (0.14 sec), and a large R in V1 and V2 (at downward-pointing arrows), with a late peak of R (0.09 sec) indicating a right bundle branch block. In Figure 9B, taken one day after 9A, the axis of QRS had shifted from –16°, as shown in Figure 9A, to –76°, indicating the development of a left anterior fascicular block in addition to a right bundle branch block (bifascicular block). (The leads are recorded as in Figure 1.)

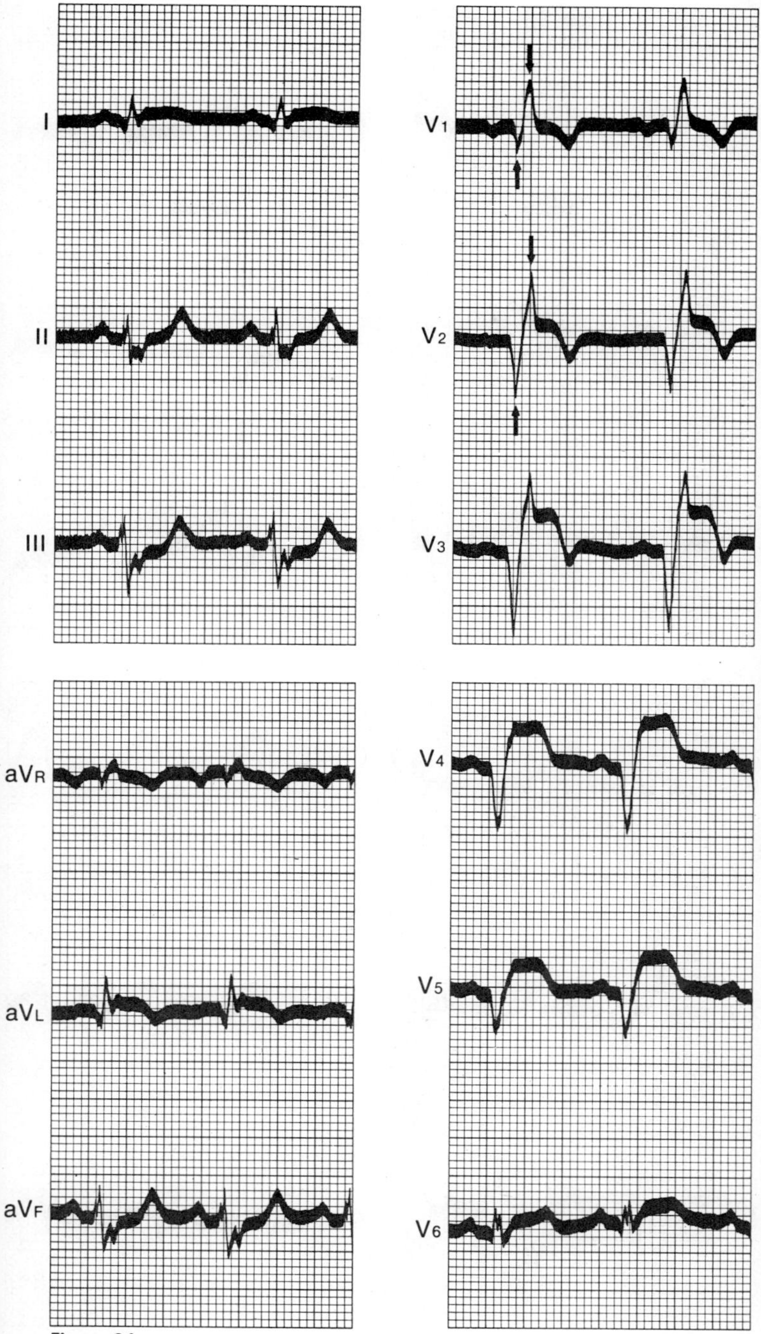

Figure 9A

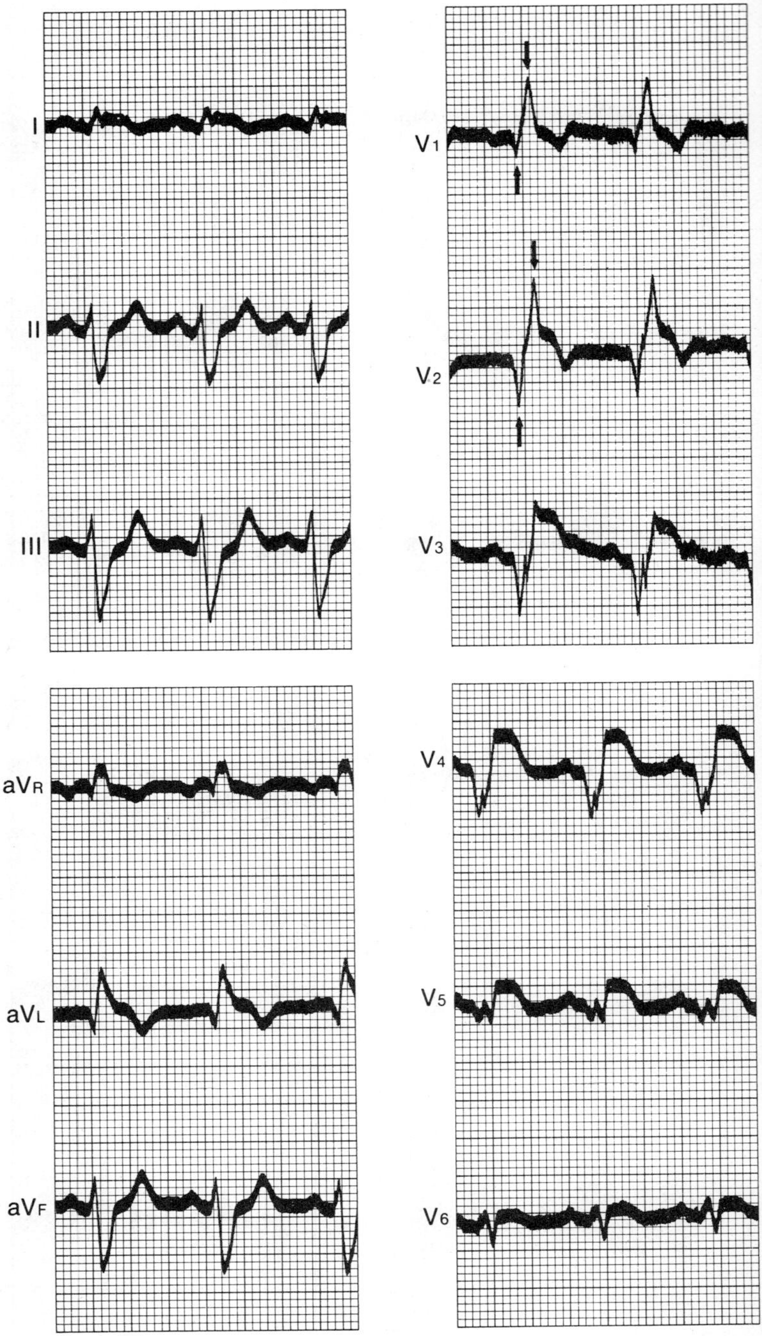

Figure 9B

inscribed counterclockwise, a characteristic feature of infarction of the lateral wall.

With extensive anterior wall infarction involving the entire anterior wall and adjacent interventricular septum, the changes represent the sum of anteroseptal and anterolateral infarctions, with a total loss of anterior forces. In the transverse plane the initial deflection and efferent limbs are inscribed posteriorly and to the right, and the loop is usually clockwise. In the right sagittal plane the entire loop is located posteriorly and may be inscribed clockwise or counterclockwise. In the frontal plane there is usually a counterclockwise loop.

With high lateral infarction, forces in the high lateral wall (normally directed superiorly and leftward) are lost, and thus the vector loop is directed inferiorly and to the right. This is best seen in the frontal plane, where the initial deflection and efferent limb are inscribed inferiorly and to the right. Although the QRS loop is usually vertical, it is inscribed counterclockwise.

With inferior (diaphragmatic) infarction and loss of inferior forces, the vector is directed superiorly, and this is seen in the sagittal and frontal planes. The transverse plane QRS loop is normal. In the right sagittal plane the initial deflection is directed anteriorly and superiorly—the characteristic finding in this infarct—and the efferent limb is usually inscribed clockwise. In the frontal plane there is an abnormal superior displacement of the early portion of the QRS loop, and the duration of these superior forces often exceeds 0.025 sec. Both this superior initial part and the efferent limb are inscribed in a clockwise direction, and the afferent limb and terminal deflection are inferior to the efferent limb.

With inferolateral infarction there is loss of both inferior and leftward forces, and the QRS loop is directed superiorly and rightward. These changes are best seen in the frontal plane. In the transverse plane the loop is counterclockwise. The initial portion is directed to the right and anteriorly, and the efferent loop proceeds leftward. The afferent and terminal portions are largely unaffected. In the right sagittal plane the alterations of the QRS loop are similar to those described for inferior infarction. The loop may be clockwise, counterclockwise, or present a figure-of-eight pattern. In the frontal plane the initial deflection is oriented superiorly and rightward, and this force is of increased duration and magnitude. The efferent limb moves leftward, and the loop is inscribed clockwise.

True posterior wall infarction is difficult to diagnose. Vectorcardiography is helpful in this regard. Normally, the true posterior (dorsal paravertebral) area is the last region of the left ventricle to be activated; with loss of those forces, alteration is in the late QRS vectors, which are displaced in an anterior direction. Transverse and sagittal planes best reflect these changes. In the transverse plane there is anterior displacement of the QRS loop. The initial deflection is normally written to the right and anteriorly. The efferent limb moves leftward and remains anterior throughout its course. The anterior displacement of the afferent limb and terminal deflection is, however, the major characteristic, and commonly there is a counterclockwise QRS loop. The right sagittal plane displays the anterior displacement of the QRS loop, consisting almost exclusively of the afferent limb, with the initial deflection and efferent limb unchanged and a clockwise rotation of the loop. In the frontal plane there are no detectable changes.

The complications of myocardial infarction include arrhythmias, shock, ventricular failure, atrioventricular and intraventricular conduction disturbances, rupture of the myocardium or a papillary muscle, hemopericardium, myocardial fibrosis, ventricular asynergy, ventricular aneurysm, and mural thrombosis.

Ultrasound may be helpful in detecting abnormalities of septal or left ventricular wall motion or thickness and in demonstrating a ventricular aneurysm. Cross-sectional examination is much more sensitive than M-mode technique for the latter. Complications of myocardial infarction such as ventricular septal rupture, flail mitral leaflet, or pericardial fluid can also be detected in some patients by echocardiography.

ONE OF THE FOLLOWING CRITERIA IS REQUIRED FOR THE DIAGNOSIS OF A RECENT (ACUTE) MYOCARDIAL INFARCTION.

1. The following abnormalities in the electrocardiogram even in the absence of symptoms or abnormalities in serum enzymes: large Q waves associated with changes in the S–T segments and T waves in specific and appropriate leads which indicate the location of the infarct; serial S–T segment and T wave changes which are specifically located, but which occur without abnormal Q waves may also be used for the diagnosis, but are less reliable.
2. The following abnormalities of the electrocardiogram coupled with specific enzyme alterations: serial T waves changes, without elevation of S–T segments or abnormal Q waves in appropriate leads indicating specific locations of the infarct. The T wave changes must be localized and not widespread.
3. In the earliest stages of myocardial infarction, a compatible history and characteristic enzyme changes without the electrocardiographic abnormalities described, provided these electrocardiographic changes subsequently appear within two to three weeks.

ONE OF THE FOLLOWING CRITERIA IS REQUIRED FOR THE DIAGNOSIS OF A PREVIOUS (OLD) MYOCARDIAL INFARCTION IN THE ABSENCE OF A DOCUMENTED PREVIOUS MYOCARDIAL INFARCTION.

1. Abnormal Q waves in appropriate electrocardiographic leads, indicating specific locations of the infarct, or abnormally small R waves in two or more adjacent V leads.
2. Arteriographic evidence of coronary occlusion or narrowing and ventricular asynergy or ventricular wall abnormality not due to ischemia alone.
3. Ventricular aneurysm in the absence of chest trauma.

2.5.4 MYOCARDIAL FIBROSIS

Replacement of the myocardium by fibrous tissue can occur in a wide variety of disorders and may be local or diffuse, minute or massive, and subendocardial, transmural, or subepicardial. Fibrosis is most often seen in patients with impaired coronary arterial flow and consequent myocardial necrosis. It may also be encountered in patients with healed myocarditis of rheumatic or other origin. Fibrosis, often with considerable hypertrophy of the heart, has also been found in some patients in whom there is no evidence of coronary arterial disease or preceding inflammation.

Ventricular fibrosis may lead to ventricular failure, cardiac dilatation, or asynergy. If it involves the conduction system, various forms of conduction abnormalities may result. Fibrosis of a papillary muscle, following a transmural or subendocardial infarction, may cause mitral regurgitation.

Although myocardial fibrosis is a common accompaniment of many cardiac disorders, there are no signs or symptoms particular to it, and hence it is rarely recognized clinically, unless it results from a myocardial infarction or myocarditis due to progressive systemic sclerosis.

THE FOLLOWING CRITERIA ARE REQUIRED FOR THE DIAGNOSIS OF MYOCARDIAL FIBROSIS.

Evidence of a myocardial infarction in the past, or of myocarditis due to progressive systemic sclerosis or other types of myocarditis known to result in fibrosis.

2.5.5 MYOCARDITIS

2.5.5.1 HYPERSENSITIVITY

Myocarditis associated with hypersensitivity reactions, with or without accompanying vascular lesions, can occur in association with sensitivity reactions to drugs or heterologous serum. Eosinophils may predominate, or the reaction may consist principally of histiocytes and neutrophils. The principal clinical manifestations are the appearance of cardiac enlargement, ventricular failure, arrhythmias, and nonspecific changes in the final ventricular deflections (S–T and T).

THE FOLLOWING CRITERIA ARE REQUIRED FOR THE DIAGNOSIS OF MYOCARDITIS ASSOCIATED WITH HYPERSENSITIVITY REACTIONS.

Evidence of hypersensitivity reactions or systemic eosinophilia unrelated to any other obvious cause and one or more of the principal clinical manifestations previously described.

2.5.5.2 Infective Myocarditis

Myocarditis can occur in association with infectious diseases of bacterial, fungal, rickettsial, viral, or parasitic origin. The lesions may consist of focal abscesses in which specific organisms may be present; or they may consist of focal or diffuse interstitial infiltration of histiocytes, lymphocytes, or polymorphonuclear leukocytes between the muscle fibers and in the perivascular connective tissue. Varying degrees of myocardial injury from fatty change to frank necrosis of the muscle cells can result.

In certain diseases, such as those produced by diphtheria toxin, *Trypanosoma cruzi* (*Chagas' disease*), and *Toxoplasma* (toxoplasmosis), the primary damage is to the myofiber itself, resulting in necrosis of muscle, with a secondary inflammatory response. Rarely, in the course of hematogenous disseminated tuberculosis or secondary or tertiary syphilis, focal granulomatous myocardial lesions occur. *Plasmodium,* usually *falciparum* and rarely *vivax,* can in severe cases produce capillary thrombi, with ischemic changes in the muscle. Healing occurs by fibrous replacement of areas of necrosis.

The clinical manifestations are protean and range from transitory nonspecific electrocardiographic changes to rapid or sudden death. Cardiac dilatation, ventricular failure, shock, conduction disturbances, sinus tachycardia or bradycardia, and atrial or ventricular arrhythmias can be encountered. The electrocardiogram may show abnormal S–T and T waves. Serum levels of intracellular enzymes may become increased. Constitutional and specific manifestations of the basic infection (fever, leukocytosis, increased erythrocyte sedimentation rate, and positive blood cultures) are usually present.

During the course of any infection associated with fever, ventricular dilatation and arrhythmias may develop in patients with preexisting heart disease (rheumatic, atherosclerotic, hypertensive, and other types). These abnormalities result from metabolic changes associated with fever and are not attributable to a direct effect of the infection on the heart.

THE FOLLOWING CRITERIA ARE REQUIRED FOR THE DIAGNOSIS OF INFECTIVE MYOCARDITIS.

The presence of an infection, as demonstrated by appropriate clinical and laboratory findings, and evidence of one or more of the following: appearance of cardiac enlargement, ventricular failure, shock, conduction defects, arrhythmias, or transient abnormal changes in the S–T segments or T waves.

2.5.5.3 Isolated Myocarditis (Fiedler's Myocarditis, Idiopathic Myocarditis)

Isolated myocarditis, a form of heart disease which is of unknown cause, occurs principally in adult males. There is cardiac enlargement and diffuse myocardial inflammation. Disseminated areas of necrosis of myofibers with histiocytic reaction and areas of replacement fibrosis may be present. Wide bands of lymphocytes, histiocytes, plasma cells, and occasionally numbers of eosinophils may separate and replace muscle fibers.

In some instances of isolated myocarditis the reaction is characterized by the presence of large numbers of giant cells. Some appear to be of muscular origin; others are of the Langhans type. They may make up part of a diffuse reaction or may be arranged in discrete granulomas in association with lymphocytes and mononuclear cells arrayed about areas of necrosis of variable size. No organisms are demonstrable. The terms *nonspecific granu-*

lomatous myocarditis and *giant cell myocarditis* are also employed to designate this form of disease.

The clinical course is marked by the appearance of considerable cardiac enlargement and ventricular failure, with rapid progression to death. The diagnosis is rarely made prior to death.

2.5.5.4 Lupus Myocarditis

The myocarditis of systemic lupus erythematosus is a focal interstitial lesion. The cellular infiltrate consists of polymorphonuclear leukocytes and macrophages, as well as plasma cells and lymphocytes. Deposition of fibrin in association with infiltrates may produce a lesion with superficial resemblance to Aschoff's bodies, but true rheumatic granulomata are not seen. Areas of myocardial necrosis have been described, but when present, seem to be secondary to vasculitis with obliteration. The arteritis is necrotizing in type, with fibrinoid mural changes and associated leukocytic infiltration. Thrombosis may be superimposed on these lesions.

THE CRITERIA REQUIRED FOR THE DIAGNOSIS OF LUPUS MYOCARDITIS ARE GIVEN IN 1.31.

2.5.5.5 Progressive Systemic Sclerosis (Scleroderma)

Myocardial involvement in progressive systemic sclerosis may take the form of interstitial fibrosis with encroachment on and replacement of myofibers. There is often associated intimal fibrosis of small arteries, but this lesion is not constant, nor is it so located as to explain the myocardial scarring.

Interstitial fibrosis may be extensive enough to produce ventricular failure through loss of myofibers or disturbances in ventricular filling. The fibrosis may also involve the conduction system. More commonly, progressive systemic sclerosis produces pulmonary heart disease by extensive interstitial fibrosis of the lungs, with obliterative disease of the pulmonary vasculature.

THE CRITERIA FOR THE DIAGNOSIS OF MYOCARDITIS DUE TO PROGRESSIVE SYSTEMIC SCLEROSIS ARE GIVEN IN 1.23.

2.5.5.6 Rheumatic Myocarditis

The anatomic hallmark of rheumatic heart disease is Aschoff's nodule. This is a focal, granulomatous lesion occurring in close proximity to blood vessels and consisting of a central core of swollen fibrinoid material surrounded by large, often multinucleated basophilic cells with large vacuolated nuclei having a prominent nucleolus (Aschoff's cells), a sprinkling of smaller mononuclear cells, and occasionally a few polymorphonuclear leukocytes. Evolutionary changes occur with the passage of time. The nodule is gradually replaced by connective tissue and after several months becomes a fibrous scar.

Aschoff's nodules are usually most abundant in the myocardium of the left ventricle and interventricular septum and less common in the right ventricle. They also occur in the atrial myocardium and left atrial appendage. Lesions morphologically resembling Aschoff's nodules have been observed at other sites, such as the valves, pericardium, pleura, around the joints, and in the adventitia of the major blood vessels.

In addition to the pathognomonic Aschoff's nodule, active rheumatic myocarditis is characterized by edema of the interstitial connective tissue and a variable cellular exudate consisting of lymphocytes, polymorphonuclear leukocytes, Anitschkow's myocytes, and sometimes plasma cells and eosinophils. The cardiac muscle fibers may occasionally show degenerative changes or frank necrosis. As the acute stage of the process subsides, the edema and cellular infiltrate disappear, leaving behind small focal interstitial and myocardial scars.

Active rheumatic myocarditis is manifested clinically by an increase in heart size and by the appearance of ventricular failure, conduction disturbances, or atrial arrhythmias.

THE FOLLOWING CRITERIA ARE REQUIRED FOR THE DIAGNOSIS OF MYOCARDITIS DUE TO RHEUMATIC FEVER.

A change in heart size or the appearance of ventricular failure in association with one or more of the fol-

lowing: evidence of infection with β-hemolytic streptococcus of group A or one of the other major or minor criteria of rheumatic fever.

2.5.5.7 RHEUMATOID MYOCARDITIS

Rheumatoid granulomata consisting of central areas of fibrinoid necrosis surrounded by palisaded rows of macrophages can occasionally be seen in the myocardium of patients with widespread joint involvement. The lesions rarely produce clinical evidence of cardiac involvement. The latter can be suspected if ventricular failure appears in a patient with active rheumatoid arthritis.

2.5.5.8 SARCOIDOSIS

Involvement of the myocardium in sarcoidosis may occasionally occur in the course of the generalized disease. There is replacement of myofibers by discrete and conglomerate epithelioid tubercles, which are noncaseous. These lesions are characteristically made up of closely aggregated epithelioid cells with multinucleated giant cells. Replacement of myofibers is irregular, and the conduction system may be involved. Enlargement of the heart is observed in instances where replacement is extensive. Hypertrophy of residual fibers is present.

Sarcoid heart disease is to be distinguished from that form of granulomatous disease which involves only the heart. This latter disease, characterized by a more diffuse type of reaction, with less of a tendency to form discrete well-defined granulomas, is best classified as isolated myocarditis, granulomatous type.

THE CRITERIA REQUIRED FOR THE DIAGNOSIS OF MYOCARDITIS DUE TO SARCOIDOSIS ARE GIVEN IN 1.28.

2.5.6 NEOPLASM

Primary intramural tumors of the heart are rare. They may be benign or malignant and may arise from any of the tissues that make up the cardiac wall. Tumors may originate in adipose tissue (lipoma and liposarcoma), fibrous tissue (fibroma and fibrosarcoma), vessels (lymphangioma, hemangioma, and angiosarcoma) and striated muscle (rhabdomyosarcoma). The tumors displace and replace muscle fibers and may involve the conducting system, impinge on the cardiac chambers, occlude valve orifices, and produce protruding surface masses.

Metastatic tumor in the myocardium is fairly common. Carcinoma of the lung is the most frequent source of such involvement, probably because of its high incidence and its intrathoracic location. However, all malignant tumors can involve the myocardium, including malignant lymphoma. Although multiple nodules may replace cardiac muscle, they are rarely extensive enough to affect myocardial function.

Myocardial tumors may cause cardiac arrhythmias or disturbances in conduction. They may also interfere with valve function or, more rarely, result in ventricular failure. Roentgenograms may show nonspecific cardiac enlargement. Occasionally, the heart shape may be so deformed as to suggest a mass. Echocardiography may be helpful in diagnosing the presence of pericardial fluid or an atrial myxoma. Angiocardiography or coronary arteriography may outline the tumor mass and its blood supply.

THE CRITERIA FOR THE DIAGNOSIS OF NEOPLASMS OF THE MYOCARDIUM ARE GIVEN IN 1.19.

2.5.7 RUPTURE OF THE MYOCARDIUM: FREE WALL, INTERVENTRICULAR SEPTUM, OR A PAPILLARY MUSCLE

Rupture or perforation of the myocardium may result from trauma or myocardial infarction. There is usually an abrupt appearance of one or more of the following: left ventricular failure, pulmonary congestion, hemopericardium, pericardial tamponade, shock, or ventricular septal defect. Rupture of a papillary muscle may produce evidence of mitral regurgitation.

Cardiac rupture due to infarction usually occurs between the fourth to seventh days after the original injury and is unusual after two weeks. Perforation of the interventricular septum may follow anteroseptal or posteroseptal myocardial infarction in the first two weeks of illness and is suggested by the sudden appearance of the harsh pansystolic murmur of ventricular septal defect, often accompanied by a thrill, at the left lower sternal border. Rupture of a papillary muscle due to infarction may also occur in the first two weeks of illness and usually produces mitral regurgitation of a severe degree and the rapid appearance of pulmonary edema. It is usually associated with the appearance of a loud apical systolic murmur.

Perforation of the heart by a cardiac catheter may not be attended by an abnormality of cardiac function until the catheter is withdrawn and bleeding occurs into the pericardial sac. It can be suspected when blood cannot be withdrawn through the catheter. Pacemaker wires may also perforate the heart.

ONE OF THE FOLLOWING CRITERIA IS REQUIRED FOR THE DIAGNOSIS OF RUPTURE OF THE MYOCARDIUM: FREE WALL, INTERVENTRICULAR SEPTUM, OR A PAPILLARY MUSCLE.

1. **Demonstration of the lesion at operation.**
2. **Radiographic evidence of a cardiac catheter or a pacemaker wire lying in the pericardial sac.**
3. **Contrast material appearing in the pericardial sac after intravascular injection of contrast material.**
4. **Abrupt appearance of ventricular septal defect in a patient with a recent anteroseptal or posteroseptal myocardial infarction.**
5. **Abrupt appearance of severe mitral regurgitation in a patient with a recent myocardial infarction.**

2.5.8 VENTRICULAR ANEURYSM

Myocardial infarction is the commonest cause of aneurysm formation, but trauma may produce it. Aneurysms vary in size from a few centimeters to as large as half of the ventricle. The commonest locations are apical, posterior, and, much more rarely, septal. Often a thrombus adheres to the wall of the ventricle and may partially or completely fill the pouch. In many instances, however, the lining is white, smooth or corrugated, and glistening. Pericardial adhesions often form over it. Rupture of a cardiac aneurysm is rare. The wall of the aneurysm consists of dense scar, with occasional groups or bands or muscle fibers and thickened endocardium, and it may be calcified.

The physiologic consequence of aneurysm of the heart is asynergy. If the asynergic area is small, asynergy may be inapparent, but if large, it can produce intractable ventricular failure, cardiac arrhythmias, or systemic emboli. The paradoxical expansion during systole may produce papillary muscle dysfunction, causing mitral regurgitation.

A double apical impulse may be felt, the added impulse coming before the normal apical thrust. An aneurysm can sometimes be noted on an ordinary chest film as a bulge along the ventricular border, but more frequently is identified on fluoroscopy by the typical paradoxical or reduced motion of the ventricular wall. Ventriculography is required for its demonstration in most instances. Persistent elevation of the S–T segments in the anterior, posteroinferior, or septal leads after myocardial infarction suggests the presence of a ventricular aneurysm, although these elevations occur in only two-thirds of patients with the lesion. Ultrasound, particularly with cross-sectional imaging, can help evaluate wall thickness and motion and, in certain cases, demonstrate ventricular aneurysm.

THE FOLLOWING CRITERION IS REQUIRED FOR THE DIAGNOSIS OF AN ANEURYSM OF THE HEART.

Radiologic demonstration of the aneurysm, usually by ventriculography.

2.6 Diseases of the Pericardium

2.6.1 CYSTS

True cysts of the pericardium are coelomic or mesodermal in origin and are lined by a single layer of cuboidal cells. These may be completely separated from the pericardial cavity or may communicate as a cystic diverticulum. More rarely, bronchial, teratomatous, or angiomatous cysts may occur. Cysts usually manifest themselves as roentgenographic abnormalities—a rounded paracardiac mass (most commonly in the regions of the right or left cardiophrenic angles). Mediastinal and pulmonary tumors must be excluded. Demonstration of clear fluid on needle aspiration of a paracardiac mass strongly suggests pericardial cyst.

ONE OF THE FOLLOWING CRITERIA IS REQUIRED FOR THE DIAGNOSIS OF PERICARDIAL CYST.

1. Demonstration of the characteristic histopathologic lesion on biopsy of the cyst.
2. Demonstration of the smooth walls of a pericardial cyst by erect and decubitus roentgenograms after replacement of cystic fluid with air.

2.6.2 FIBROSIS, CALCIFICATION, OR BOTH

Pericarditis may lead to fibrosis of the pericardium; when tuberculosis is the etiologic factor, or when the pericarditis has a large hemorrhagic component, calcification may ensue. When there is extensive involvement of pericardium and epicardium by fibrinous inflammation, healing may result in partial or complete obliteration of the pericardial cavity by fibrous adhesions. This usually has no functional significance. When healing of pericarditis results in the encasement of the heart in a thick, rigid fibrous coat, with or without calcification, pericardial restriction may result. This functional abnormality is dependent upon the presence of widespread involvement of the pericardium.

ONE OF THE FOLLOWING CRITERIA IS REQUIRED FOR THE DIAGNOSIS OF FIBROSIS OR CALCIFICATION OF THE PERICARDIUM.

1. Radiographic evidence of calcification of the pericardium.
2. Evidence of pericardial restriction in the absence of neoplastic disease and pericardial fluid.

2.6.3 HEMOPERICARDIUM

Blood in the pericardial sac may be caused by trauma or may follow rupture of a myocardial infarct or of a dissecting hematoma of the aorta. Rupture of coronary arteries may also produce hemopericardium. Hemorrhagic pericardial fluid may also be present in the post-pericardiotomy and post-myocardial infarction syndromes. Perforation of a cardiac chamber during cardiac catheterization can lead to hemopericardium. Hemopericardium may also result from blood dyscrasias, anticoagulant therapy, tumor, or pericarditis. Considerable bleeding into the pericardial sac may cause cardiac tamponade.

THE CRITERIA REQUIRED FOR THE DIAGNOSIS OF HEMOPERICARDIUM ARE THE SAME AS THOSE REQUIRED FOR THE DIAGNOSIS OF PERICARDIAL EFFUSION EXCEPT THAT BLOOD WILL BE FOUND ON ASPIRATION.

2.6.4 NEOPLASM

Primary neoplasms of the pericardium are extremely rare. All varieties of connective tissue tumors have been described, some of which, however, probably arise in the myocardium or other neighboring structures and extend into the pericardium. They may cause abnormal cardiac shadows on roentgenographic examination. Primary mesothelioma of the pericardium produces pericardial effusions which are usually hemorrhagic.

Secondary neoplasms involve the pericardium by direct extension from the myocardium, lung, mediastinum, and mediastinal lymph nodes. Blood or lymph-borne metastatic nodules can also reach the pericardial connective tissues. Secondary tumors frequently evoke a hemorrhagic pericardial effusion.

These tumors can produce roentgenographic abnormalities which may be better demonstrated by the introduction of gas or radiopaque contrast material into the pericardium.

THE CRITERIA FOR THE DIAGNOSIS OF NEOPLASMS OF THE PERICARDIUM ARE GIVEN IN 1.19.

2.6.5 PERICARDIAL EFFUSION (HYDROPERICARDIUM)

Pericardial effusion may be caused by pericarditis, tumor, or trauma. Chronic effusions are seen in patients with uremia undergoing dialysis, those with thoracic tumors undergoing chemotherapy or radiation, rheumatoid arthritis, systemic lupus erythematosus, progressive systemic sclerosis, and myxedema. In myxedema it may contribute to the syndrome of myxedema heart disease. It may also occur in diseases in which extracellular fluid volume is increased, as in combined ventricular failure.

Pericardial fluid can muffle heart sounds or be associated with a pericardial friction rub. Serial chest roentgenograms can demonstrate a rapid change in the cardiac silhouette due to the accumulation of fluid. Fluid often causes a symmetrical enlargement of the cardiac silhouette, with obliteration of the outlines of individual cardiac chambers and great vessels.

Gradual accumulation of large quantities of fluid may be accommodated by a slowing distending pericardium with evidence of pericardial restriction appearing late. Rapid accumulation of fluid leads to cardiac tamponade.

ONE OF THE FOLLOWING CRITERIA IS REQUIRED FOR THE DIAGNOSIS OF PERICARDIAL EFFUSION.

1. Demonstration of pericardial fluid by direct aspiration, either percutaneously or at the thoracotomy.
2. Demonstration by angiocardiography that the distance between the outer borders of contrast medium in the right atrium and the overlying cardiac shadow is greater than 5 mm.
3. Demonstration by echocardiography of an abnormal layer of fluid over the dorsal or ventral cardiac walls.
4. Demonstration by radionuclide scanning of an increased distance between radioactivity in the lungs and in the right atrium in the absence of pleural thickening or effusion.
5. Demonstration by coronary arteriography of an in-

creased distance between the opacified vessel and the adjacent outer border of the pericardial shadow.

2.6.6 PERICARDITIS

Inflammation of the pericardium results in a localized or widespread deposition of fibrin, which may be scant or dense. The quality of the cellular reaction depends on the inciting organism. The pericardial sac may contain little fluid. However, there may be sufficient serous, purulent, or sanguineous fluid to alter the cardiac silhouette or produce pericardial restriction. The most superficial layers of the subepicardial myocardium may be involved in the disease process and give rise to electrocardiographic abnormalities.

Specific causes of pericarditis include bacteria, viruses, and fungi. Bacterial infection may be secondary to septicemia or regional inflammation (pulmonary, pleural, mediastinal). Penetrating chest wounds, perforation of the esophagus, or descending infection originating in the neck may result in bacterial pericarditis. Infection of the pericardium by bacteria usually results in a purulent pericarditis. Tuberculous pericarditis results from extension of pulmonary or pleural foci, from caseous mediastinal lymph nodes, or in the course of miliary tuberculosis. The manifestations of tuberculous pericarditis may vary from a few scattered miliary tubercles to extensive pericardial thickening, caseation, and obliteration of the pericardial sac by tuberculous granulation tissue. Large effusions may be encountered. Healing is often accompanied by calcification and may result in pericardial restriction.

Viral pericarditis, which is not associated with other demonstrable heart disease, occurs chiefly in young adults and is commonly associated with pneumonitis and pleuritis. In infants, children, and young adults the Coxsackie B virus has been isolated from pericardial fluid and from stools. Death from this infection is rare in adults and children, but in newborn infants, in whom myocarditis usually also occurs, it is not uncommon.

Noninfective pericarditis is seen in rheumatic fever,

systemic lupus erythematosus, rheumatoid arthritis, progressive systemic sclerosis, uremia, and following myocardial infarction.

In rheumatic fever, pericarditis almost always occurs in conjunction with myocardial and endocardial lesions. The pericarditis is usually fibrinous, but may be serofibrinous. In rheumatic fever, systemic lupus erythematosus, and rheumatoid arthritis the lesion ranges from fibrinous exudate to obliterative fibrosis.

Uremic pericarditis occurs terminally in chronic renal disease in the form of a mild fibrinous inflammation. It has, however, been shown to be reversible in the course of treatment of uremic patients by dialysis. In more severe lesions the exudate may be hemorrhagic and may show partial organization. The lesion is nonspecific histologically, and the identification of its uremic origin depends upon the demonstration of renal disease sufficient to cause renal failure.

Pericarditis may occur following myocardial infarction, but usually is more or less limited to the epicardial surface overlying the zone of infarction, but may occasionally be diffuse. It is generally fibrinous in character. In extensive myocardial infarction, a hemorrhagic exudate may cover the entire pericardium. Local adhesions or more widespread obliteration of the pericardial sac may follow healing.

Inflammatory reactions of the pericardium may occur in the absence of identifiable cause: idiopathic (benign) pericarditis, following pericardiotomy (postpericardiotomy syndrome) or as a late consequence of myocardial infarction (post-myocardial infarction syndrome). In these conditions, fluid accumulation in the pericardium is rarely large.

The onset of pericarditis may be insidious or abrupt and marked by fever and dull or sharp precordial or substernal pain radiating to the neck or shoulders. Characteristically, the pain is relieved by sitting up and leaning forward. In the more indolent forms, such as tuberculous and uremic pericarditis, the patient may be free of pain.

The characteristic physical finding is a friction rub, which may be heard throughout the cardiac cycle or may be present only in systole or in diastole. Leukocytosis and a rapid erythrocyte sedimentation rate are common findings.

Electrocardiograms recorded early in the course may show elevation of the S–T segments in two or three of the standard leads and in some or all of the V leads. Subsequently, these segments return to the baseline, and the T waves become flattened and then inverted throughout the electrocardiogram, with the exception of lead aVR. In contradistinction to myocardial infarction, pericarditis does not produce abnormal Q waves or loss of R wave voltage in the V leads. The cardiac silhouette is usually not enlarged unless there is coexisting heart disease or the effusion is greater than 250 ml.

Echocardiography can be useful in demonstrating pericardial fluid, and may, on occasion, show evidence of constriction.

ONE OF THE FOLLOWING CRITERIA IS REQUIRED FOR THE DIAGNOSIS OF PERICARDITIS.

1. **Pericardial friction rub.**
2. **Chest pain and characteristic electrocardiographic findings or evidence of pericardial fluid.**
3. **Direct aspiration of fibrinous, serofibrinous, or purulent fluid.**

2.6.7 PNEUMOPERICARDIUM

Air in the pericardial sac, demonstrable by radiography, is the result of communication with the lung or gastrointestinal tract or, rarely, may result from infection of the pericardium by gas-forming organisms. Fistula formation between the esophagus and pericardial sac may result from peptic ulceration, traumatic rupture, or perforation by tumor. Only rarely will mediastinal emphysema be associated with pneumopericardium. This occurs almost exclusively following pericardiotomy or in infants after forced positive-pressure breathing. Therapeutic or diagnostic pericardial tap may, of course, introduce air into the cavity.

ONE OF THE FOLLOWING CRITERIA IS REQUIRED FOR THE DIAGNOSIS OF PNEUMOPERICARDIUM.

1. Roentgenographic demonstration of gas within the pericardial sac. This may be difficult to differentiate from mediastinal emphysema unless gas can be seen around the roots of the great vessels.
2. Rarely, radiopaque material can be demonstrated roentgenographically to enter the pericardium from the esophagus, stomach, chest wall, or a bronchus and thereby indicate a pericardial fistula.
3. Direct demonstration of gas within the pericardium at thoracotomy.

2.6.8 CONGENITAL ABSENCE OF THE LEFT PERICARDIUM

Most congenital pericardial defects are left-sided; complete absence of the left pericardium is commoner than partial left-sided defects. The anomaly may be isolated or occur with other cardiovascular malformations or with pectus excavatum. Usually, there are no symptoms associated with absent left pericardium; occasionally, chest pain occurs with changing posture or respiratory infection.

In complete absence of the left pericardium, the chest roentgenogram in the frontal view shows the heart displaced into the left chest, usually with its right border overlying the spine. The pulmonary artery segment is slightly prominent, and an unusually sharp cleft is seen separating the main pulmonary artery from the aortic arch. With partial left-sided defects, which are usually located just inferior and anterior to the left hilus, herniation of the left atrial appendage through the defect often produces an unusually pulsatile mass density in the left infrahilar region. Occasionally, bronchogenic cysts are associated with these partial defects.

When there is complete absence of the left pericardium the electrocardiogram may show sinus bradycardia, right axis deviation, and low voltage of the QRS complexes in the right precordial leads.

Pneumothorax has been employed as a diagnostic procedure: Air injected into the left pleural space can separate the heart from the dome of the diaphragm in the frontal view (due to the absence of the left pericardium) and, in the left lateral decubitus position, air from the left pleural space may enter the right pleural space or the right pericardium. At times, the roentgenographic findings are so suggestive of this defect that additional diagnostic studies may not be indicated.

ONE OF THE FOLLOWING CRITERIA IS REQUIRED FOR THE DIAGNOSIS OF CONGENITAL ABSENCE OF THE LEFT PERICARDIUM.

1. **Radiologic findings as described.**
2. **Demonstration of air entering the pericardial space after induction of left pneumothorax.**
3. **Observation at thoracotomy.**

2.7 Anomalies of Cardiac Position

2.7.1 DEXTROCARDIA

Dextrocardia is an anomaly in which the heart lies predominantly in the right chest. It may be a primary developmental anomaly or it may result from congenital or acquired abnormalities of the chest wall, spine, lungs, or diaphragm.

The nomenclature used to describe the various types of primary congenital positional abnormalities is related to (1) the position of the right atrium and abdominal viscera and (2) the direction of the bending of the bulboventricular loop during embryologic development, which determines the position of the ventricles relative to each other. For example, the normal rightward bending of this loop (concordant bending relative to atrial and visceral situs) determines that the right ventricle is on the right of the left ventricle.

In normal development, the liver, great veins, and right atrium lie on the right side of the body; this position is termed situs solitus. The bulboventricular loop, which lies distal to the atria, initially bends to the right (concordant dextro [D] loop), and then the entire ventricular region of the heart later shifts to the left to form the normal left-sided heart.

When the liver and right atrium develop on the left, situs inversus, a mirror image of normal relationships is present. The bulboventricular loop initially bends to the left (concordant levo [L] loop), and the entire ventricular region later shifts to the right to produce mirror-image dextrocardia.

When bulboventricular loop formation is discordant to viscero-atrial situs (L-loop in situs solitus and D-loop in situs inversus), transposition of the great arteries is regularly present (this combination of anomalies is usually called *corrected transposition of the great arteries*); additional intracardiac malformations are common. Abdominal heterotaxy, or the development of viscero-atrial sinus ambiguus, is often associated with complex intracardiac defects as well as dextrocardia. Midline liver, asplenia, polysplenia and bilateral lung symmetry are common in this circumstance.

Angiocardiography is essential for the recognition of the morphologic patterns of development in dextrocardia, the position of the great vessels, and associated intracardiac defects.

2.7.1.1 Dextrocardia with Situs Inversus

Dextrocardia with situs inversus most commonly results from concordant L-loop bulboventricular development with situs inversus of the abdominal viscera (liver and great veins on the left and stomach on the right). This form of dextrocardia (mirror-image), which represents the normal cardiac position for situs inversus, is infrequently associated with intracardiac defects. Since the right atrium and sino-atrial node are on the left (on the same side as the liver), and the left ventricle is on the right, the electrocardiogram characteristically shows a negative P, QRS, and T in lead I.

Dextrocardia with situs inversus occasionally results from discordant D-loop bulboventricular development. In this circumstance, complex intracardiac malformations associated with cyanosis or veno-arterial shunting are usually encountered. Ectopic atrial rhythms are often noted on the electrocardiogram.

THE FOLLOWING CRITERIA ARE REQUIRED FOR THE DIAGNOSIS OF DEXTROCARDIA WITH SITUS INVERSUS.

Radiologic evidence of the heart in the right chest and evidence of complete abdominal situs inversus.

2.7.1.2 DEXTROCARDIA WITH SITUS SOLITUS

Dextrocardia with situs solitus may result from either (1) failure of expected leftward shift of the normal concordant D bulboventricular loop in situs solitus or (2) inappropriate initial development, that is, discordant L-loop bending of the bulboventricular region, with expected late shift of the ventricular region into the right chest. When the latter mechanism is present, intracardiac defects are frequently encountered.

THE FOLLOWING CRITERIA ARE REQUIRED FOR THE DIAGNOSIS OF DEXTROCARDIA WITH SITUS SOLITUS.

Radiologic evidence of the heart in the right chest and evidence of abdominal situs solitus.

2.7.2 LEVOCARDIA WITH SITUS INVERSUS

A left-sided heart represents a positional abnormality when it is associated with situs inversus of the abdominal viscera. It may result from failure of rightward shift of a concordant L-loop of the bulboventricular region or from an inappropriate discordant D-loop bulboventricular development. The right atrium, like the liver, is on the left. The P wave in the electrocardiogram is frequently inverted in lead I.

THE FOLLOWING CRITERIA ARE REQUIRED FOR THE DIAGNOSIS OF LEVOCARDIA WITH SITUS INVERSUS.

Radiologic evidence of the heart in the left chest and evidence of complete abdominal situs inversus.

2.8 Anomalies of the Aorta and Aortic Arch System

2.8.1 COARCTATION OF THE AORTA

Localized narrowing of the aorta most often occurs at the junction of the arch and descending aorta. It may lie proximal, opposite, or distal to the ductus arteriosus, which may be patent or closed. The aortic obstruction appears to be caused by a curtain-like infolding of the media toward the lumen, which is thereby narrowed and eccentrically located.

A systolic pressure gradient develops across the obstruction, causing the blood pressure in the upper extremities to be significantly higher than that in the lower extremities. Femoral pulses may be weak or absent, and recordings of femoral pulses show a delayed systolic upstroke. Arterial hypertension in the upper extremities may be progressive with advancing age; its absolute level may be modified by the development of collateral vessels which bypass the obstructed segment from proximal to distal aorta.

Characteristically, there is a harsh systolic murmur in the back overlying the site of coarctation. Additional murmurs may be heard over the anterior chest, which are caused by commonly associated lesions, such as a bicuspid aortic valve.

Chest roentgenograms in the frontal view with the esophagus filled with barium may show indentations of the esophagus simulating the letter E which are caused by irregularities and post-stenotic dilatation of the aorta. Beyond early childhood, notching of the inferior margins of the ribs from collateral circulation may be seen on chest films.

ONE OF THE FOLLOWING CRITERIA IS REQUIRED FOR THE DIAGNOSIS OF COARCTATION OF THE AORTA.

1. **A significant difference in systolic blood pressure between the upper and lower extremities, the pressure in the arms being higher.**
2. **Angiographic demonstration.**

2.8.2 RIGHT AORTIC ARCH

A right aortic arch is frequently associated with congenital intracardiac defects; it occurs in about one-third of the patients with tetralogy of Fallot. The ascending aorta and aortic arch normally pass anterior to the right pulmonary artery and right main stem bronchus, but instead of crossing to the left in front of the trachea, as with left aortic arch, remain to the right of the trachea and esophagus, leading to a right upper descending aorta. The aorta often descends on the right to the level of the diaphragm, then crosses the midline to the left, and passes through a left-sided hiatus, resulting in an abdominal aorta in the expected position. Most commonly, the branches of the arch are in a mirror-image relationship to normal; the first branch is a left innominate artery, after which the right common carotid and right subclavian arteries arise separately. The majority of patients have a left ductus arteriosus connecting the left innominate artery with the left pulmonary artery.

A right aortic arch by itself does not produce symptoms. However, when right aortic arch occurs in the absence of associated congenital heart disease, an aberrant left subclavian artery is nearly always present. This combination typically causes a large retro-esophageal defect, with considerable anterior displacement of both the esophagus and trachea. The retro-esophageal component, including the distal arch, the aberrant left subclavian artery, and a ligamentum arteriosum (from the aorta or left subclavian artery) to the left pulmonary artery, forms a vascular ring which may cause tracheal or esophageal obstruction.

The right aortic arch produces an indentation or indentations on the right of the esophagus and displaces the trachea to the left.

ONE OF THE FOLLOWING CRITERIA IS REQUIRED FOR THE DIAGNOSIS OF RIGHT AORTIC ARCH.

1. **Radiographic evidence of the aortic arch being on the right of the trachea or barium-filled esophagus.**
2. **Angiographic demonstration.**

2.8.3 VASCULAR RING

Variations in the development and arrangement of the aortic arch system may result in the encirclement of the trachea and esophagus. In all these anomalies, the trachea and esophagus, which normally lie posterior to the vascular structures, are surrounded by vessels. Two common patterns are: (1) a double aortic arch, consisting of a right and left aortic arch, which unite and continue as the descending aorta; and (2) a right aortic arch with retroesophageal segment, a left ligamentum arteriosum, and left-sided descending aorta.

Symptoms may occur if the ring is "tight" with respiratory distress, stridor, and brassy cough noted in early infancy. Dysphagia may first become apparent in early adult life.

ONE OF THE FOLLOWING CRITERIA IS REQUIRED FOR THE DIAGNOSIS OF VASCULAR RING.

1. **Evidence on chest roentgenogram of an indentation on the posterior wall of the barium-filled esophagus in the lateral view. In the frontal projection, appropriate lateral indentation(s) on the barium-filled esophagus made by the aortic arches or possibly by the ligamentum arteriosum.**
2. **Angiographic demonstration.**

2.9 Anomalies of the Pulmonary Arteries

2.9.1 PULMONARY ARTERIOVENOUS FISTULA

Congenital pulmonary arteriovenous fistula results from the persistence of fetal anastomotic capillaries which divert pulmonary arterial blood to the pulmonary veins along a path that fails to traverse the alveolar capillary bed. Such communications tend to increase in size, and the walls of the supplying artery become thin, tortuous, and dilated as an increasing volume of blood flows through this path of least resistance. The veins draining the anastomoses distend and become varicose. The walls separating varicosities atrophy, leaving large, blood-filled cavities partly divided by septa which are the original walls. When such fistulae exist between a large artery and vein, anastomotic arteries also contribute flow to the "feeder" artery and themselves tend to become dilated. Hence a large arteriovenous anastomosis, once established, is a slowly expanding lesion.

These malformations may be solitary or multiple, involving one or both lungs, and may represent but one manifestation of generalized hereditary telangiectasis (Osler-Rendu-Weber disease). On occasion, these fistulae occur as a fine microscopic network of capillaries rather than as the larger cavernous lesions previously described. Subpleural fistulae may rupture into the pleural cavity, while intrapulmonary lesions frequently rupture and cause hemoptysis.

The clinical consequences of this disorder depend upon the magnitude of total shunt flow across the lungs, regardless of the size of individual lesions. Systemic arterial blood oxyhemoglobin unsaturation, cyanosis, clubbing, and secondary polycythemia appear when shunt flow exceeds approximately 20 percent of total pulmonary blood flow. Overall resistance to pulmonary blood flow is not increased in the presence of these lesions, and right ventricular hypertrophy is rare. Infective end angiitis occasionally develops within the lesion and can result in metastatic cerebral and other systemic abscesses. These lesions may also permit systemic embolization or may manifest themselves solely as abnormal densities in the chest roentgenogram.

ONE OF THE FOLLOWING CRITERIA IS REQUIRED FOR THE DIAGNOSIS OF PULMONARY ARTERIOVENOUS FISTULA.

1. **Angiographic demonstration of the arteriovenous fistula during the stage of pulmonary arterial filling.**

2. Demonstration of right-to-left intrapulmonary shunt by appropriate indicator-dilution techniques in the presence of normal levels of pulmonary blood flow and pulmonary arterial pressure.

2.9.2 PULMONARY VASCULAR SLING

The left pulmonary artery takes origin from the right pulmonary artery and crosses the mediastinum between the trachea (just above its bifurcation) and esophagus to enter the left lung.

Evidence of respiratory distress and frequent pulmonary infections, especially of the right lung, may occur in infancy.

A chest roentgenogram in the lateral view with a barium-filled esophagus shows a persistent anterior indentation of the esophagus just above the level of tracheal bifurcation. A selective pulmonary arteriogram outlines the aberrant origin and course of the left pulmonary artery.

THE FOLLOWING CRITERION IS REQUIRED FOR THE DIAGNOSIS OF PULMONARY VASCULAR SLING.

A selective pulmonary arteriogram demonstrating the aberrant origin and course of the left pulmonary artery.

2.9.3 PERIPHERAL PULMONARY ARTERIAL STENOSIS

Localized constriction may occur at the origin of the right or left pulmonary artery, or multiple sites of narrowing may exist peripherally throughout their distal courses. Both entities are frequently associated with pulmonary valvular stenosis. Multiple peripheral constrictions are common in the post-rubella syndrome. Supravalvular aortic stenosis is sometimes associated with these lesions.

Systolic murmurs, and occasionally diastolic ones, may be widely transmitted over the anterior or posterior chest wall. Pressure gradients within the pulmonary vessels may be demonstrated by catheterization. Selective injection of contrast material in the main pulmonary artery reveals the location of the narrowed sites.

THE FOLLOWING CRITERION IS REQUIRED FOR THE DIAGNOSIS OF PERIPHERAL PULMONARY ARTERIAL STENOSIS.

Angiographic demonstration of localized or multiple constrictions in right, left, or both pulmonary arteries.

2.10 Anomalies of the Coronary Arteries

2.10.1 ANOMALOUS ORIGIN OF THE LEFT CORONARY ARTERY FROM THE PULMONARY ARTERY

The left coronary artery usually arises between the pulmonary valve and the bifurcation of the main pulmonary artery and passes to the myocardium with the same pattern of branching as a "normal" left coronary artery. The direction of blood flow through an anomalously arising left coronary artery usually changes in the first few months of life as the high pulmonary arterial pressure, present at birth, falls toward normal. Initially, blood flows from the main pulmonary artery into the left coronary artery and its distal branches to perfuse the subjacent myocardium. As pulmonary arterial pressure falls and intercoronary anastomotic channels develop between the right and left coronary arteries, blood from the aorta may then flow from the right coronary artery to the left coronary and enter the pulmonary artery. This bypass, acting like an arteriovenous fistula, may cause ischemia of the left ventricular myocardium.

The occurrence of symptoms depends on the extent of ischemia resulting from inadequate perfusion of the left ventricular myocardium. Extreme pallor and restlessness may develop in a previously thriving infant and may be likened to angina. Frequently, a shocklike picture occurs around 3 months of age, with the sudden onset of ventricular failure, attributed to myocardial infarction, which may lead to death. Those infants in whom adequate collateral circulation develops may show no symptoms, and the lesion may not be recognized until childhood.

The electrocardiogram may show S–T and T wave changes and the presence of deep Q waves in leads I, aVL, V5, and V6 resembling anterolateral myocardial infarction. The chest roentgenogram shows marked cardiomegaly, predominantly of the left ventricle.

Murmurs are absent in early infancy. An apical systolic murmur compatible with mitral regurgitation may develop in late infancy or childhood secondary to papillary muscle infarction. In children in whom an extensive flow from the aorta to the pulmonary artery has developed, a continuous murmur may be audible over the midprecordium.

Selective retrograde aortography or coronary arteriography will reveal that only the right coronary artery arises from the aorta. Contrast material may be visualized in the anastomotic channels which enter the left coronary artery and drain into the pulmonary artery. Right heart catheterization may demonstrate a left-to-right shunt at the level of the pulmonary artery.

ONE OF THE FOLLOWING CRITERIA IS REQUIRED FOR THE DIAGNOSIS OF ANOMALOUS ORIGIN OF THE LEFT CORONARY ARTERY FROM THE PULMONARY ARTERY.

1. **Demonstration by selective aortography of the right coronary artery arising from the aorta through which contrast material flows via anastomotic channels to the left coronary artery, which empties into the pulmonary artery.**
2. **Demonstration by pulmonary arteriography of the left coronary artery arising anomalously.**

2.10.2 CORONARY ARTERIAL FISTULA TO A CARDIAC CHAMBER

Either of the coronary arteries, most commonly the right, arising normally from the aorta may make a direct communication with any one of the cardiac chambers, usually a right-sided one. The artery proximal to the fistulous connection is usually wide and tortuous. The physiologic effect of a communication between a coronary artery and the right heart is that of left-to-right shunt at the level of the right atrium or ventricle. The level of the shunt may be detected during right heart catheterization.

A continuous systolic and diastolic murmur, with the diastolic component frequently the louder, is present over the mid-precordium or slightly to the right of the sternum.

The defect is best visualized by selective coronary arteriography or retrograde aortography showing contrast material shunting from an unusually large coronary artery into a particular cardiac chamber.

THE FOLLOWING CRITERION IS REQUIRED FOR THE DIAGNOSIS OF CORONARY ARTERIAL FISTULA TO A CARDIAC CHAMBER.

Demonstration by selective coronary arteriography or aortography of a fistula connecting a coronary artery and a cardiac chamber.

2.11 Communications Between the Great Arteries

2.11.1 AORTICOPULMONARY WINDOW

Aorticopulmonary window, a rare localized defect in the walls of the ascending aorta and main pulmonary artery, permits communication of the great vessels just distal to their respective semilunar valves. Aorticopulmonary window mimics the clinical findings and physiologic derangements of patent ductus arteriosus; however, the left-to-right shunt is frequently larger, and pulmonary hypertension is usually present. The continuous systolic and diastolic murmur may be more intense and widespread than in patent ductus arteriosus. The pulse pressure is usually widened.

At cardiac catheterization the catheter may pass from the main pulmonary artery to the ascending aorta. Following injection of contrast material into the root of the aorta, the main pulmonary artery is opacified.

ONE OF THE FOLLOWING CRITERIA IS REQUIRED FOR THE DIAGNOSIS OF AORTICOPULMONARY WINDOW

1. **Passage of a catheter from the main pulmonary artery into the ascending aorta.**
2. **Direct opacification of the main pulmonary artery when contrast material is selectively injected into the root of the aorta.**

2.11.2 PATENT DUCTUS ARTERIOSUS

This persistent fetal communication between the pulmonary artery and aorta is usually several millimeters in length at birth. It is most commonly a left-sided structure which connects the proximal portion of the left pulmonary artery to the descending aorta just distal to the origin of the left subclavian artery. In the fetus, blood flows from the pulmonary artery into the descending aorta; postnatally, if the channel fails to close spontaneously, blood usually flows from the systemic (aortic) circuit into the pulmonary circuit. Reversal of flow with right-to-left shunting may occur when pulmonary arterial pressures exceed those in the systemic arterial bed.

Symptoms and signs vary with the size of the ductus and the volume and direction of the extracardiac shunt. Although in a small number of infants, left ventricular failure may develop from a large shunt from the aorta into the pulmonary artery, the majority grow and develop normally and are asymptomatic in childhood and early adult life. Infective endocarditis is a potential complication.

The characteristic continuous murmur is maximal in the second left intercostal space and is crescendo during systole and decrescendo during diastole. When severe pulmonary hypertension is present, and flow through the ductus is small, one or both components of the murmur may be absent.

The electrocardiogram and the chest roentgenogram may be normal when the shunt is small. With a large left-to-right shunt the electrocardiogram may indicate left or combined ventricular hypertrophy. In this circumstance, the chest roentgenogram may show prominence of the main and left pulmonary artery segments and increased peripheral pulmonary vascular markings; the heart size is usually increased due to left atrial and left ventricular enlargement.

While direct visualization of the patent ductus by ultrasound is not currently possible, an increased ratio of the left atrial dimension to aortic dimension usually indicates a large left-to-right shunt.

During right heart catheterization, the catheter may be manipulated through the ductus into the descending aorta, or a left-to-right shunt demonstrated at the level of the pulmonary artery, or both. Selective retrograde aortography reveals opacification of the pulmonary arteries when contrast material is injected just below the arch of the aorta.

ONE OF THE FOLLOWING CRITERIA IS REQUIRED FOR THE DIAGNOSIS OF PATENT DUCTUS ARTERIOSUS.

1. **Passage of a catheter from the left pulmonary artery into the descending aorta.**
2. **Opacification of the pulmonary arteries via a patent ductus arteriosus following selective retrograde aortography.**

2.11.3 TRUNCUS ARTERIOSUS

A single large arterial vessel, truncus arteriosus, gives rise to the coronary, pulmonary, and aortic arch branches and continues as the descending aorta. The truncus takes origin from both ventricles. A common semilunar valve and a large ventricular septal defect are integral parts of the malformation. Variations occur in the site of origin and size of the pulmonary arteries which emerge from the lateral or posterior walls of the truncus. The right and left pulmonary arteries arise either from a common pulmonary trunk immediately above the truncal valve, or separately from the ascending portion of the truncus.

When one or both pulmonary arteries are absent, the blood supply to the lungs sometimes may be asymmetric and derived from branches of the brachiocephalic vessels or from the descending aorta through bronchial collateral vessels.

The physiologic derangements and clinical picture depend on the magnitude of the aortic-to-pulmonary shunt, the presence of anatomic changes in the pulmonary vascular bed, and the relation between the systemic and pulmonary blood flow. Although systemic arterial oxyhemoglobin unsaturation is always present, it may be minimal when pulmonary blood flow is markedly increased.

A loud systolic murmur is usually present along the left sternal border. A high-pitched, decrescendo diastolic murmur may be heard in the same area when there is truncal valve dilatation and regurgitation. A loud second sound, often single, may be present. The electrocardiogram and chest roentgenogram offer no specific clues to the diagnosis of truncus arteriosus. By ultrasound examination a single large great vessel may be identified, but the technique has not been helpful in further delineation of the various types of truncal abnormalities.

Right heart catheterization usually permits passage of the catheter from the right ventricle to the ascending truncus and frequently into each of the pulmonary arteries. The blood pressure in the right ventricle and frequently in the pulmonary arteries reaches levels encountered in the systemic arterial bed. A left-to-right shunt may be detected at the ventricular level or in the pulmonary arteries. Truncal or systemic arterial oxyhemoglobin unsaturation varies from mild (90 percent) to severe.

Contrast visualization studies are essential to the delineation of the anomaly. Although right ventricular injection of contrast material may establish the diagnosis of truncus arteriosus, additional selective injections into the ascending truncus are frequently required to localize clearly the sites of origin of the pulmonary arteries.

THE FOLLOWING CRITERION IS REQUIRED FOR THE DIAGNOSIS OF TRUNCUS ARTERIOSUS.

Demonstration by selective aortic root aortography or right ventriculography of a single large ascending vessel, or truncus, which gives origin both to the aorta and the pulmonary arteries.

2.11.4 AORTIC ORIGIN OF THE RIGHT PULMONARY ARTERY

In this vascular malformation the right lung receives its sole arterial blood supply from a large vessel arising from the ascending aorta, and the left lung receives the entire right ventricular output. It is probably derived from embryologic failure of migration of the right sixth aortic arch to join its counterpart on the left before the truncus is divided into the aorta and pulmonary artery. The lesion is not infrequently complicated by a coexisting patent ductus arteriosus.

Although this anomaly may be accompanied by ventricular failure and death in infancy, it may also occur in asymptomatic adults. Clinical findings are not distinctive, although they may suggest truncus arteriosus.

Selective injection of contrast material into the right ventricle delineates a single pulmonary artery going to the left lung; following opacification of the ascending aorta, the anomalous large vessel going to the hilus of the right lung will be visualized at about the same time as the left pulmonary artery. Retrograde aortography provides optimal visualization of the origin and course of the right pulmonary artery.

THE FOLLOWING CRITERION IS REQUIRED FOR THE DIAGNOSIS OF AORTIC ORIGIN OF THE RIGHT PULMONARY ARTERY.

Angiographic demonstration of a single large vessel arising from the ascending aorta passing to the

hilus of the right lung, with the left pulmonary artery arising from the right ventricle.

2.12 Transposition Complexes

2.12.1 COMPLETE TRANSPOSITION OF THE GREAT ARTERIES

The most common transposition complex, referred to as complete transposition of the great arteries (or vessels), designates the aorta arising anteriorly from the right ventricle and the pulmonary artery arising relatively posteriorly from the left ventricle. Because the origins of the great arteries are transposed, the systemic and pulmonary circuits are basically separate: systemic venous blood is directed into the aorta, and pulmonary venous blood is directed into the pulmonary artery. Postnatal survival depends upon the presence of other anomalies which, alone or in combination, permit flow of oxygenated blood into the systemic circulation; that is, communications at the atrial or ventricular level or through a patent ductus arteriosus. A variety of additional malformations may coexist, such as pulmonary valvular stenosis, coarctation of the aorta, or single ventricle.

Cyanosis appears early and becomes progressively more intense in the first few weeks of life, especially when the ventricular septum is intact. Most infants with complete transposition of the great arteries succumb in the first six months of life from hypoxemia and ventricular failure unless therapeutic enlargement of an atrial communication has been accomplished. The prognosis for immediate survival is improved in those with an associated ventricular septal defect, although progressive pulmonary vascular disease is a liability in this group.

Systolic murmurs are usually present, but are not specific. The electrocardiogram is abnormal and may show right, left, or combined ventricular enlargement. The chest roentgenogram may be of diagnostic importance and usually reveals the following: an ovoid, or egg-shaped, cardiac contour (in about 70 percent), often with a narrow superior mediastinal (vascular) pedicle, progressive cardiac enlargement in early infancy, and increased pulmonary vascular markings.

Severe systemic arterial oxyhemoglobin unsaturation may occur, with values under 30 percent, in infants with an intact ventricular septum. Injection of contrast material into the right ventricle permits visualization, particularly in the lateral view, of the anteriorly arising aorta and identifies the relationship between the great arteries, their semilunar valves, and their respective ventricles. Anatomic details of associated malformations, such as ventricular septal defect or pulmonary valvular stenosis, may be enhanced by additional selective injection of contrast material into the left ventricle.

Ultrasound, especially cross-sectional imaging, may be very helpful in showing the abnormal spatial orientation of the aorta and pulmonary artery in either short axis or long axis scans.

THE FOLLOWING CRITERION IS REQUIRED FOR THE DIAGNOSIS OF COMPLETE TRANSPOSITION OF THE GREAT ARTERIES.

Angiocardiographic demonstration of the aorta arising from the right ventricle and receiving the systemic venous return, while the pulmonary artery arises from the left ventricle.

2.12.2 CONGENITALLY CORRECTED TRANSPOSITION OF THE GREAT ARTERIES

This entity consists of ventricular inversion and transposition of the pulmonary artery and aorta in their anteroposterior relations. Ventricular inversion results in the right-sided venous ventricle having the morphologic structure of the left ventricle and the left-sided systemic ventricle resembling the right ventricle; it derives from discordant L-loop bulboventricular development in the presence of a normal, or situs solitus, position of the abdominal viscera. Typically, the pulmonary artery arises medially and posteriorly from the right-sided venous ventricle, and the aorta ascends anteriorly and laterally from the left-sided systemic ventricle. The atrioventricular valves are inverted with the ventricles. Hence the valve on the right is bicuspid and resembles a mitral valve, and that on the left is tricuspid. Intracardiac blood flows and pressures are normal unless there are additional malformations such as ventricular septal defect.

The clinical course and findings mimic those of the associated intracardiac defect, if present. In the absence of other malformations, bradycardia at birth or developing in childhood may be the only clue to the underlying anomaly. Murmurs are not present unless there is left-sided atrioventricular valvular regurgitation. A loud second sound at the left base represents aortic valve closure.

The electrocardiogram frequently shows atrioventricular conduction defects, including complete atrioventricular heart block. A Q wave is often present in right precordial leads and absent in the left precordial leads.

The chest roentgenogram may show straightening or a long convexity of the upper left heart border due to the laterally placed ascending aorta. The heart may be in the left chest or midline in position.

THE FOLLOWING CRITERION IS REQUIRED FOR THE DIAGNOSIS OF CONGENITALLY CORRECTED TRANSPOSITION OF THE GREAT ARTERIES.

Angiocardiographic demonstration of ventricular morphology, with the pulmonary artery arising medially (and posteriorly from a smooth-walled, right-sided (anatomic left) ventricle and the aorta arising on the left and anteriorly from a trabeculated, left-sided (anatomic right) ventricle.

2.12.3 DOUBLE-OUTLET RIGHT VENTRICLE

In double-outlet right ventricle, both the aorta and pulmonary artery take origin from the morphologic right ventricle. Neither semilunar valve is in fibrous continuity with the mitral valve. A ventricular septal defect is an integral part of the anomaly and is the only outlet for blood from the left ventricle. Variations in the anomaly may be identified by the position of the ventricular defect relative to that of the semilunar valves and the location of the conus or infundibulum. The Taussig-Bing malformation is a form of transposition of the great arteries complicated by a double-outlet right ventricle with a subpulmonary ventricular septal defect.

The hemodynamic and clinical picture of double-outlet right ventricle resembles that of ventricular septal defect. If, however, there is associated obstruction to pulmonary blood flow, the lesion may mimic tetralogy of Fallot. The electrocardiogram frequently shows a left or superior QRS axis in the range of $-30°$ to $-170°$.

Cardiac catheterization may reveal a left-to-right shunt at the ventricular level and increased pulmonary artery pressure; the aortic or systemic arterial oxyhemoglobin saturation may be normal from direct streaming of left ventricular blood into the aorta. In right ventricular infundibular stenosis or pulmonary vascular disease, systemic arterial oxyhemoglobin unsaturation may be present.

The diagnosis rests upon filling of both great arteries by contrast material following injection into the right ventricle and visualization of an aortic valve which lies abnormally high and at the same level as the pulmonary valve. Additional selective injections of contrast material into the aorta or left ventricle may be needed to clarify the relationship and origin of the great arteries.

THE FOLLOWING CRITERION IS REQUIRED FOR THE DIAGNOSIS OF DOUBLE-OUTLET RIGHT VENTRICLE.

Angiocardiographic demonstration that both great arteries arise from the right ventricle, with the aortic valve lying in an abnormally high position, and with both semilunar valves separated from the anterior leaflet of the mitral valve by muscular (or conal) tissue.

2.13 Defects at the Atrial Level

2.13.1 PATENT FORAMEN OVALE

The foramen ovale is a slitlike opening in the atrial septum at the site of the foramen secundum (or fossa ovalis), which has a flaplike rim of septal tissue overhanging its left side. It is an important aperture during fetal life, permitting shunting of inferior vena caval blood, which has a high oxygen content, from the right atrium to the left atrium. At or soon after birth, the left atrial pressure rises, and the flap, or valve, is pushed tightly against the septum, functionally closing the foramen ovale. Anatomic or probe patency usually occurs for several months and may persist into adult life in 20 to 30 percent of persons. Occasionally, a cardiac catheter advanced through the inferior vena cava may cross the atrial septum through the foramen ovale and enter the left atrium.

An isolated patent foramen ovale is of no clinical significance. If, however, right atrial pressure is increased because of associated malformations, such as tricuspid atresia or severe pulmonary valvular stenosis with an intact ventricular septum, a right-to-left shunt may occur through the foramen ovale into the left atrium.

THE FOLLOWING CRITERIA ARE REQUIRED FOR THE DIAGNOSIS OF PATENT FORAMEN OVALE.

Passage of a catheter from the right to the left atrium or angiographic demonstration of a right-to-left shunt at the atrial level in the absence of specific findings compatible with the diagnosis of an atrial septal defect of an ostium secundum or primum type.

2.13.2 ATRIAL SEPTAL DEFECT (OSTIUM SECUNDUM)

Atrial septal defect (ostium secundum), a common type of interatrial communication, usually occurs in the region of the fossa ovalis and is separated from the atrioventricular valves by a rim of septal tissue. The size of the defect may range from 0.5 to 3.0 cm or more. It is usually a single opening, although bands of septal tissue may divide it into multiple apertures. When the location of the defect is high—near the superior vena cava (sinus venosus defect)—some of the pulmonary veins, particularly from the right lung, may drain anomalously into the right atrium or the proximal portion of the superior vena cava. Blood is usually shunted through the defect from the left to the right atrium in the presence of normal, or only slightly elevated, right heart pressure.

Symptoms and signs vary with the size of the defect and the volume and direction of intracardiac shunting. A left-to-right shunt at the atrial level may not occur in early infancy until the pulmonary vascular resistance falls toward normal because of maturation of the pulmonary vascular bed. Slow weight gain may be noted in those in whom extremely large left-to-right atrial shunts develop. The majority of children and young adults have moderate shunts and are asymptomatic. In those few in whom increased pulmonary vascular resistance develops in late childhood or adult life, right-to-left shunting may occur and cyanosis ensues.

Murmurs characteristic of atrial septal defect are related to increased blood flow across the tricuspid and pulmonic valves: a mid-diastolic murmur at the lower left sternal border and a more prominent systolic ejection murmur at the upper left sternal border. The second sound in the pulmonic area is widely split and usually fixed. With right-to-left shunting at the atrial level, the pulmonic component of the second sound is very loud and may be followed by a decrescendo diastolic murmur of pulmonary valvular regurgitation.

The electrocardiogram usually reveals right axis deviation and right ventricular conduction delay of the right bundle branch type, with an rsR′ pattern in the right precordial leads. Prolongation of the P–R interval is occasionally noted. Atrial arrhythmias, notably atrial fibrillation, may occur in older children and adults.

The chest roentgenogram may show mild to moderate cardiac enlargement, particularly involving the right atrium and right ventricle, and prominent pulmonary vascular markings.

With significant shunting (1.5:1), echocardiography characteristically demonstrates a dilated right ventricular dimension and abnormal septal motion. While these abnormalities are not specific for an atrial septal defect, a normal examination is considered reliable evidence against a significant shunt.

Right heart catheterization reveals a left-to-right shunt at the atrial level, with normal or elevated pulmonary arterial pressure.

ONE OF THE FOLLOWING CRITERIA IS REQUIRED FOR THE DIAGNOSIS OF ATRIAL SEPTAL DEFECT (OSTIUM SECUNDUM).

1. **A systolic ejection murmur in the pulmonary area, followed by a widely split and fixed second sound, electrocardiographic evidence of right axis deviation and rsR′ in the right precordial leads, and radiologic evidence of increased pulmonary vascular markings.**
2. **Documentation of a left-to-right shunt at the atrial level, with one or both of the following: a systolic ejection murmur in the pulmonary area, followed by a widely split second sound, or normal or right axis deviation.**
3. **Angiocardiographic demonstration of a right-to-left shunt at the atrial level, with markedly elevated pulmonary vascular resistance.**

2.13.3 ENDOCARDIAL CUSHION DEFECT (OSTIUM PRIMUM AND ATRIOVENTRICULAR CANAL DEFECTS)

Abnormalities in the development of the endocardial cushions and the regions immediately adjacent produce characteristic defects of the atrial septum, ventricular septum, and atrioventricular valves. These defects may occur together or singly and range in complexity from the so-called partial form of atrioventricular canal, or persistent ostium primum atrial defect with cleft mitral valve, to the complete form of atrioventricular canal, in which there is a common atrioventricular valve (formed by contiguity of the mitral and tricuspid apparatus), with an ostium primum defect above and a subjacent ventricular defect. The ostium primum defect occupies the lowermost portion of the atrial septum, so that no rim of tissue exists below it. A cleft of the anterior leaflet of the mitral valve is almost always present, and the septal leaflet of the tricuspid valve is frequently deformed. These atrioventricular valvular malformations also occur when no atrial septum is present, as in single, or common, atrium.

The ostium primum defect permits a left-to-right shunt at the atrial level. Often, though not invariably, mitral regurgitation occurs through the cleft anterior leaflet. In the complete form of atrioventricular canal, additional left-to-right shunting may occur at the ventricular level or from left ventricle to right atrium. Pulmonary hypertension and increased pulmonary vascular resistance may develop early in the complete forms of atrioventricular canal and result in bidirectional or right-to-left shunting.

The majority of patients with ostium primum defect and cleft mitral valve without mitral regurgitation have a clinical course similar to that of ostium secundum atrial septal defect. Ventricular failure may occur in infancy or early childhood in those with severe mitral regurgitation or in those with a common atrioventricular valve. Survival beyond childhood is uncommon with the complete forms of atrioventricular canal. The incidence of trisomy 21, or mongolism, is high in all varieties of endocardial cushion defect.

The murmurs associated with ostium primum defect are similar to those found in secundum atrial defect, but an apical systolic murmur may also be heard in the presence of mitral regurgitation.

The electrocardiogram is invaluable in the diagnosis of endocardial cushion defects since it characteristically shows left axis deviation or a superior QRS axis, usually between $-40°$ and $-180°$, with vectorcardiographic display of a counterclockwise loop in the frontal plane. Right bundle branch block is usually seen. Prolongation of the P–R interval is common. In addition, right, left, or biventricular enlargement may be present.

Selective left ventriculography shows specific deformity of the left ventricular outflow tract related to the abnormality of insertion of the anterior leaflet of the mitral valve.

Echocardiographic findings in ostium primum may include right ventricular dilatation and abnormal septal motion similar to that seen with ostium secundum. However, the abnormal insertion of the anterior leaflet of the mitral valve is reflected in mitral valve echoes which are very close to the septum in both systole and diastole. With more complex defects, the tricuspid valve echoes may appear to blend with the septum or may appear to blend with those of the mitral valve as a single, multileaflet atrioventricular valve with but a remnant of intraventricular septum visible.

ONE OF THE FOLLOWING CRITERIA IS REQUIRED FOR THE DIAGNOSIS OF ENDOCARDIAL CUSHION DEFECT (OSTIUM PRIMUM AND ATRIOVENTRICULAR CANAL DEFECTS).

1. **Electrocardiographic evidence of a left or superior QRS axis and left-to-right shunt at the atrial level.**
2. **Angiocardiographic demonstration of characteristic left ventricular outflow tract deformity.**

2.13.4 SINGLE (COMMON) ATRIUM

In single atrium, the atrial septum is absent, but there are two atrial appendages. A left superior vena cava, as well as a right superior vena cava, is frequently present. A single sino-atrial node is usually present on the right, but may be bilateral. Functionally, a left-to-right shunt predominates, the magnitude being dependent on the relationship of the pulmonary-to-systemic resistance.

A single atrium is encountered mainly in two circumstances: (1) abnormalities of cardiac position associated with discordant viscero-atrial situs and bulboventricular looping and (2) endocardial cushion defects with cleft mitral valve or common atrioventricular valve.

The clinical picture resembles that of large atrial septal defects of the secundum or primum types. Ectopic atrial rhythms are occasionally noted.

THE FOLLOWING CRITERIA ARE REQUIRED FOR THE DIAGNOSIS OF SINGLE (COMMON) ATRIUM.

Angiocardiographic demonstration of a single large atrial chamber receiving both systemic and pulmonary venous blood, usually in association with a diagnosis of anomalous cardiac position or endocardial cushion defect.

2.13.5 COR TRIATRIATUM

Cor triatriatum is an unusual congenital anomaly in which there is failure of the pulmonary veins to be directly incorporated into the definitive left atrium, emptying instead to an atrium-like chamber above the left atrium. The two chambers communicate through an opening which, if narrow, causes obstruction to pulmonary venous flow, with altered dynamics simulating those of mitral obstruction. An atrial septal defect with communication between the right atrium and the left atrium sometimes coexists.

Tachypnea and evidences of respiratory distress may be the major findings in infancy or early childhood. An apical systolic or diastolic murmur may be audible. Electrocardiograms usually indicate right ventricular enlargement. Chest roentgenograms may show pulmonary venous congestion.

During right heart catheterization the catheter may pass across the atrial septum to the left atrium. If the atrial defect is above the level of the obstructing membrane, a high atrial pressure will be recorded; if the defect is between the membrane and the mitral valve, the left atrial pressure will be normal. Pulmonary arterial hypertension is usually severe, with the systolic pressure sometimes exceeding that in the systemic arterial bed.

Angiocardiography, best performed by injection into

the pulmonary artery, reveals drainage of the pulmonary veins into an accessory left atrial chamber and a linear filling defect indicating a ledge or diaphragm between the chamber and the more distal true left atrium.

THE FOLLOWING CRITERION IS REQUIRED FOR THE DIAGNOSIS OF COR TRIATRIATUM.

Angiocardiographic demonstration of the pulmonary veins draining into an accessory atrial chamber which is separated by a linear filling defect from the more distal true left atrium.

2.14 Defects at the Ventricular Level

2.14.1 VENTRICULAR SEPTAL DEFECT

Ventricular septal defects are the commonest of all congenital heart lesions, alone or in combination with other malformations. The size of an isolated ventricular septal defect is probably the most important feature in determining the hemodynamic derangements that ensue. However, the anatomic location, whether in the membranous or muscular portion of the septum or above or below the crista supraventricularis, also may influence the clinical course and surgical management. The most common defect, usually referred to as the membranous type, lies inferior to the crista and is in part overhung by the septal leaflet of the tricuspid valve. Muscular defects may occur in any portion of the muscular part of the septum; they are frequently small and may be multiple. A ventricular septal defect may decrease in size with advancing age or even close completely.

Symptoms vary with the magnitude of left-to-right shunting through the defect, which is dependent upon its size and the level of pulmonary vascular resistance. When defects are large, ventricular failure may develop during the first few months of life. When shunts are moderate in size, reduced exercise tolerance and growth impairment may occur. When shunts are small, no symptoms ensue. Pulmonary vascular resistance may increase when shunts are large; high pulmonary vascular resistance in children and young adults may cause reversal of the shunt and the appearance of cyanosis.

The physical signs usually include a harsh holosystolic murmur and thrill along the lower left sternal border. An apical mid-diastolic murmur accompanies large left-to-right shunts, which markedly increase the pulmonary venous flow traversing the mitral valve into an enlarged left ventricular chamber. The intensity of the pulmonic valve closure sound varies directly with the pulmonary arterial pressure. In the presence of cyanosis due to right-to-left shunting at the ventricular level, a decrescendo diastolic murmur may indicate pulmonary valvular regurgitation.

When the left-to-right shunt through the ventricular septal defect is small, the electrocardiogram and chest roentgenogram may be normal. However, with moderate and large shunts there is usually increased left ventricular QRS voltage in the electrocardiogram. The chest film may show enlargement of the left atrium and ventricle, a dilated pulmonary arterial segment, and increased pulmonary vascular markings. With right-to-left shunting, right ventricular hypertrophy is noted on the electrocardiogram, and the central pulmonary arteries may appear enlarged, with sparse peripheral vascular markings.

By either M-mode or cross-sectional echocardiography, the actual ventricular septal defect can rarely be visualized. Occasionally, however, evidence of hemodynamic abnormalities can be seen such as atrial or ventricular dilatation or pulmonary hypertension.

Right heart catheterization indicates the presence of a left-to-right shunt at the ventricular level, with normal or elevated pulmonary arterial pressure. No shunt will be detected if pulmonary vascular resistance is markedly increased. Occasionally, a catheter in the right ventricle will traverse the ventricular defect and enter the aorta.

Injection of contrast material into the left ventricle demonstrates a left-to-right shunt and the size and location of the defect. Following right ventricular injection, there may be reopacification of the right ventricle or pulmonary artery after the left ventricle fills. If there is severe pulmonary hypertension, selective injection into the right ventricle may demonstrate a right-to-left ventricular shunt.

ONE OF THE FOLLOWING CRITERIA IS REQUIRED FOR THE DIAGNOSIS OF VENTRICULAR SEPTAL DEFECT.

1. A harsh systolic murmur along the lower left sternal border and documentation of a left-to-right shunt at the ventricular level, with normal right ventricular pressure.
2. Demonstration of the defect by means of a left ventriculogram.
3. Documentation of a left-to-right shunt at the ventricular level, with an elevated pulmonary arterial pressure, and angiocardiographic demonstration of normally related great arteries.
4. Severe pulmonary hypertension and angiocardiographic documentation of a right-to-left shunt at the ventricular level in the absence of other malformations.

2.14.2 VENTRICULAR SEPTAL DEFECT WITH OBSTRUCTION TO RIGHT VENTRICULAR OUTFLOW

2.14.2.1 Mild or Moderate Obstruction to Right Ventricular Outflow

A ventricular septal defect, usually one of moderate or large size, may be complicated by obstruction to right ventricular outflow either at the subvalvular or valvular level. There may be hypertrophy of the crista supraventricularis or occasionally pulmonary valvular stenosis. The presence of mild to moderate obstruction to right ventricular outflow effects a rise in right ventricular pressure and a reduction in the flow from left to right through the ventricular septal defect. In some instances the muscular hypertrophy is progressive and may develop into severe obstruction, presenting the clinical picture of tetralogy of Fallot.

The signs differ from those of isolated ventricular septal defect due to the associated right ventricular obstruction. A loud, coarse, ejection systolic murmur may be heard along the entire left sternal border and may be well transmitted under the clavicles. The murmur is usually associated with a thrill. The second heart sound at the pulmonic area is usually of normal intensity. The electrocardiogram usually shows a right ventricular hypertrophy pattern; the chest roentgenogram shows only a modest increase in pulmonary vascularity.

In addition to a left-to-right shunt at the ventricular level, a systolic pressure gradient usually in excess of 20 mm Hg is recorded across the right ventricular outflow tract, the pulmonary valve, or both.

Angiocardiography permits visualization of the narrowed right ventricular outflow tract or pulmonary valvular obstruction.

THE FOLLOWING CRITERIA ARE REQUIRED FOR THE DIAGNOSIS OF VENTRICULAR SEPTAL DEFECT WITH MILD OR MODERATE OBSTRUCTION TO RIGHT VENTRICULAR OUTFLOW.

Documentation of a left-to-right shunt at the ventricular level and measurement of a systolic pressure gradient between the body of the right ventricle and the pulmonary artery or angiographic demonstration of obstruction.

2.14.2.2 Severe Obstruction to Right Ventricular Outflow (Tetralogy of Fallot)

The combination of a ventricular septal defect, usually of large size, and severe obstruction to right ventricular outflow comprises the two critical anatomic components of tetralogy of Fallot. The ventricular defect usually lies below the crista supraventricularis. Obstruction to right ventricular outflow is most frequently due to narrowing of the infundibulum associated with muscular hypertrophy and may be progressive. In addition, there may occasionally be pulmonary valvular stenosis, hypoplasia of the pulmonary anulus, or constriction at the origin of the right or left pulmonary artery.

The two other features included in the designation of tetralogy of Fallot are overriding of the aorta and right ventricular hypertrophy, both of which are of secondary importance. The aorta arises from both ventricles above the large ventricular defect, with considerable variation in the degree of its dextroposition or overriding of the right ventricle. Since the systolic pressures in the body of the right ventricle and aorta are always equal, and the right ventricular outflow tract is obstructed, the direction of the right-to-left shunt is determined physiologically rather than anatomically. Additional anomalies encountered in tetralogy of Fallot include a right aortic arch, present in about one-third of cases, and an aberrant branching of the right coronary artery, with a large anterior descending vessel crossing the outflow tract of the right ventricle. The coexistence of a patent ductus arteriosus permits survival in those with pulmonary atresia.

Signs and symptoms vary with the severity of obstruction of the right ventricular outflow tract. Cyanosis may be present at birth or develop sometime after infancy. Clubbing of the digits eventually accompanies the cyanosis. Breathlessness with exertion may be manifested in infancy by distress during crying. Hypoxic "spells" with loss of consciousness may ensue. Breathlessness or extreme fatigue with exercise in childhood may be relieved by a squatting posture. Ventricular failure does not occur except in infants with associated pulmonary atresia. Cerebral complications, which include thrombosis or profound hypoxia, may be life-threatening or cause death.

A systolic thrill and harsh ejection systolic murmur are usually present at the mid- and upper left sternal border. The murmur is related to the systolic pressure gradient at the site or sites of right ventricular outflow obstruction. When pulmonary atresia exists, no systolic murmur is audible. The pulmonic component of the second sound is diminished or absent; the aortic valve closure sound may be prominent along the left sternal border.

By ultrasound, a large and somewhat anteriorly displaced aorta can be seen and, in contrast to other ventricular septal defects, a discontinuity between the aorta and intraventricular septum can often be seen. Thickening of the anterior right ventricular wall and possible dilatation of the right ventricle with normal septal motion may also be seen.

The electrocardiogram shows right axis deviation and moderate to severe right ventricular hypertrophy. The chest roentgenogram reveals a small or normal-sized heart, usually with uplifted apex (boot-shaped contour) due to right ventricular hypertrophy and a relatively concave pulmonary artery segment. The pulmonary arteries are small, and the peripheral vascular markings are usually diminished. The aortic knob may be seen at the right base.

A systolic pressure gradient exists between the body of the right ventricle and the outflow tract, and an additional distal gradient may occasionally be found at the level of the pulmonary valve. The pulmonary arterial pressure may be normal, but is usually reduced. The systolic pressure in the right ventricle equals that in the aorta, which is frequently entered by passage of a catheter through the large ventricular septal defect. Systemic arterial oxyhemoglobin saturation is always reduced.

Angiocardiography with selective injection into the right ventricle demonstrates early opacification of the aorta as contrast material passes directly from the right ventricle into the aorta. It also indicates the site or sites of right ventricular outflow tract obstruction and the size of the pulmonary arteries.

THE FOLLOWING CRITERION IS REQUIRED FOR THE DIAGNOSIS OF VENTRICULAR SEPTAL DEFECT WITH SEVERE OBSTRUCTION TO RIGHT VENTRICULAR OUTFLOW (TETRALOGY OF FALLOT).

Angiocardiographic demonstration, following selective right ventricular injection, of early opacification of the left ventricular outflow tract and aorta in addition to the site or sites of right ventricular outflow tract obstruction.

2.14.3 LEFT VENTRICULAR TO RIGHT ATRIAL COMMUNICATION

Left ventricular to right atrial communication is an uncommon defect. Two types occur: (1) a defect in that part of the membranous portion of the ventricular septum which enters into the formation of the floor of the right atrium and (2) a defect in the ventricular septum posterior to the crista supraventricularis, associated with a cleft or a double orifice of the tricuspid valve. In the latter situation, left ventricular blood may be ejected through the right ventricle directly into the right atrium. An extra opening of the tricuspid valve or adhesions between the edges of the ventricular septal defect and those of the cleft often permit a direct channel from left ventricle to right atrium.

The clinical picture, including a systolic thrill and murmur along the left sternal border, is identical with that noted with a ventricular septal defect, usually one of small or moderate size.

The electrocardiogram often shows tall P waves, suggesting right atrial enlargement. The chest roentgenogram may show prominence of the right atrium. The pulmonary vascular markings are increased. Right heart catheterization documents a left-to-right shunt at the atrial level. Selective left ventriculography demonstrates shunting from the left ventricle to the right atrium.

THE FOLLOWING CRITERION IS REQUIRED FOR THE DIAGNOSIS OF LEFT VENTRICULAR TO RIGHT ATRIAL COMMUNICATION.

Demonstration by left ventriculography of a normal left ventricular outflow tract and direct communication or shunt into the right atrium.

2.14.4 SINGLE (COMMON) VENTRICLE

Morphologically, single ventricle usually resembles a large left ventricle into which both atrioventricular valves empty; the outflow tract of the underdeveloped right ventricle is represented by the infundibulum. The aorta and pulmonary artery are usually transposed, with the aorta arising anteriorly above the infundibular chamber. In the circumstances of ventricular inversion, single ventricle may also occur.

As a result of admixture of right and left atrial blood in the single ventricle, there may be evidence of a left-to-right shunt at the ventricular level, and of a right-to-left shunt as revealed by a reduction in oxyhemoglobin saturation in the systemic arterial circulation. The relative magnitude and direction of the shunt depends on the pulmonary vascular resistance and the presence or absence of obstruction at the outlet of either the aorta or pulmonary artery.

The clinical features are variable, depending on the relative magnitude of pulmonary blood flow and associated defects. Cyanosis is usually obvious, since the most frequently encountered situation is that of single ventricle with transposition of the great arteries and increased pulmonary vascular resistance. Auscultation, electrocardiography, and roentgenography offer no particular clues to the anatomic situation.

Specific diagnosis can only be afforded by angiocardiography. Particularly valuable is the selective injection of contrast media into the left atrium through the usually present atrial communication. Opacification of the common ventricular chamber reveals a large, relatively smooth, finely trabeculated ventricle, which resembles the left ventricle. Following opacification of the large ventricular chamber, there may be dense opacification of an anterior infundibular chamber, from which the aorta may arise in a transposed position.

THE FOLLOWING CRITERION IS REQUIRED FOR THE DIAGNOSIS OF SINGLE (COMMON) VENTRICLE.

Selective angiocardiographic demonstration of a ventricular chamber receiving both atrioventricular valves.

2.15 Malformations of the Aortic Valve

2.15.1 AORTIC LEAFLET, ANULAR, OR COMMISSURAL DEFORMITIES CAUSING REGURGITATION

Defects of the aortic valve resulting in regurgitation are less frequently observed than those causing obstruction. Bicuspid aortic valves may become incompetent with advancing age, due to cusp distortion. Aortic regurgitation may occur with ventricular septal defect, most often due to prolapse of the right coronary cusp. In rare instances, distortion of a single leaflet or commissure may impair cusp apposition.

The symptoms and signs will be affected by the associated defects and by the degree of regurgitation. A high-pitched, decrescendo diastolic murmur is heard at the right base and transmitted down the left sternal border. An aortic ejection sound is frequently present. Widening of the pulse pressure and radiographic and electrocardiographic evidence of left ventricular hypertrophy will vary with the severity of the regurgitant volume. Echocardiographic signs are discussed in Section 3.3.2.

Retrograde aortography with selective injection at the aortic root best demonstrates the degree of regurgitation and may outline the precise type of valve deformity present.

THE FOLLOWING CRITERIA ARE REQUIRED FOR THE DIAGNOSIS OF AORTIC LEAFLET, ANULAR, OR COMMISSURAL DEFORMITIES CAUSING REGURGITATION.

A decrescendo diastolic murmur at the right base or left sternal border, either dating from infancy or early childhood or noted in association with another congenital defect, and demonstration of aortic valvular regurgitation by selective retrograde aortography.

2.15.2 AORTIC ATRESIA

With aortic atresia, a fibrous membrane without an orifice constitutes the valve area; the ascending aorta is almost invariably hypoplastic. The mitral valve is small but structurally normal and communicates with a diminutive blind left ventricular cavity. An interatrial communication permitting a left-to-right shunt is essential for survival. The right ventricle therefore supplies both the pulmonary circulation and, through a patent ductus arteriosus, the systemic circulation.

Atresia of the aortic valve is one of the variants in the so-called hypoplastic left heart syndrome. This designation refers to a group of lesions which include varying degrees of mitral and aortic valve obstruction, a small left ventricle, and a hypoplastic ascending aorta.

Symptoms and signs are usually severe and progressive and result from pulmonary venous congestion and right ventricular failure, with inadequate systemic arterial perfusion and shock. Respiratory distress, pallor, and poor peripheral pulses are striking. Death almost invariably occurs during the first two weeks of life. Murmurs are nonspecific and unimpressive. The pulmonic component of the second heart sound is very loud.

The electrocardiogram shows a right axis deviation and right ventricular hypertrophy. The chest roentgenogram may show cardiac enlargement due to right atrial and right ventricular dilatation; the pulmonary artery may be dilated. Pulmonary venous congestion is prominent. A very hypoplastic left ventricle may be seen by echocardiography, although the atretic valve is usually not well visualized.

Cardiac catheterization demonstrates a left-to-right shunt at the atrial level, a systemic pressure in the right ventricle, and patency of the ductus arteriosus by passage of a catheter through it.

After selective left atrial injection, angiocardiography demonstrates the blind left ventricular cavity and the passage of contrast material into the right atrium. Additional right ventricular or pulmonary artery injection permits visualization of retrograde aortic flow to the level of the atretic valve through a patent ductus arteriosus.

THE FOLLOWING CRITERION IS REQUIRED FOR THE DIAGNOSIS OF AORTIC ATRESIA.

Angiocardiographic demonstration of a small left ventricular chamber which does not opacify the aorta, and retrograde aortic flow to the level of the aortic valve.

2.15.3 AORTIC VALVULAR STENOSIS

Aortic valvular stenosis is a common type of valve defect which may occur in three major anatomic forms according to the nature of commissural fusion and the number of apparent leaflets present: (1) a dome-shaped malformation due to varying degrees of fusion of the three commissures producing a central orifice; (2) a unicuspid valve resulting from complete fusion of two commissures, usually leaving a single commissure which produces an eccentric orifice; and (3) a bicuspid valve may be only mildly obstructive in early childhood, but may become progressively narrowed by thickening and calcification and cause obstruction in adult life. Mild regurgitation may be associated with any of these types of malformations.

With mild and moderate stenosis, symptoms may be lacking. With severe obstruction in early infancy, left ventricular failure may rapidly develop. In the older age group with severe obstruction, fatigue, chest pain, or syncope may occur; left ventricular failure is usually preceded by cardiomegaly. Sudden death may be preceded by electrocardiographic evidence of severe left ventricular hypertrophy, with S–T segment and T wave changes.

A loud, harsh ejection systolic murmur accompanied by a thrill may be present at the right base and is transmitted to the brachiocephalic vessels. An ejection click is frequently audible. A narrow pulse pressure may be noted with moderate or severe obstruction.

The electrocardiogram usually is normal in mild obstruction. Evidence of left ventricular hypertrophy and S–T segment and T wave changes in the left precordial leads may occur with increasing obstruction.

The chest roentgenogram shows a normal heart size, with some dilatation of the ascending aorta. Left ventricular enlargement may be apparent with severe obstruction or left ventricular failure.

A systolic gradient is present across the aortic valve. This may range from 10 mm Hg with minimal obstruction to over 200 mm Hg with extreme obstruction.

By ultrasound, an eccentricity of the aortic valve echo in diastole or multiple diastolic echoes may suggest the diagnosis of a bicuspid valve. Although evidence of thickened valve leaflets and restricted leaflet motion may be seen by echocardiography, quantitation of the degree of stenosis is not at present possible by the M-mode technique. Further, in children with severe aortic stenosis without fibrosis or calcification, the valve echoes may appear normal.

Selective left ventriculography permits visualization of the nature and the site of obstruction.

THE FOLLOWING CRITERIA ARE REQUIRED FOR THE DIAGNOSIS OF AORTIC VALVULAR STENOSIS.

A harsh ejection systolic murmur at the right base dating from infancy or early childhood and evidence of aortic valvular obstruction.

2.15.4 SUBVALVULAR AORTIC STENOSIS

A fibrous ridge or diaphragm may be present a few millimeters to several centimeters below a normal aortic valve. Clinically, this type of discrete obstruction may be indistinguishable from that due to valvular stenosis, except that no ejection click is audible, and dilatation of the ascending aorta is not prominent. Discrete subvalvular aortic stenosis must be distinguished from diffuse, fixed, tunnellike obstruction of the left ventricular outflow tract and from diffuse obstruction caused by a hypertrophied septum abutting the anterior leaflet of the mitral valve during systole. This abnormality can, in certain cases, be seen by echocardiography.

At cardiac catheterization it is sometimes possible to

determine that the site of obstruction is below the valve. Left ventriculography may demonstrate that the stenotic site is below a normally moving valve. However, when the fibrous diaphragm is close to the valve, it may be difficult to distinguish it from valvular stenosis.

THE FOLLOWING CRITERION IS REQUIRED FOR THE DIAGNOSIS OF SUBVALVULAR AORTIC STENOSIS.

Evidence of a localized obstruction below the valve.

2.15.5 SUPRAVALVULAR AORTIC STENOSIS

Supravalvular aortic stenosis is a localized or diffuse narrowing of the aorta originating just above the level of the coronary arteries at the superior margin of the sinuses of Valsalva. It may occur with or without peripheral pulmonary arterial stenosis in a familial or sporadic form. The anomaly may be identified with idiopathic infantile hypercalcemia when associated defects include mental retardation, elfin facies, strabismus, dental abnormalities, and peripheral pulmonary and systemic arterial stenoses.

The symptoms are similar to those of aortic valvular stenosis. Although the systolic thrill and ejection murmur at the right base may be indistinguishable from those of valvular or supravalvular stenosis, the aortic closure sound is frequently accentuated, and an ejection click is uncommon. Inequality in the brachial arterial pressures may be noted, the right more often being higher than the left.

The electrocardiograms and chest roentgenograms resemble those of aortic valvular stenosis. The defect may be seen echocardiographically. A systolic pressure gradient is present above the valve. Left ventriculography permits visualization of the supravalvular aortic obstruction. The coronary arteries, located proximal to the stenosis, are usually prominent vessels. Selective injection of contrast material into the main pulmonary artery may permit demonstration of associated peripheral pulmonary arterial stenosis.

THE FOLLOWING CRITERION IS REQUIRED FOR THE DIAGNOSIS OF SUPRAVALVULAR AORTIC STENOSIS.

Angiographic demonstration of obstruction distal to the aortic valve.

2.16 Malformations of the Mitral Valve

2.16.1 MITRAL LEAFLET, ANULAR, OR COMMISSURAL DEFORMITIES CAUSING REGURGITATION

Isolated malformations of the mitral valve are uncommon; more often, these malformations are associated with other defects, such as endocardial cushion defect with a cleft in the anterior leaflet, congenitally corrected transposition of the great arteries with abnormality of the left-sided atrioventricular valve, or anomalous origin of the left coronary artery from the pulmonary artery, causing infarction of a papillary muscle. The rare isolated deformities of the mitral valve causing regurgitation include clefts in the anterior or posterior leaflet, separation of the commissures with dilatation of the anulus, an accessory orifice in one of the cusps, anomalies of the chordae tendineae or their insertion, and prolapsing of a cusp associated with papillary muscle dysfunction.

The symptoms and signs vary with the severity of the valvular defect. Left ventricular failure with pulmonary edema may occur early in severe cases; milder cases may have exertional breathlessness. A blowing apical systolic murmur present from early infancy usually distinguishes these lesions from acquired mitral valvular deformity, notably that secondary to rheumatic valvulitis. At the apex a prominent systolic click may be heard when papillary muscle dysfunction permits billowing of a leaflet.

The electrocardiogram may show a broad P wave, with usually a normal QRS axis and left ventricular hypertrophy. Progressive T wave changes may develop in papillary muscle dysfunction with inversion in leads II, III, aVF, and over the left precordium.

The chest roentgenogram may show left atrial and

left ventricular enlargement. The left atrium may be enormous in severe cases. Echocardiographic manifestations are discussed in Section 3.3.4.

The pulmonary arterial wedge pressure is usually elevated, and there is a tall V wave in the left atrial pressure tracing.

Significant regurgitation into the left atrium may be demonstrated by injection of contrast material into the left ventricle. Cineangiocardiographic techniques may permit precise identification of the valve dysfunction.

THE FOLLOWING CRITERIA ARE REQUIRED FOR THE DIAGNOSIS OF MITRAL LEAFLET, ANULAR, OR COMMISSURAL DEFORMITIES CAUSING REGURGITATION.

A blowing apical systolic murmur first noted in infancy or early childhood, and angiocardiographic demonstration of mitral regurgitation in the absence of congenitally corrected transposition of the great arteries and anomalous origin of the left coronary artery.

2.16.2 MITRAL ATRESIA

With mitral atresia, only a blind dimple is seen at the site of the mitral valve. It is usually associated with aortic valvular hypoplasia or atresia and an atrial septal defect. Usually, the interatrial communication is small, so that the left-to-right shunt is limited, and pulmonary venous congestion occurs. When the great arteries are normally related, some of the blood from the pulmonary artery may pass through a patent ductus arteriosus to the systemic arterial bed or through a ventricular septal defect to the left ventricle and then to the aorta. Occasionally, mitral atresia may coexist with single ventricle and complete transposition of the great arteries.

Severe respiratory distress, present from birth, is the dominant finding. Pallor or mild to moderate cyanosis may develop. Pulmonary venous congestion and right ventricular failure are usually progressive. Death usually occurs in infancy or childhood.

Murmurs are nonspecific. When present, they are related to the associated defects. The pulmonic valve closure sound is usually very loud.

The electrocardiogram reveals marked right axis deviation and right ventricular hypertrophy. The chest roentgenogram shows enlargement of the right heart chambers and pulmonary venous congestion. Left atrial pressure is elevated, and there is severe pulmonary hypertension. There is failure of the left ventricle to opacify after selective injection of contrast material into the left atrium.

THE FOLLOWING CRITERION IS REQUIRED FOR THE DIAGNOSIS OF MITRAL ATRESIA.

Angiocardiographic demonstration of failure to opacify the left ventricle after injection of contrast material into the left atrium.

2.16.3 MITRAL STENOSIS

Mitral stenosis, an uncommon congenital lesion, may result from a fusion of the two leaflets at the commissures and a shortening of the chordae tendineae, often creating a funnel-shaped mitral valve. Malformation of the mitral valve causing obstruction must be considered in the differential diagnosis of cor triatriatum. Congenital mitral stenosis is frequently associated with other defects, particularly aortic stenosis, coarctation of the aorta, and patent ductus arteriosus.

Symptoms of respiratory distress dominate the clinical picture. An apical diastolic murmur, usually with presystolic accentuation, is audible from early infancy. The loud pulmonary valve closure sound reflects the severe pulmonary hypertension which is commonly present.

The electrocardiogram shows broad P waves, right axis deviation, and right ventricular hypertrophy. The chest roentgenogram shows left atrial enlargement, a prominent pulmonary arterial segment, and right ventricular enlargement. Pulmonary venous congestion may be present. Echocardiographic criteria are similar to those of acquired mitral stenosis.

There is a diastolic pressure gradient across the mitral valve, and the pressures in the left atrium and pulmonary circulation are elevated. There may be a prominent A wave in the left atrial pressure curve.

Selective angiocardiography with injection of contrast material into the pulmonary artery may show delayed emptying of an enlarged left atrium.

THE FOLLOWING CRITERIA ARE REQUIRED FOR THE DIAGNOSIS OF MITRAL STENOSIS.

An apical diastolic murmur dating from infancy or early childhood and evidence of mitral valvular obstruction.

2.17 Malformations of the Pulmonary Valve

2.17.1 ABSENT PULMONARY VALVE

In absent pulmonary valve, the sinuses of Valsalva or cusps have not developed, and only a rim of irregular fibrous tags exists. The hypoplastic valve ring is frequently obstructive. This may occur as an isolated lesion, but is more often associated with a ventricular septal defect and right ventricular outflow tract obstruction. Pulmonary regurgitation invariably results.

Evidence of respiratory distress and right ventricular failure often dominate the picture in early infancy. A medium to low-pitched diastolic murmur along the upper left sternal border is usually present. Additional murmurs vary, depending on the frequently associated ventricular septal defect and the presence or absence of right ventricular outflow tract obstruction.

The electrocardiogram demonstrates right ventricular hypertrophy. The chest roentgenogram frequently shows striking enlargement of the pulmonary arterial trunk and its main branches. Sometimes these vessels may be aneurysmally dilated and cause bronchial compression.

There is low diastolic pressure in the pulmonary artery, with a normal or low systolic pressure and an elevated end-diastolic pressure in the right ventricle.

Injection of contrast material into the pulmonary artery demonstrates the pulmonary valvular regurgitation.

THE FOLLOWING CRITERIA ARE REQUIRED FOR THE DIAGNOSIS OF ABSENT PULMONARY VALVE.

A normal or low pulmonary arterial systolic pressure and angiocardiographic demonstration of pulmonary regurgitation.

2.17.2 PULMONARY ATRESIA WITH INTACT VENTRICULAR SEPTUM

In pulmonary atresia with intact ventricular septum, there is no patency of the valve, which is represented by a fibrous diaphragm from the upper aspect of which three equidistant raphes radiating to the pulmonary arterial wall may be visible. The pulmonary trunk distal to the atretic valve may be somewhat narrower than normal, but its two major branches are usually of normal size. The size of the right ventricular cavity is usually small, and the wall is markedly hypertrophied. If, however, the tricuspid valve is of normal size, the right ventricular chamber may be either normal in size or enlarged. In all instances of pulmonary atresia an interatrial communication is present, permitting a right-to-left shunt. The lungs are perfused via a patent ductus arteriosus.

The symptoms and signs are severe: marked cyanosis and difficulty in breathing are present soon after birth. The absence of a murmur in the presence of ischemic lung fields suggests the diagnosis.

The electrocardiogram shows diminished right ventricular forces. Both the electrocardiogram and chest roentgenogram may be similar to those seen with tricuspid atresia; differentiation between the two conditions can be made only by further laboratory studies.

Passage of a catheter from the right atrium into the right ventricle distinguishes this lesion from tricuspid atresia.

Angiocardiography demonstrates the size of the right

ventricular lumen, the atretic pulmonic valve, and the right-to-left atrial shunt.

THE FOLLOWING CRITERION IS REQUIRED FOR THE DIAGNOSIS OF PULMONARY ATRESIA WITH INTACT VENTRICULAR SEPTUM.

Angiocardiographic demonstration of a blind right ventricular outflow tract with an intact ventricular septum.

2.17.3 PULMONARY VALVULAR STENOSIS WITH INTACT VENTRICULAR SEPTUM

Pulmonary valvular stenosis with intact ventricular septum is a common lesion, which, in mild form, usually shows a partial fusion of one or more commissures of a bicuspid or tricuspid valve. In severe stenosis the commissures are poorly developed, and the valve cusps form a dome-shaped diaphragm with a small central orifice. Right ventricular hypertrophy is present, varying directly with the severity of the obstruction. Subvalvular hypertrophy of the crista supraventricularis develops with the more severe degrees of stenosis. Right atrial enlargement may occur, and a right-to-left shunt through a patent foramen ovale may develop with severe obstruction.

No symptoms may be present with mild and even moderate stenosis. However, with severe obstruction, breathlessness and cyanosis with exertion are common, and right ventricular failure may ensue. The physical signs include a prominent left parasternal impulse, a systolic thrill at the left base, a loud, harsh ejection systolic murmur maximal in the first and second left intercostal spaces, and a delayed, low-intensity pulmonic valve closure sound. A systolic click is frequently audible in the pulmonic area.

With mild stenosis the electrocardiogram may be normal. With moderate obstruction the electrocardiogram usually shows right axis deviation and evidence of right atrial and right ventricular hypertrophy. With very severe obstruction, extreme R wave voltage in the right precordial leads may be accompanied by deep T wave inversion.

The chest roentgenogram may be normal with mild stenosis, but may show evidence of right ventricular enlargement with the more severe lesions. Post-stenotic dilatation of the main or left pulmonary artery or both is common.

Cardiac catheterization documents right ventricular hypertension and a systolic pressure gradient across the pulmonary valve, with normal or low pulmonary arterial pressure.

Selective angiocardiography from the right ventricle allows precise visualization of the site of obstruction and absence of shunting at the ventricular level.

THE FOLLOWING CRITERIA ARE REQUIRED FOR THE DIAGNOSIS OF PULMONARY VALVULAR STENOSIS WITH INTACT VENTRICULAR SEPTUM.

An ejection systolic murmur at the upper left sternal border and evidence of pulmonary valvular obstruction and an intact ventricular septum.

2.18 Malformations of the Tricuspid Valve

2.18.1 TRICUSPID ATRESIA

With tricuspid atresia no valve elements are visible, and only a dimple may be seen in the floor of the right atrium. Survival demands that an interatrial communication exist, which may be either a secundum atrial defect or, more frequently, a patent foramen ovale. Right atrial blood is shunted to the left atrium and mixes with the pulmonary venous blood, which flows to the left ventricle; its subsequent course varies with the associated anomalies. Most often, the great arteries are normally related (in 70 percent), and blood is shunted through a small ventricular septal defect into a hypoplastic right ventricle and out through a small pulmonic valve and trunk to the lungs. When the great arteries are transposed (in 30 percent), so that the pulmonary artery arises from the left ventricle, blood flow to the lungs is increased unless subpulmonic stenosis is present.

Cyanosis usually exists from birth. A systolic murmur at the left sternal border is audible if pulmonary valvular stenosis or a ventricular septal defect is present.

The electrocardiogram is of great diagnostic importance, showing left axis deviation, tall peaked P waves, and increased left ventricular QRS voltage for the age level.

The chest roentgenogram usually shows a small or normal-sized heart with a prominent right atrial border and an enlarged left ventricle. Pulmonary vascular markings are usually diminished since pulmonary valvular stenosis or right ventricular outflow obstruction is commonly present. The hypoplastic right ventricle may be detected by echocardiography.

The right atrial pressure is elevated. A cardiac catheter cannot be passed into the right ventricle, but may enter the left atrium.

Selective angiocardiography from the right atrium demonstrates all the contrast material passing from the right atrium to the left atrium and into the left ventricle. Its course thereafter is determined by the associated lesions.

THE FOLLOWING CRITERIA ARE REQUIRED FOR THE DIAGNOSIS OF TRICUSPID ATRESIA.

Failure of a cardiac catheter to enter the right ventricle from the right atrium, and angiocardiographic demonstration of the entire right atrial contents flowing into the left atrium and left ventricle.

2.18.2 DOWNWARD DISPLACEMENT OF THE TRICUSPID VALVE (EBSTEIN'S MALFORMATION)

In downward displacement of the tricuspid valve, portions of the valve, usually the septal and posterior leaflets, may be attached to the right ventricular wall at varying distances between the anulus fibrosus and the apex. The downwardly displaced leaflets divide the right ventricle into a large proximal atrialized portion and a small-volume distal portion, which functions as the ejectile chamber. The right atrium is usually large. The pulmonary valve is normal, and the pulmonary artery is of normal or small caliber. A patent foramen ovale is usually present, although a secundum atrial septal defect may occur.

The symptoms and signs vary with the severity of the tricuspid regurgitation and the capacity of the distal portion of the right ventricle. When the small right ventricular ejectile chamber causes an obstruction to forward flow, a rise in right atrial pressure results, and blood is shunted from right to left at the atrial level, producing cyanosis. Right ventricular failure may occur when considerable tricuspid regurgitation exists.

A blowing systolic murmur, and often an early low-pitched diastolic murmur, may be heard over the lower precordium. Prominent third and fourth heart sounds are common.

The electrocardiogram usually shows tall, peaked P waves and right ventricular conduction delay, usually with low voltage in the right precordial leads. The Wolff-Parkinson-White syndrome may occur. Atrial arrhythmias are common.

The chest roentgenogram may show a relatively normal to massively enlarged cardiac silhouette. The pulmonary vascularity is normal or reduced. Echocardiography may demonstrate delayed tricuspid closure (50 msec. after mitral closure) and a leftward displacement of the tricuspid valve with simultaneous recording of mitral and tricuspid valve motion.

Right atrial pressure is usually elevated; the right ventricular and pulmonary arterial systolic pressures are either normal or low. Cardiac catheterization may show that the tricuspid valve is displaced to the left of the spine.

Angiocardiography demonstrates an enlarged right atrium and an abnormal division of the right ventricle into an "atrialized" segment proximal to the displaced tricuspid leaflets and a small ejectile chamber distal to them.

THE FOLLOWING CRITERIA ARE REQUIRED FOR THE DIAGNOSIS OF DOWNWARD DISPLACEMENT OF THE TRICUSPID VALVE (EBSTEIN'S MALFORMATION).

Angiocardiographic demonstration of an enlarged right atrium, a small right ventricular ejectile chamber and evidence of displacement of the tricuspid valve to the left.

2.18.3 TRICUSPID STENOSIS

Isolated stenosis resulting from congenital fusion of the tricuspid leaflets is an uncommon malformation. More often, a narrowing of the tricuspid valve orifice is associated with hypoplasia of the right ventricle or pulmonary valvular obstruction or both. The elements of the valve are identifiable, but smaller than normal or even diminutive.

When tricuspid stenosis occurring as an isolated lesion is mild, symptoms are usually absent. With severe stenosis, increasing right atrial pressure may cause systemic venous congestion and hepatomegaly or a right-to-left shunt through a patent foramen ovale. When pulmonary valvular obstruction coexists, its signs dominate the clinical picture.

A low-pitched diastolic murmur may be heard along the lower sternal border. The electrocardiogram usually shows peaked P waves and decreased right ventricular voltage. The chest roentgenogram shows right atrial enlargement and sometimes diminished pulmonary vascularity.

A diastolic pressure gradient is present across the tricuspid valve, and the right atrial pressure is elevated. There is delayed emptying of a dilated right atrial chamber through a small tricuspid orifice into the right ventricular cavity, which is usually small.

ONE OF THE FOLLOWING CRITERIA IS REQUIRED FOR THE DIAGNOSIS OF TRICUSPID STENOSIS.

1. **Evidence of a diastolic pressure gradient across the tricuspid valve.**

2. Angiocardiographic demonstration of a narrowed tricuspid orifice.

2.19 Anomalies of Venous Drainage

2.19.1 ANOMALOUS PULMONARY VENOUS DRAINAGE

2.19.1.1 TOTAL

In total anomalous pulmonary drainage, the pulmonary veins from the right and left lungs may terminate directly in the right atrium or coronary sinus, or enter a common pulmonary vein and drain via a vertical vein into the left innominate vein, or drain below the diaphragm into a tributary of the inferior vena cava. These locations are sometimes referred to as cardiac, supracardiac, or infracardiac to designate respectively the anatomic type of total anomalous pulmonary venous drainage. An atrial septal defect, or patent foramen ovale, is an integral part of the anomaly, permitting some of the admixed pulmonary and systemic venous blood in the right atrium to flow into the left atrium. Systemic arterial oxyhemoglobin unsaturation is always present and ranges from minimal to severe. Pulmonary hypertension is frequent. In occasional circumstances, the pulmonary venous pressure is elevated because of anatomic obstruction or compression of the pulmonary veins.

Tachypnea and signs of right ventricular failure may occur in the neonatal period, especially when the drainage of the pulmonary veins is below the diaphragm or in other locations when there is obstruction of the pulmonary veins. Cyanosis may be present. Systolic murmurs are frequently heard along the left sternal border, but are nonspecific. The second sound in the pulmonic area is usually widely split and fixed.

The electrocardiogram usually reveals tall P waves and right ventricular preponderance. Atrial tachycardia or flutter may occur. The chest roentgenogram shows markedly increased pulmonary vascular markings, occasionally with pulmonary venous engorgement. Prominent convex vascular shadows are present bilaterally at the base of the heart in the supracardiac type of anomalous drainage, in which the pulmonary veins enter a left vertical vein, which in turn drains into the left innominate vein, the right superior vena cava, and the right atrium.

Right heart catheterization reveals an elevated oxygen content in the right atrium or in one of the venae cavae. Pulmonary arterial pressure may approximate that in the systemic arterial tree, particularly in early infancy. Selective angiocardiography performed from the pulmonary artery delineates the pathways of anomalous pulmonary venous return.

THE FOLLOWING CRITERION IS REQUIRED FOR THE DIAGNOSIS OF TOTAL ANOMALOUS PULMONARY VENOUS DRAINAGE.

Angiocardiographic visualization of anomalous pathways of pulmonary venous drainage from the right and left lungs.

2.19.1.2 Partial

In partial anomalous pulmonary drainage, some of the pulmonary veins from one or more lobes, usually of the right lung, may drain directly into the right atrium, superior vena cava, innominate vein, or inferior vena cava. Frequently, an ostium secundum atrial defect is present; with a sinus venosus type of atrial defect, partial anomalous pulmonary vein drainage into the right superior vena cava is common.

The clinical and laboratory findings, including echocardiographic signs, are similar to those of an ostium secundum atrial septal defect. Right heart catheterization may reveal an elevated oxygen content in the superior or inferior cava in addition to a left-to-right shunt at the atrial level. Selective angiocardiography from the pulmonary artery may delineate the sites of partial anomalous pulmonary vein drainage.

ONE OF THE FOLLOWING CRITERIA IS REQUIRED FOR THE DIAGNOSIS OF PARTIAL ANOMALOUS PULMONARY VENOUS DRAINAGE.

1. Elevated oxygen content in the superior or inferior vena cava.
2. Angiocardiographic visualization of partial anomalous pulmonary vein drainage.

2.19.2 PERSISTENT LEFT SUPERIOR VENA CAVA

The most common malformation involving the major central systemic veins is the presence of bilateral superior venae cavae, usually called *persistent left superior vena cava*. The latter vein usually terminates in the coronary sinus, through which blood is delivered to the right atrium. A venous bridge in the superior mediastinum commonly exists between the left and right upper venous systems. Occasionally, the right superior vena cava is absent. Persistent left superior vena cava may occur with any other cardiovascular defect and is particularly frequent with tetralogy of Fallot.

The chest roentgenogram may reveal a vertical shadow at the upper left border of the cardiac silhouette lateral to the aorta and pulmonary artery.

THE FOLLOWING CRITERION IS REQUIRED FOR THE DIAGNOSIS OF PERSISTENT LEFT SUPERIOR VENA CAVA.

Angiographic visualization of a left-sided superior vena cava.

2.19.3 AZYGOS CONTINUATION OF THE INFERIOR VENA CAVA

The inferior vena cava may fail to take a normal position with respect to the liver and becomes continuous with the azygos vein, which drains into the superior vena cava and thence into the right atrium. It may occur without heart disease, though more frequently it is associated with lesions such as ventricular septal defect or complex abnormalities of cardiac position and abdominal visceral situs especially as seen in the polysplenia syndrome.

The chest roentgenogram in the frontal projection may show a right-sided mediastinal mass in the angle between the trachea and the right main stem bronchus. This shadow is produced by the azygos vein, the lateral margin of which can often be followed inferiorly in the right paravertebral region.

When a venous catheter is passed from a lower extremity to the right atrium, it can be seen on fluoroscopy in the lateral view to pass behind the heart and then bend forward as it enters the superior vena cava; the configuration of the catheter resembles that of a "candy cane."

ONE OF THE FOLLOWING CRITERIA IS REQUIRED FOR THE DIAGNOSIS OF AZYGOS CONTINUATION OF THE INFERIOR VENA CAVA.

1. Angiographic visualization of the abnormal venous channel.
2. Demonstration of a catheter from a lower extremity vein ascending behind the heart and reaching the superior vena cava along the expected course of the azygos vein.

The Physiologic Cardiac Diagnosis

3

NOMENCLATURE

3.1 Normal and Abnormal Rhythms
- 3.1.1 Sinus Mechanisms
  - 3.1.1.1 Normal sinus rhythm
  - 3.1.1.2 Sinus tachycardia
  - 3.1.1.3 Sinus bradycardia
  - 3.1.1.4 Sinus arrhythmia
  - 3.1.1.5 Sinus arrest
  - 3.1.1.6 Sinoventricular rhythm
  - 3.1.1.7 Dysfunction of the sino-atrial node (sick sinus syndrome)
- 3.1.2 Atrial Mechanisms
  - 3.1.2.1 Atrial premature contraction
  - 3.1.2.2 Atrial rhythm
  - 3.1.2.3 Atrial tachycardia
  - 3.1.2.4 Atrial flutter
  - 3.1.2.5 Atrial fibrillation
- 3.1.3 Atrioventricular Junctional Mechanisms
  - 3.1.3.1 Atrioventricular junctional escape beat
  - 3.1.3.2 Atrioventricular junctional rhythm
  - 3.1.3.3 Atrioventricular junctional premature contraction
  - 3.1.3.4 Atrioventricular junctional tachycardia
- 3.1.4 Supraventricular Mechanisms
  - 3.1.4.1 Supraventricular premature contraction
  - 3.1.4.2 Supraventricular rhythm
  - 3.1.4.3 Supraventricular tachycardia

- 3.1.5 Ventricular Mechanisms
  - 3.1.5.1 Ventricular premature contraction
  - 3.1.5.2 Ventricular rhythm (idioventricular rhythm)
  - 3.1.5.3 Ventricular tachycardia
  - 3.1.5.4 Ventricular fibrillation
- 3.1.6 Rhythms from Artificial Pacing
  - 3.1.6.1 Atrial rhythm from artificial pacing
  - 3.1.6.2 Ventricular rhythm from artificial pacing
- 3.1.7 Malfunction of Electronic Pacemaker Systems

3.2 Disturbances in Conduction

- 3.2.1 Sino-atrial Exit Block
- 3.2.2 Intra-atrial Block
- 3.2.3 Atrioventricular Conduction Disturbances
  - 3.2.3.1 Incomplete atrioventricular block
    - 3.2.3.1.1 Prolonged P–R interval (first degree atrioventricular block)
    - 3.2.3.1.2 Incomplete atrioventricular block with periodically dropped beats (second degree atrioventricular block)
      - 3.2.3.1.2.1 Type I (Wenckebach periods)
      - 3.2.3.1.2.2 Type II (Mobitz block)
      - 3.2.3.1.2.3 Incomplete atrioventricular block with 2:1 atrioventricular response (2:1 atrioventricular block)

- 3.2.3.2 Complete atrioventricular block (third degree atrioventricular block)
- 3.2.3.3 Adams–Stokes syndrome

3.2.4 Atrioventricular Dissociation

3.2.5 Intraventricular Conduction Defects

- 3.2.5.1 Monofascicular block
  - 3.2.5.1.1 Right bundle branch block
  - 3.2.5.1.2 Left bundle branch block
  - 3.2.5.1.3 Anterior fascicular block
  - 3.2.5.1.4 Posterior fascicular block
- 3.2.5.2 Bifascicular block
  - 3.2.5.2.1 Right bundle branch block and left main stem bundle branch block
  - 3.2.5.2.2 Right bundle branch block and incomplete left bundle branch block
  - 3.2.5.2.3 Right bundle branch block and anterior fascicular block
  - 3.2.5.2.4 Right bundle branch block and posterior fascicular block
  - 3.2.5.2.5 Anterior fascicular block and posterior fascicular block
- 3.2.5.3 Trifascicular (multifascicular) block
  - 3.2.5.3.1 Right bundle branch block, anterior fascicular block, and posterior fascicular block
  - 3.2.5.3.2 Right bundle branch block, anterior fascicular block, and incomplete posterior fascicular block
  - 3.2.5.3.3 Right bundle branch block, posterior fascicular block, and incomplete anterior fascicular block

3.2.5.3.4 Right bundle branch block, incomplete anterior fascicular block, and incomplete posterior fascicular block
3.2.5.3.5 Right bundle branch block, anterior fascicular block, and incomplete left bundle branch block
3.2.5.3.6 Right bundle branch block, posterior fascicular block, and incomplete left bundle branch block
3.2.5.3.7 Anterior fascicular block, posterior fascicular block, and incomplete right bundle branch block
3.2.5.4 Diffuse intraventricular (myofibrillar) block
3.2.5.5 Rarer forms of intraventricular conduction defects
3.2.6 Anomalous Atrioventricular Conduction (Ventricular Preexcitation)
3.3 Disturbances in Supravalvular, Valvular, or Subvalvular Function
3.3.1 Aortic Obstruction
3.3.1.1 Supravalvular obstruction
3.3.1.2 Valvular obstruction
3.3.1.3 Subvalvular obstruction
3.3.2 Aortic Regurgitation
3.3.3 Mitral Obstruction
3.3.4 Mitral Regurgitation
3.3.5 Pulmonic Obstruction
3.3.5.1 Valvular obstruction
3.3.5.2 Subvalvular obstruction
3.3.6 Pulmonic Regurgitation
3.3.7 Tricuspid Obstruction
3.3.8 Tricuspid Regurgitation
3.3.9 Malfunction of Prostheses and Homografts

- 3.3.10 Prolapse of Valves
  - 3.3.10.1 Prolapse of the aortic valve
  - 3.3.10.2 Prolapse of the mitral valve
- 3.4 Disturbances in Myocardial Function
  - 3.4.1 Ventricular Failure
    - 3.4.1.1 Left ventricular failure
    - 3.4.1.2 Right ventricular failure
  - 3.4.2 Ventricular Asynergy
  - 3.4.3 Pericardial Restriction
  - 3.4.4 Myocardial Restriction
  - 3.4.5 Cardiogenic Shock
- 3.5 Disturbances in Intravascular Pressures
  - 3.5.1 Pulmonary Arterial Hypertension
  - 3.5.2 Pulmonary Venous Hypertension
  - 3.5.3 Systemic Arterial Hypertension
  - 3.5.4 Pulmonary Circulatory Congestion
  - 3.5.5 Systemic Circulatory Congestion
- 3.6 Abnormal Communications in the Heart or Great Vessels
  - 3.6.1 Intracardiac Shunts
    - 3.6.1.1 Left-to-right shunts
    - 3.6.1.2 Right-to-left shunts
  - 3.6.2 Extracardiac Shunts
    - 3.6.2.1 Left-to-right shunts
    - 3.6.2.2 Right-to-left shunts
- 3.7 Anginal Syndrome

CRITERIA

3.1 Normal and Abnormal Rhythms

3.1.1 SINUS MECHANISMS

Sinus mechanisms originate within the sino-atrial node and probably represent phasic discharges from specialized pacemaker (P) cells.

3.1.1.1 Normal Sinus Rhythm

Normal sinus rhythm is a regular rhythm at a rate of 60 to 100 per minute, and the cycle length (P to P interval) does not vary by more than 10 percent. The P wave or atrial deflection is upright in leads I, II, aVF, V4, V5, and V6 and negative in aVR (Fig. 10). The P wave is followed by the ventricular deflections, QRS–T (unless there is atrioventricular block), and the P–R interval is of normal duration.

3.1.1.2 Sinus Tachycardia

Sinus tachycardia is a regular sinus rhythm at a rate exceeding 100 per minute. It may be induced by any condition or agent that abolishes or decreases vagal tone, or stimulates sympathetic tone, or both. Emotion, anxiety, exercise, thyrotoxicosis, hypotension, hypoxia, hyperthermia, anemia, hemorrhage, infections, certain neuroses, and neurocirculatory asthenia (vasomotor instability) are frequent causes. Ventricular failure and diseases of the pericardium, myocardium, or endocardium are often accompanied by sinus tachycardia. Certain drugs, such as atropine, epinephrine, isoproterenol, nicotine, lysergic acid diethylamide (LSD), marijuana, cocaine, heroin, and morphine can elicit this response.

Palpitations may or may not be experienced with this tachycardia.

3.1.1.3 Sinus Bradycardia

Sinus bradycardia is a regular sinus rhythm at a rate less than 60 per minute. The cause is usually an increase in vagal tone, but it may also result from primary depression of the sino-atrial node. The vagus center may be stimulated by central nervous system diseases such as meningitis or increased intracranial pressure due to tumor or hemorrhage; or reflexly by pain, gastrointestinal disturbances, pressure on the carotid sinus or the eyeballs, or stimulation of the posterior pharynx. Prolonged hypotension or severe hypothermia may cause bradycardia. Certain inhalation anesthetics and beta-adrenergic blocking agents are also the cause of bradycardia. Sinus bradycardia occurs during normal rest or sleep, in young athletes, in persons convalescing from infectious diseases, and in patients with jaundice.

Sinus bradycardia, if persistent and uninfluenced by sympathomimetic maneuvers or agents, and especially if it is present when one would usually expect sinus tachycardia, may indicate that disease of the sino-atrial node is present.

Severe bradycardia with rates between 40 and 50 per minute produces symptoms of underperfusion of the vital organs, such as dizziness, edema, oliguria, and fatigue while syncope and convulsions occur at rates usually under 20 per minute.

3.1.1.4 Sinus Arrhythmia

Sinus arrhythmia is an irregular sinus rhythm with the cycle lengths (the P to P intervals) varying by 10 percent or more (Fig. 11). The arrhythmia is usually phasic, increasing in rate during inspiration and decreasing during expiration. Unless there is atrioventricular block, each P wave, which has a normal duration, is followed by a QRS–T complex after a normal P–R interval.

There are seldom any symptoms due to sinus arrhythmia.

3.1.1.5 Sinus Arrest

Sinus arrest (Fig. 12) can result from digitalis, quinidine, reserpine, excess potassium, vagotonia, or intrinsic disease of the sino-atrial node. During sinus rhythm there is periodic failure of impulse formation within the primary pacemaker, the sino-atrial node. A P wave and its accompanying QRS–T complex fail to appear at the expected time. The resulting pause is usually slightly shorter than two normal cardiac cycles and is not an exact multiple of the P to P cycle length, in contrast to sino-atrial exit block. If the sinus pause is long, escape beats may appear.

If the pause is long and no escape rhythm takes over, the symptoms of hypoperfusion of vital organs similar to those seen with sinus bradycardia occur. Such long pauses

---

Figure 10. *Normal sinus rhythm.* Each of the leads is recorded separately, and the standardization is 1 mv = 10 mm in all twelve leads.

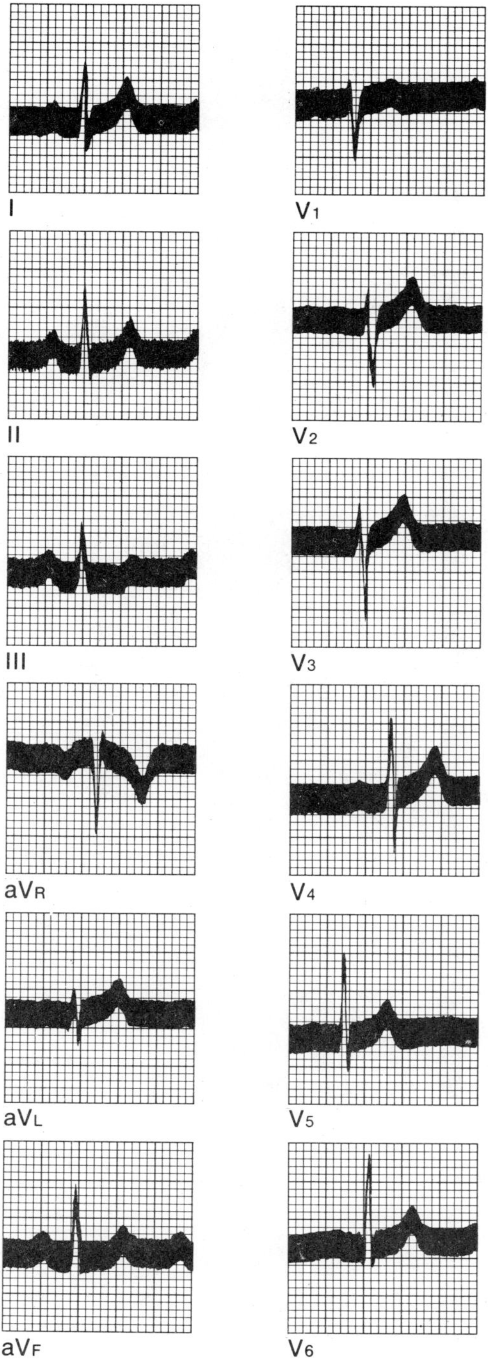

Figure 10

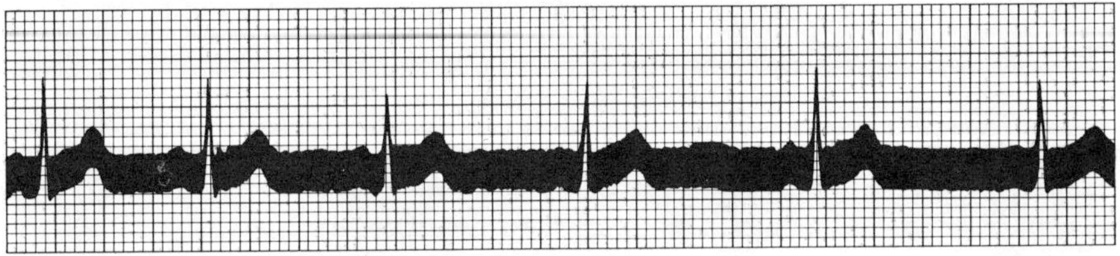

Figure 11. *Sinus arrhythmia.* Lead I is shown. Minor variations in the shape of the P wave, as seen here, are not unusual in this rhythm.

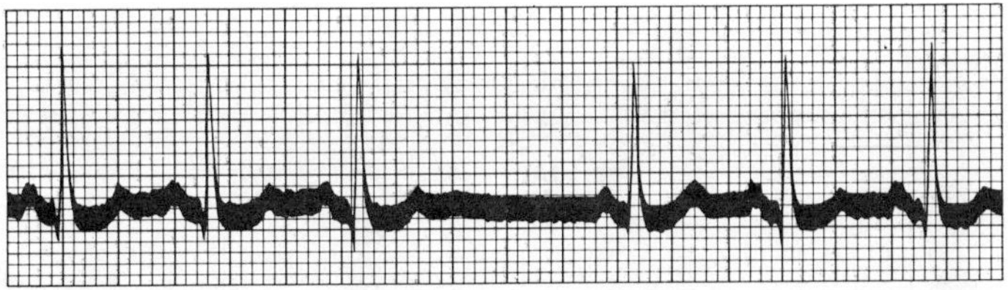

Figure 12. *Sinus arrest.* Lead II is shown. An absent sinus beat is seen after the third P–QRS–T. The small positive deflection following the third T wave is a U wave, a normal finding obscured by the onset of the P wave in other beats.

are seen in the carotid sinus syndrome, in which a very sensitive carotid sinus is mechanically stimulated and produces sinus arrest.

3.1.1.6 Sinoventricular Rhythm

Sinoventricular rhythm is most commonly produced by severe hyperpotassemia. It results from a specific depression of atrial myocardial cells, so that they cannot respond to or accept the excitation process from the sino-atrial node and interatrial tracts. The sino-atrial node, whose pacemaker function is not impaired, delivers the impulse over the intact specific atrial internodal tracts to the atrioventricular node and junctional tissue. Because of atrial electrical silence, there are no P waves seen in this unusual form of sinus rhythm. A sequence of normal ventricular (QRS–T) complexes without preceding P waves is characteristic of this arrhythmia. The heart rate can be altered by any of the maneuvers which ordinarily increase or decrease normal sinus rhythm, in contrast to the situation in atrioventricular junctional rhythm.

No symptoms apart from those due to hyperpotassemia are present, as the rate is normal and regular.

3.1.1.7 Dysfunction of the Sino-atrial Node (Sick Sinus Syndrome)

Disturbances in the function of the sino-atrial node can be found in atherosclerotic heart disease with or without myocardial infarction and in rheumatic and congenital heart disease, as well as in a variety of inflammatory conditions, pericarditis, cardiomyopathies, or surgical injury to the nodal tissue. It may also result from fibrotic or sclerotic lesions localized in the nodal area. Digitalis and excessive vagal discharge may disturb the function of the sino-atrial node, but since their effects are temporary, the resulting disturbances are excluded from the syndrome.

Malfunction of the sino-atrial node may be manifested in a number of ways: (1) persistent, severe (50 per minute or less), or unexpected sinus bradycardia, which is often the earliest sign of a failing sino-atrial node; intermittent but atropine and exercise resistant bradycardia can also occur early in the disease; (2) short periods of sinus arrest, with escape rhythms supervening that are usually atrial or junctional rhythms, but occasionally are ventricular; (3) long periods of sinus arrest without escape rhythms (implying co-existent infra nodal disease) and hence asystolic periods leading to cardiac arrest; (4) inability of the heart to resume sinus rhythm after cardioversion from atrial fibrillation or flutter; (5) chronic atrial fibrillation occurring with a slow ventricular response which cannot be related to the effects of digitalis; atrial fibrillation permanently replaces sinus rhythm, which cannot be generated by the sino-atrial node, and the slow ventricular rate is due to coexisting atrioventricular node dysfunction, producing atrioventricular block; (6) episodes of sino-atrial exit block not related to drug therapy.

This syndrome is often characterized by periods of sinus bradycardia alternating with periods of ectopic tachycardias, such as atrial tachycardia, atrial flutter or fibrillation or AV junctional tachycardia. The symptoms of such periods are dizziness, faintness, syncopal attacks, and palpitations, and, if the episodes of slow or fast rate are frequent, ventricular failure may appear. Sudden death can occur if asystole is prolonged. Prolonged electrocardiographic monitoring may be necessary to establish the periodic abnormalities which together make up the syndrome of dysfunction of the sino-atrial node. Provocative testing of nodal function can be achieved by the administration of atropine and isoproterenol, to which the response is weak, and by atrial pacing, which in some cases may produce overdrive suppression of the failing sino-atrial nodal pacemaker. This suppression is expressed as an unduly prolonged recovery time of the sino-atrial node; there is a delayed or late resumption of sinus rhythm after atrial pacing ceases.

3.1.2 ATRIAL MECHANISMS

Atrial mechanisms originate within the atrial cavities, possibly in specialized cell populations rather than in the working atrial myocardial cells.

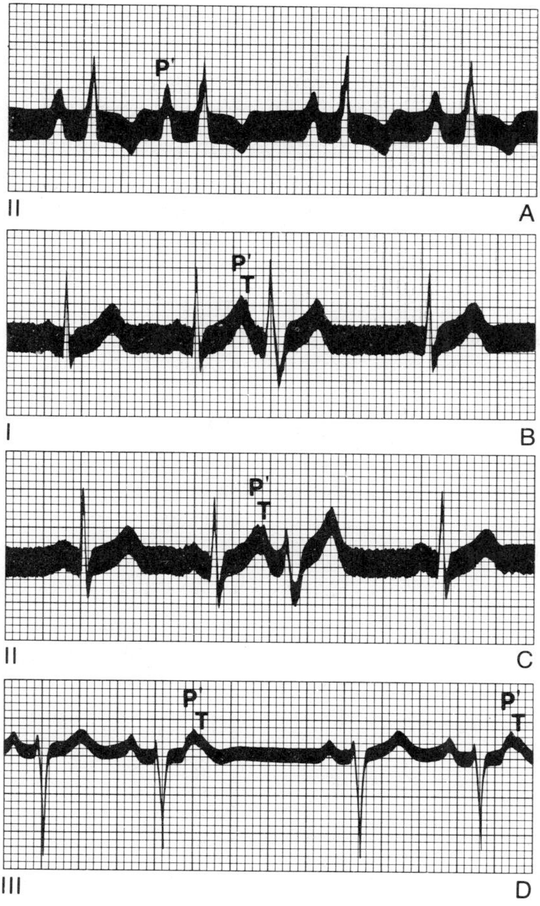

Figure 13. *Atrial premature contractions.* The leads recorded are indicated in Roman numerals on the left. In B, C, and D, the P′ wave of the atrial premature contraction falls within the preceding T wave, deforming it, as can be seen by comparing it with the T wave of the sinus beats. In A, the P wave of the premature beat is seen separately and is different from those of the sinus beats. In D, the P wave is blocked; it is not followed by a QRS complex. The ventricular complex (QRS) may be the same as the sinus beat as seen in A, or aberrant, that is, wider and notched or showing a right bundle branch block, as seen in B and C.

3.1.2.1 Atrial Premature Contraction

Atrial premature contractions (Fig. 13) can be found in normal hearts, in inflammatory or degenerative myocardial diseases, especially rheumatic and atherosclerotic, in ventricular failure, and in conditions stimulating the release of endogenous catecholamines such as anxiety, fatigue, and disturbed psychologic states. Sympathomimetic drugs, digitalis, tobacco, caffeine, hypokalemia, hypoxia, and disturbances in the central nervous system, gastrointestinal, or genitourinary tracts can cause these premature contractions. In hyperthyroidism and in rheumatic or atherosclerotic heart disease, they often precede the onset of atrial fibrillation or flutter.

The symptoms of these, and indeed of all, premature contractions is usually a sensation in the chest of an irregular heartbeat in the form of a choking sensation or thump.

The premature atrial contraction (Fig. 13A) is an early ectopic beat which produces a P wave, the shape of which is different from the P wave of the sinus beats; the P–R interval is usually longer than that of the sinus beat. The ventricular complex which follows the P wave may be either normal (Fig. 13A) or somewhat different, due to aberrant conduction (Fig. 13B and C). If the atrial impulse does not reach the ventricles, no QRS complex follows the P wave, and the beat is termed *blocked atrial premature contraction* (Fig. 13D). If the premature beats have P waves of differing shapes, they are termed *multifocal atrial premature contractions.*

3.1.2.2 Atrial Rhythm

Atrial rhythm is a relatively slow and regular rhythm (Fig. 14), usually between 50 and 80 per minute, which arises as an escape rhythm when sinus rhythm fails. The

---

Figure 14. *Atrial rhythm.* The P waves (marked P in II, III, aVR) are negative in leads II, III, and aVF and positive in aVR. The rate is 72 per minute. There are also diffuse S–T depressions and low T waves. (The leads are recorded as in Figure 1.)

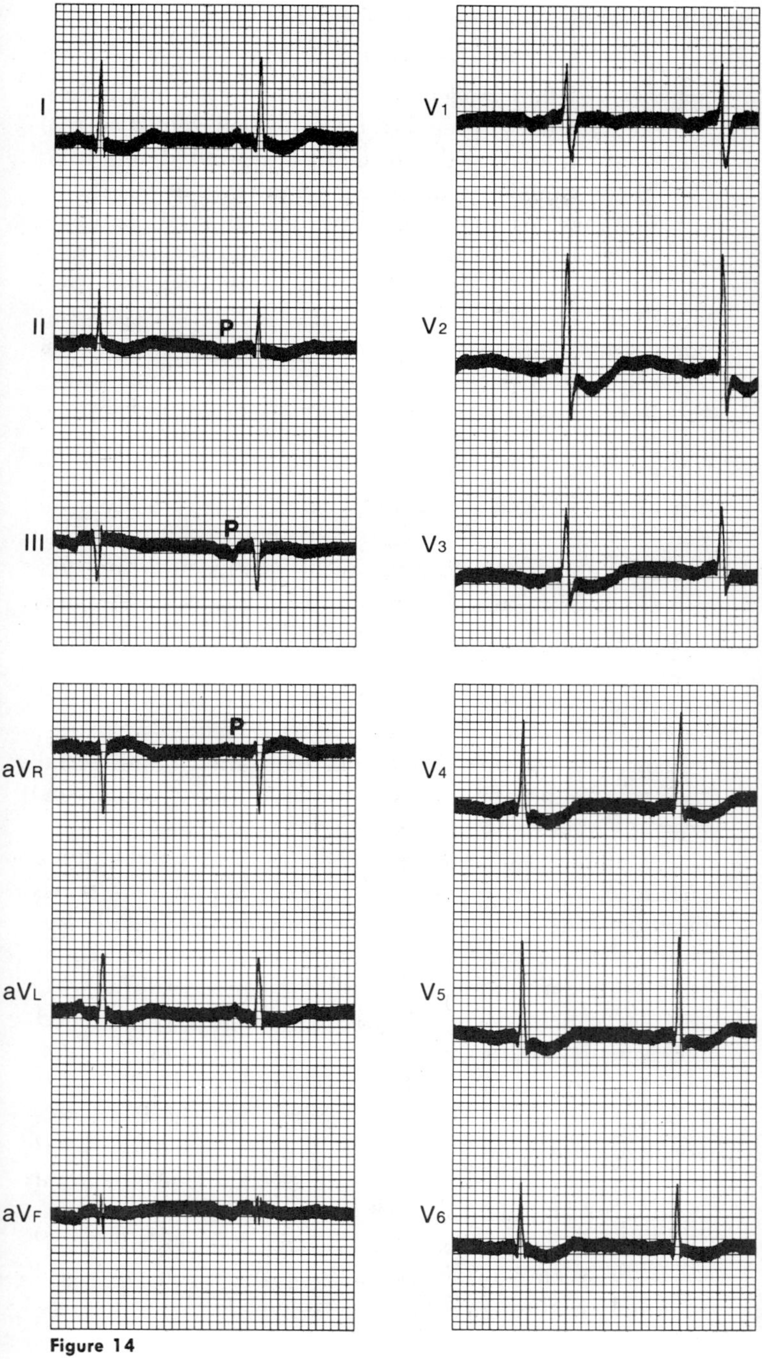

Figure 14

appearance often is identical to that of atrial premature contractions in that there is a P wave followed by a normal QRS–T complex; but the form of the P wave differs from that of the sinus beat, and the P–R interval is also different. The P waves may be negative in leads II, III, and aVF and positive in aVR. If the polarity of the P wave is normal, it may be difficult to distinguish this rhythm from sinus rhythm unless previous electrocardiograms showing sinus rhythm are available for comparison, or the onset of the slow atrial pacemaker is seen after a sinus pause. Single escape beats may also occur after such pauses.

3.1.2.3 Atrial Tachycardia

Atrial tachycardia (Figs. 15A and 15B) may be seen in normal hearts, in rheumatic or atherosclerotic heart disease, and in subjects with the Wolff-Parkinson-White syndrome. It may also be caused by digitalis excess and hypopotassemia, as well as the conditions which produce atrial premature contractions.

The symptoms of this tachycardia are usually limited to a feeling of palpitation, but may include faintness, nausea, and, rarely, chest pain. In infants, rapid atrial tachycardia may be a serious disturbance initiating ventricular failure and may be fatal if untreated.

In the electrocardiogram, there is a rapid and regular succession of P waves whose form differs from the P wave of sinus rhythm (Fig. 15A). The P waves are usually upright in leads I and II but occasionally are negative. There may be a normal or prolonged P–R interval. The QRS complex can be normal or slightly aberrant (longer and different in contour) than during sinus rhythm. There is an isoelectric or flat baseline between P waves. The P–R interval and atrial rate may be such that the P wave is superimposed on the preceding T wave, and thus the P wave may be difficult to identify. Special leads are then needed to identify this tachycardia. Atrial tachycardia usually has a rate between 140 and 200, with every P wave conducted to the ventricle (1:1 response). Vagal stimulation through carotid massage, the Valsalva maneuver, or emesis often converts this tachycardia to sinus rhythm.

Atrial tachycardia with 2:1 atrioventricular block (Fig. 15B) is often produced by digitalis excess.

3.1.2.4 Atrial Flutter

Atrial flutter (Fig. 16) is almost always associated with organic heart disease and is most frequently seen in rheumatic or atherosclerotic heart disease or conditions which cause atrial enlargement. It can also occur in the Wolff-Parkinson-White syndrome, hyperthyroidism, and atrial septal defect. It may complicate acute myocardial infarction, pulmonary embolization, acute pericarditis, restrictive pericardial disease, or severe hypoxia, or may develop after intrathoracic operations. Infiltration of the atria by tumor tissue is another cause for this arrhythmia.

The symptoms are related to the fall in cardiac output which occurs with the onset of atrial flutter and to the rapid ventricular rate. These include nausea, faintness, fatigue, palpitations, and occasionally chest pain and ventricular failure.

Atrial activity is represented in the electrocardiogram by regular biphasic oscillations (F waves), which are of uniform shape and occur at rates between 200 and 400 per minute (Figs. 16A and 16B). The ventricular response, with a normal QRS complex, is usually at half this rate, as a 2:1 atrioventricular block exists (Fig. 16A). An atrial rate of 300, with an extremely regular ventricular rate of 150, is the classic form of this arrhythmia. The F waves are best seen in leads II, III, aVF, and V1. There is no isoelectric baseline, as the atrial oscillations have a continuous sawtooth appearance. There may be a varying degree of atrioventricular block, with 2:1, 3:1, 4:1 ratios appearing successively and producing an irregular ventricular rate (Fig. 16B). Rarely, atrial flutter waves conduct at a 1:1 atrioventricular ratio, and a very rapid ventricular rate ensues. Vagal stimulation does not convert atrial flutter, as it may with atrial tachycardia, but may increase the atrioventricular block from 2:1 to 4:1 or more and

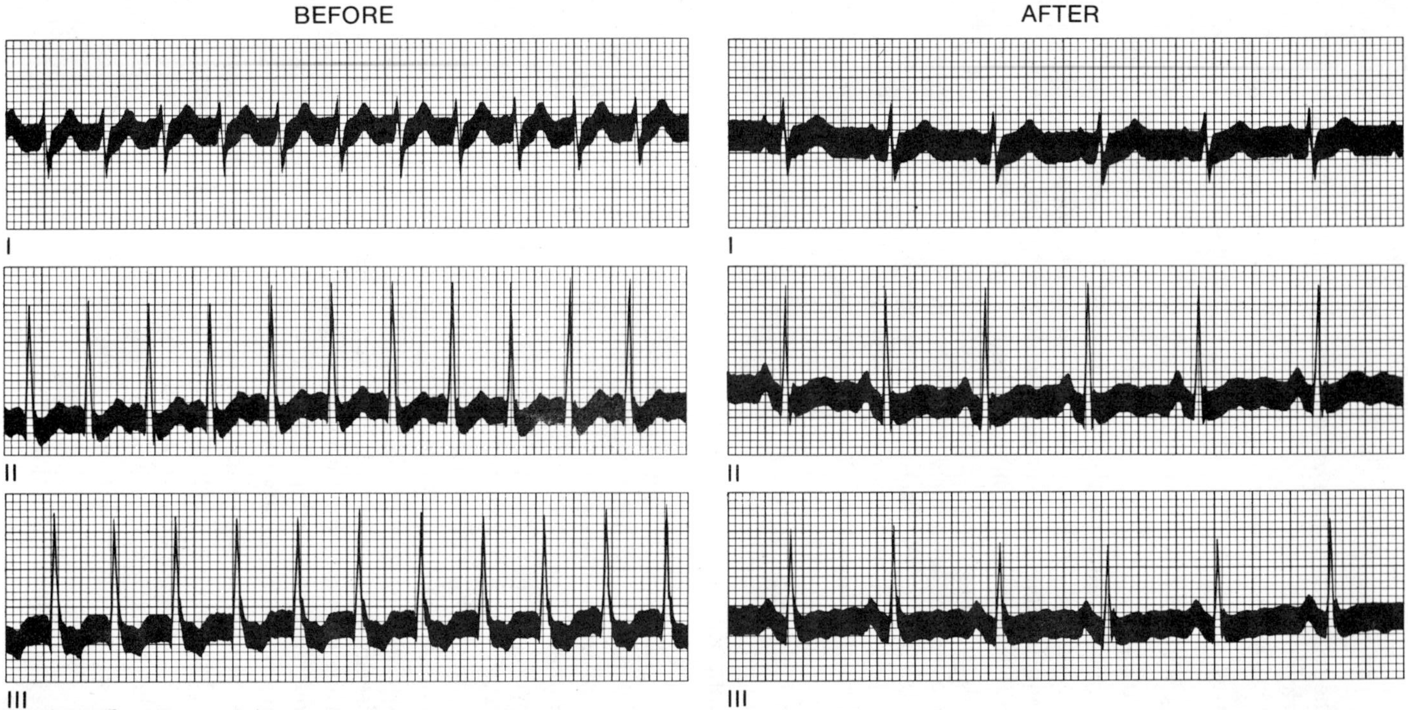

Figure 15A

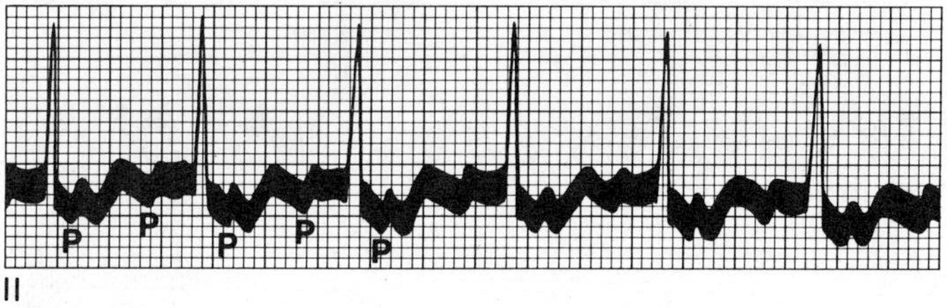

Figure 15B

Figure 15A. *Atrial tachycardia* (left) and sinus rhythm after conversion (right). This regular tachycardia at 187 per minute has P wave falling within the T waves, which can best be seen in lead III, where the negative P deforms the S–T segment, and by comparison with the tracing after conversion to sinus rhythm (on the right). The QRS is normal.

Figure 15B. *Atrial tachycardia with 2:1 atrioventricular block.* The P waves are marked in lead II.

Figure 16A. *Atrial flutter with 2:1 atrioventricular block.* The flutter waves (marked F) seen in lead II are regular and identical. They occur at a rate of 300 per minute; with 2:1 atrioventricular block, there is a regular ventricular rate of 150 per minute. The F waves have a sawtooth biphasic appearance.

Figure 16B. *Atrial flutter with variable atrioventricular block.* The atrioventricular response is variable (3:1, 4:1); hence the ventricular rate is irregular. Note that the flutter waves are best seen in the leads II, III, aVR, and aVF. The slight variations in the form of the QRS complexes are due to the presence of simultaneous flutter waves, which deform the complexes. (Each lead is recorded separately.)

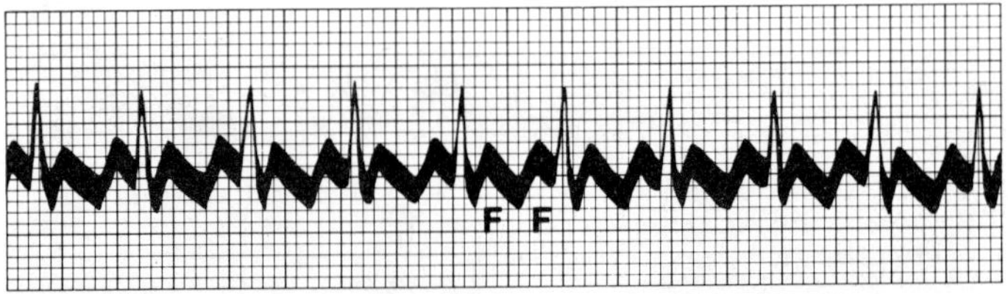

Figure 16A

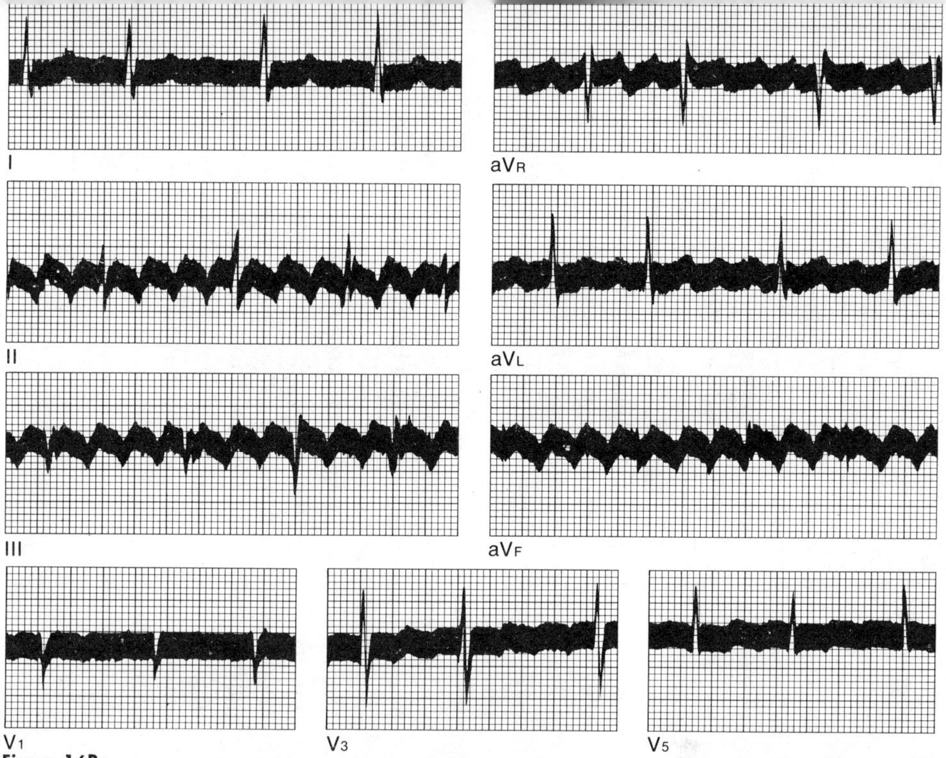

Figure 16B

allow flutter waves to become clearly visible. Occasionally, special leads (esophageal or intra-atrial) will be required to identify the flutter waves.

It is rare for atrial flutter to become a chronic arrhythmia.

3.1.2.5 Atrial Fibrillation

In contrast to atrial flutter, atrial fibrillation may occur in otherwise normal hearts in paroxysmal form. In diseased hearts, however, it often becomes a chronic arrhythmia. The causes and symptoms are similar to those of atrial flutter.

P waves are absent, and atrial oscillations are usually small and irregular in shape and duration; when seen, they occur at a rate of 450 to 600 or more per minute (Fig. 17). These are best seen in leads II, III, and V1 or special leads utilizing esophageal or intra-atrial electrodes. The ventricular deflections occur at totally irregular intervals, are usually of normal contour, but can become aberrant with rapid rates. If there is a low degree of atrioventricular block, the ventricular rate may be rapid and variable—150 to over 200 per minute. With greater atrioventricular block the rate may be slower—90 to 120 per minute. The presence of a regular ventricular rate in atrial fibrillation is due either to complete atrioventricular block with an independent lower focus controlling the ventricles or to activation of a lower center, such as junctional tissue, which fires at a faster ventricular rate than occurs in response to the atrial fibrillation and therefore controls the ventricles.

3.1.3 ATRIOVENTRICULAR JUNCTIONAL MECHANISMS

The area giving rise to atrioventricular junctional mechanisms (Figs. 18A, 18B, and 18C) includes the atrioventricular node, the nodal-bundle junction, and the common bundle of His down to the bifurcation, where the first fibers of the posterior fascicle leave the left bundle (see Fig. 24).

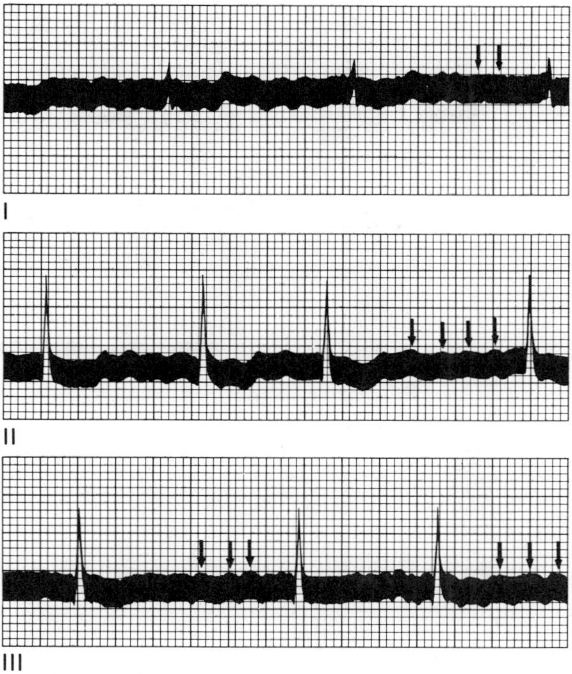

Figure 17. *Atrial fibrillation.* The atrial deflections, which are small and variable in form, are marked by arrows. The ventricular rate is totally irregular, and there are T wave abnormalities in all three leads.

3.1.3.1 Atrioventricular Junctional Escape Beat

A junctional escape beat appears and takes over both atrial and ventricular rhythms when the sino-atrial node either fails to emit one or more impulses or is depressed, so that its rate falls below that of the junctional tissue pacemaker.

3.1.3.2 Atrioventricular Junctional Rhythm

A sustained but slow junctional rhythm, with rates between 40 and 55 and, rarely, up to 80 to 90 per minute, replaces a flagging sinus rhythm or takes over the ventri-

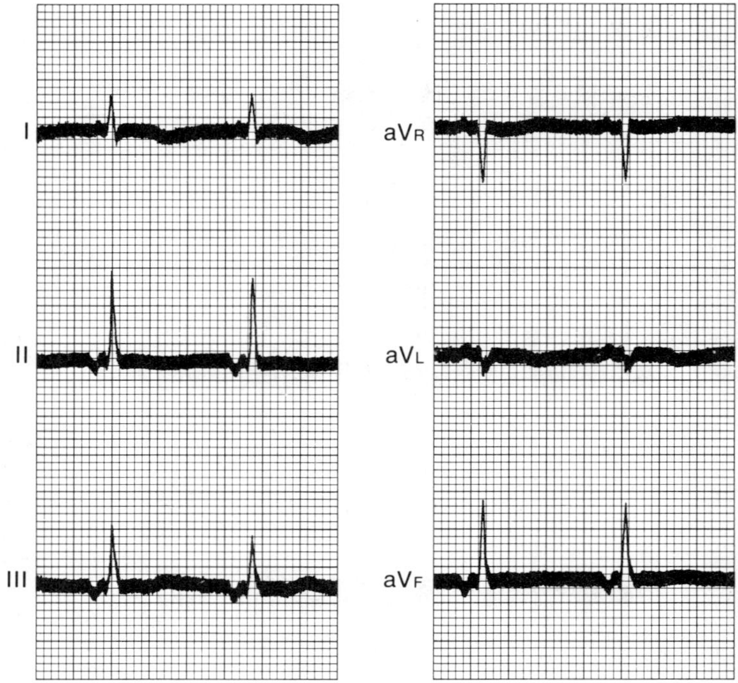

Figure 18A

Figures 18A–C. *Atrioventricular junctional mechanisms.*

Figure 18A. *Junctional rhythm.* Slow junctional rhythm (70 per minute), with negative P waves in II, III, and aVF and positive P waves in aVR. (The three standard leads and the three aV leads are recorded simultaneously with a standardization of 1 mv = 10 mm.)

Figure 18B. *Junctional premature contractions.* Three examples of atrioventricular junctional premature contractions. The upper trace has a negative P wave in front of the QRS, with a short P–R interval; the middle trace has a P (marked by an arrow) falling in the QRS; the lower trace has a negative P wave in the S–T segment.

Figure 18C. *Junctional tachycardia.* Junctional tachycardia at 187 per minute. The negative P waves (marked with P) are best seen in II, III, and aVF.

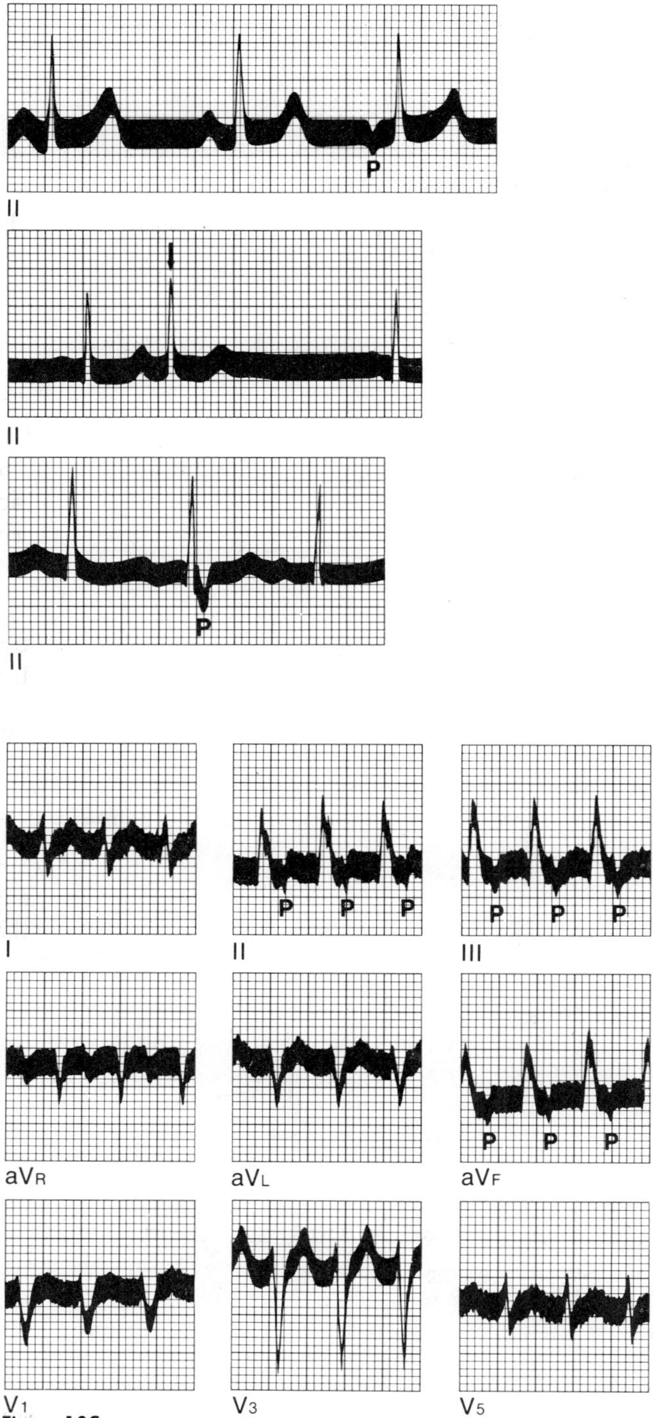

Figure 18C

cles with the onset of complete atrioventricular block. In complete atrioventricular block, when the lower pacemaker arises in the junctional tissue, it fires at 40 to 55 per minute in the adult. In children with complete atrioventricular block the junctional rate is faster, usually between 70 to 80 per minute at rest, increasing somewhat with exercise.

3.1.3.3 Atrioventricular Junctional Premature Contraction

When the junctional tissue fires early, that is, ahead of the expected sinus beat, it produces a junctional premature contraction.

3.1.3.4 Atrioventricular Junctional Tachycardia

This is a sustained and rapid regular rhythm, with a rate exceeding 100 per minute and occasionally exceeding 200 per minute.

The cause of junctional rhythms may be difficult to determine, but the tachycardias and premature contractions are seen in atherosclerotic heart disease, particularly in acute myocardial infarction, in acute rheumatic carditis, with digitalis or quinidine excess, and with hypoxia. If the rhythm is slow, there are no symptoms unless the bradycardia is extreme. In the presence of tachycardia and junctional premature contractions, palpitations are often felt.

In the junctional rhythms the P wave is inverted in leads II, III, and aVF and upright in aVR. The P wave has a constant relationship to the QRS, but may occur before, during, or after the QRS deflections. When it falls before the QRS complex, the P–R interval is short—less than 0.12 sec. When it falls during the QRS, it is difficult to find without special leads, but may appear as a notch on the R wave. When it follows the QRS, it often falls within the S–T segment and deforms it. The QRS in junctional rhythms is somewhat different in form from that occurring during sinus rhythm and is slightly longer in duration, but does not exceed 0.10 sec. Occasionally, due to ventriculo-atrial block, the retrograde atrial excitation from junctional beats does not occur, and no P waves are seen.

3.1.4 SUPRAVENTRICULAR MECHANISMS

3.1.4.1 Supraventricular Premature Contraction

3.1.4.2 Supraventricular Rhythm

3.1.4.3 Supraventricular Tachycardia

When the rhythm is regular and characterized by QRS complexes of normal duration and no atrial waves can be seen, the term *Supraventricular Mechanisms* is used to indicate that the site of ectopic activity is unknown; if the rate is less than 100, it is called supraventricular rhythm, if the rate is over 100 it is supraventricular tachycardia. If the ventricular rhythm is totally irregular, atrial fibrillation is the likely mechanism, even though no atrial activity can be demonstrated. In this instance the designation *Probable Atrial Fibrillation* is used.

3.1.5 VENTRICULAR MECHANISMS

Ventricular mechanisms (Figs. 19A–C) originate within the ventricular chambers, probably in specialized cell populations rather than in the ventricular working myocardial cells. The rhythms include ventricular premature contractions, ventricular rhythm, ventricular tachycardia, and ventricular fibrillation.

3.1.5.1 Ventricular Premature Contraction

Ventricular premature contractions may occur in health and disease and have the same general causes and symptoms as do atrial premature contractions.

The beats (Fig. 19A) are characterized by early, bizarre, and wide QRS–T complexes, greater than 0.10 sec, which are not preceded by P waves. The T wave often is opposite in direction to the QRS. The rhythm of the atria is

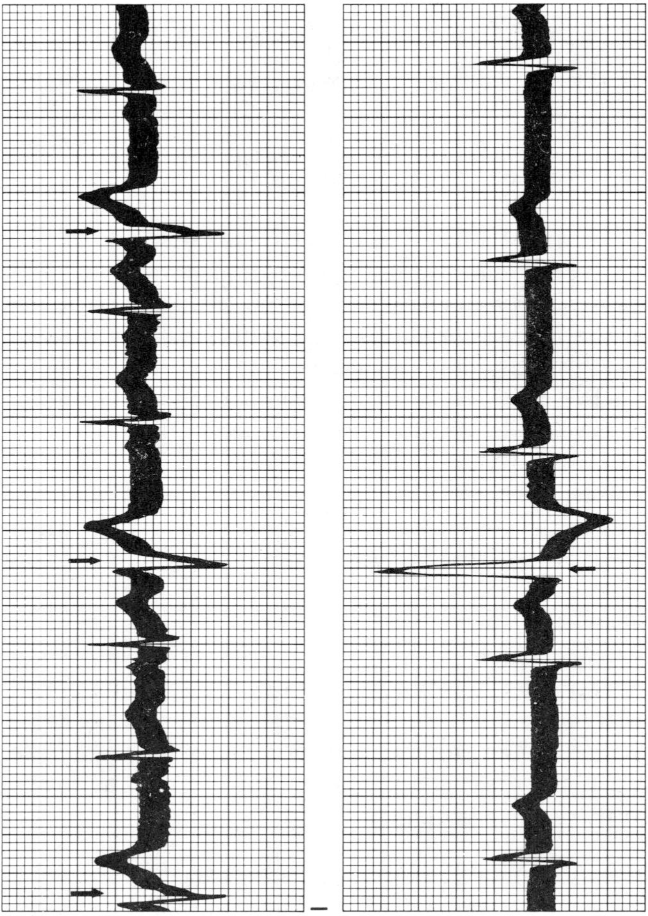

Figure 19A

seldom disturbed and is independent. There is usually a pause after the ventricular premature contraction, since the ventricles are refractory to the next sinus beat. However, if the next sinus beat is sufficiently distant from the premature beat, the ventricles can respond, and no sinus beat is dropped; such a ventricular premature contraction is called *interpolated* (Fig. 19A). It is not unusual for a ventricular premature contraction to conduct in a retrograde fashion, enter the atria, and produce a P wave which may or may not disturb the basic sinus rhythm.

Ventricular premature contractions may be uniform in contour, suggesting a single origin, or of varying contour, suggesting multifocal origins. The beats may be coupled to a preceding sinus beat by an unchanging coupling interval (fixed coupling), suggesting their dependence upon sino-atrial excitation. They may have variable coupling intervals, which suggests the presence of a stable, regularly firing, but slow ventricular rhythm (a parasystolic or independent ventricular pacemaker) rather than an occasional ectopic ventricular discharge.

3.1.5.2 Ventricular Rhythm (Idioventricular and Accelerated Idioventricular Rhythm)

The rate of this sustained but slow ventricular rhythm is usually between 25 and 50. It occasionally reaches 70 to 90 per minute and is then called *accelerated idioventricular rhythm*. It often starts spontaneously with a premature ventricular beat close to the preceding sinus beat. It may also arise when complete atrioventricular block exists. The QRS complexes, which occur regularly, are wider than 0.10 sec, are not preceded by P waves, and often the T wave is opposite in direction to the QRS. The atrial rhythm is often silenced by ventriculo-atrial conduction,

---

Figures 19A–C. *Ventricular mechanisms.*

Figure 19A. *Ventricular premature contractions.* Ventricular premature contractions are marked with arrows. The top line presents beats followed by a pause, and the bottom line, an interpolated beat.

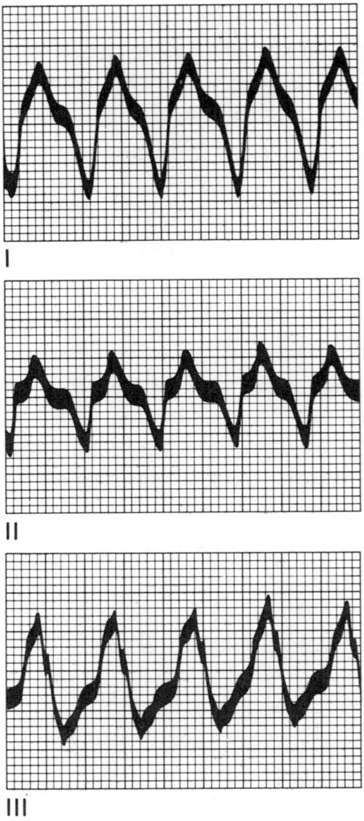

Figure 19B. *Ventricular tachycardia.* Ventricular tachycardia at 166 per minute. Atrial waves are not clearly seen. The QRS complexes, which occur regularly, are wide and bizarre, and the T waves are in a direction opposite to the QRS.

and hence no atrial waves are seen. The rhythm may be short-lived and seldom goes on to ventricular tachycardia or ventricular fibrillation. Accelerated idioventricular rhythm is often associated with myocardial infarction.

3.1.5.3 Ventricular Tachycardia

Ventricular tachycardia (Fig. 19B) is usually, but not always, seen in diseased hearts, particularly in those with coronary atherosclerosis; it is very rarely encountered in

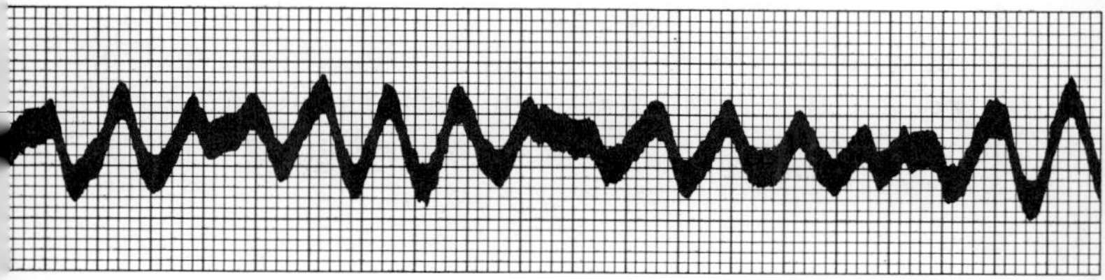

Figure 19C. *Ventricular fibrillation.* Ventricular fibrillation with wide, bizarre, and irregular QRS complexes, which have a constantly changing form.

rheumatic heart disease. It often is an expression of digitalis excess. It may lead to shock or ventricular failure. The onset of ventricular tachycardia is often the result of a ventricular premature contraction falling in the vulnerable period of the preceding supraventricular beat, during the peak of the preceding T wave. Vagal stimuli do not affect ventricular tachycardia.

Whenever three or more ventricular premature contractions occur in sequence, have approximately the same contour, and are separated by a fixed interval, ventricular tachycardia is present. The rate usually ranges from 140 to 200 per minute, but may be somewhat slower or faster. The rhythm is regular, but 0.01- to 0.02-sec variations in cycle time are seen, in contrast to such supraventricular rhythms as atrial tachycardia and atrial flutter, where the ventricular rate tends to be precisely regular.

The atrial rhythm, if recognizable, is independent of the ventricular rhythm; hence the P waves bear no relationship to the QRS complexes in this form of atrioventricular dissociation. The differential diagnosis of ventricular tachycardia from supraventricular tachycardia with aberrant, wide QRS complexes may be difficult if P waves cannot be identified.

3.1.5.4 Ventricular Fibrillation

Ventricular fibrillation (Fig. 19C) is incompatible with life unless it occurs in short bursts. It frequently is initiated by a ventricular premature contraction falling in the vulnerable period (during the peak of the T wave) of the preceding beat. It is a totally irregular rhythm, which may be slow or fast. The oscillations seen on the electrocardiogram are wide, bizarre QRS complexes whose contours are constantly changing. Atrial waves usually cannot be identified.

3.1.6 RHYTHMS FROM ARTIFICIAL PACING

3.1.6.1 Atrial Rhythm From Artificial Pacing

Direct stimulation of the atrial wall by an electrical pacemaker (asynchronous generator) produces a pacemaker artifact, or spike, which is followed by a P wave and then a QRS complex which is similar to the QRS seen in sinus rhythm. The rate can be set at will. Atrial synchronous generators are activated by spontaneous atrial impulses, which thus regulate the rate of ventricular stimulation. The P wave is followed by an electrical spike, and then the QRS complex appears.

3.1.6.2 Ventricular Rhythm From Artificial Pacing

This rhythm (Fig. 20), which is initiated by an electrical pacemaker, consists of a succession of wide, regular QRS complexes, which resemble ventricular premature contractions, but which are preceded by the electrical pacemaker artifact, or spike. The T waves are usually in a direction opposite to the QRS complexes. The pacing unit is preset for a specific rate (asynchronous ventricular generator), usually around 70 per minute, and hence the rate is fixed and uninfluenced by spontaneous rhythms. Other types of units respond only on demand, whenever the spontaneous rhythm falls below the preset rate of the

---

Figure 20. *Ventricular rhythm from artificial pacing.* The pacing artifacts, or spikes, are marked with arrows and are followed by wide QRS complexes which are upright in lead I, identifying the pacing site as the right ventricle. The pacing rate is 71 per minute. (The leads are recorded as in Figure 1.)

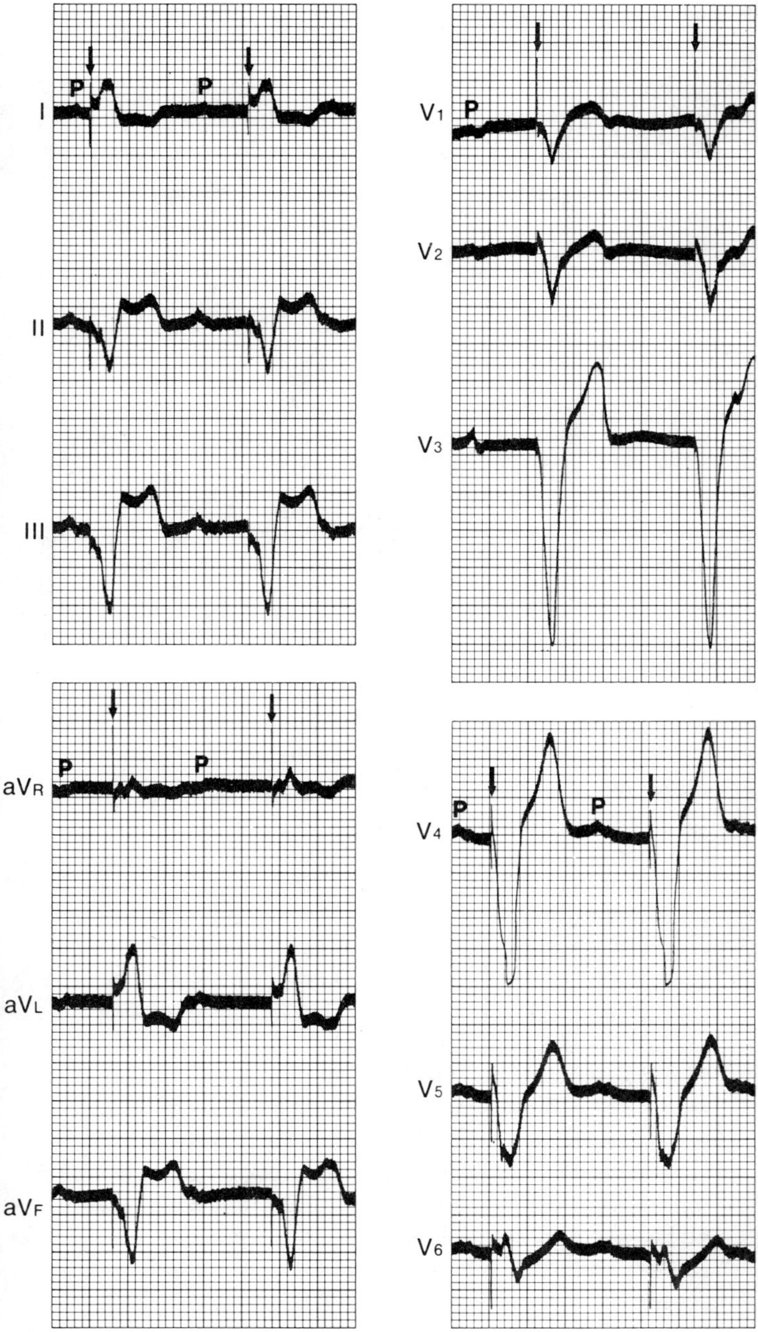

Figure 20

pacemaker. If the pacing electrode stimulates the right ventricle, as in transvenous pacing, the QRS usually will be upright in lead I, and the QRS complexes will resemble those of left bundle branch block; if the electrode lies next to the left ventricle, as occurs with an epicardial electrode, the QRS will be largely negative in lead I, and the complexes will resemble those seen in right bundle branch block.

3.1.7 MALFUNCTION OF ELECTRONIC PACEMAKER SYSTEMS

All currently used cardiac pacing systems are composed of three elements: a source of electrical energy (a pulse generator), a means by which the electrical signals are transmitted to the myocardium (an electrode), and the end organ (the heart). Effective pacing is accomplished only when each element functions properly. Thus the output and repetition rate of the generator must be sufficient to evoke physiologic myocardial responses; the transmission system must be structurally intact and the resistance within it small enough to prevent significant loss of energy at the interface between the electrode and the myocardium; and the threshold of the myocardium to excitation must be low enough to permit a response.

Malfunction of the pacemaker system may be the result of defects in one or more of these component pacing and sensing elements. Pulse generator failure occurs as a result of depletion of the energy source (battery failure) or defects in the circuits which regulate energy release, repetition rate, and the form and duration of the generator's signals. The transmission system may cause pacemaker malfunction as a result of faulty connection between the terminals of the electrode and the pulse generator; breaks in the electrode wires or their insulation; malposition of the electrode (endocardial or epicardial), causing poor contact with the myocardium (including perforation of the right ventricle); and electrochemical changes at the electrode tip, causing increased impedance to current flow. The responsiveness of the myocardium to electrical stimulation or the myocardial signal which triggers sensing may be decreased by an excessive fibro-inflammatory reaction to the electrode or by unrelated tissue injury, hypoxia, electrolyte abnormalities, or drug effects.

Gross malfunction in pacing can usually be recognized by clinical, radiologic, and electrocardiographic examinations. The exact cause of the pacing failure, including failure to sense, may be difficult to determine even if determined in both free running and magnetic modes, since defects in any of the elements of the pacing system may produce similar effects. Oscilloscopic analysis of the pacemaker pulse on an expanded time scale may provide more precise analysis. This method allows accurate measurements of the repetition rate of the generator and the amplitude, form, and duration of the signal. In some instances, identification of the cause of pacemaker malfunction requires surgical exposure of the unit and independent measurement of the output of the generator, the excitation threshold and voltage output signal of the myocardium, and of impedance in the electrode leads.

Clinical manifestations of pacemaker malfunction may include dizziness, syncope, increasing fatigue, chest pain, dyspnea, bradycardia, tachycardia, or arrhythmias. Radiologic examination may disclose malposition of the electrode tip or unusual angulation or fracture of the electrode. Deterioration of batteries may also be recognized radiographically, but this method is unreliable.

Electrocardiographic examination done regularly provides the most reliable and specific evidence of pacemaker system malfunction. While this method is limited, and more refined analyses may be obtained by additional techniques, it is the most useful procedure at the present time. It is recommended, however, that an accurate rate meter be used, in addition to the electrocardiogram, to measure the cycle length of pacemaker pulses. Conventional electrocardiographs sometimes contain a defective paper speed mechanism which may cause errors in cycle length measurement of up to 60 to 80 msec. Since early generator malfunction may be manifested by a change in cycle length as small as 2 to 4 msec, precise measurement is essential. Simple, easy to operate rate meters are commercially available. Some of these units measure pulse duration as well as rate.

The manifestations of pacemaker malfunction vary with the type of pulse generator which has been implanted. Engineering specifications provided by the manufacturer should be consulted since different generators vary somewhat in respect of the earliest signs of malfunction. The repetition rate and pulse duration of noncompetitive (demand) generators which are suppressed at the time of examination may be evaluated by conversion to the fixed rate mode with the external application of a magnet directly over the implanted generator. Asynchronous (competitive) atrial or ventricular generators normally produce continuous pulses at a preset fixed rate which is unaffected by spontaneous myocardial impulses. Excitation of the atria or ventricles occurs whenever they are nonrefractory. Atrial- or ventricular-inhibited, noncompetitive generators normally produce pulses only when the rate of spontaneous impulses falls below a preset fixed rate of the pacemaker. When the spontaneous cardiac rate exceeds the pacemaker rate, no pacemaker pulses are produced. Ventricular-synchronous, noncompetitive generators also normally produce pulses only when the rate of spontaneous impulses falls below a preset fixed rate of the pacemaker. However, spontaneous impulses initiate pacemaker impulses shortly after ventricular depolarization has begun; since the ventricles are still in their refractory phase, these pulses do not stimulate contraction.

Noncompetitive pacemakers have refractory periods during which electrical signals cannot be sensed. Atrial synchronous generators (with ventricular pacing) are activated by spontaneous atrial impulses; thus the rate of excitation of the ventricles by generator pulses varies with the atrial rate. A delay circuit defers emission of impulse by the generator for 120 to 160 msec after the atrial impulse is sensed. When the spontaneous atrial rate falls below a preset minimum, the pulse generator produces automatic ventricular signals at a fixed rate. When the spontaneous atrial rate exceeds a preset maximum, the generator responds to every second or third atrial impulse.

ONE OF THE FOLLOWING CRITERIA IS REQUIRED FOR THE DIAGNOSIS OF MALFUNCTION OF AN ELECTRONIC PACEMAKER SYSTEM.

1. Malfunction of an asynchronous ventricular pacemaker is manifested electrocardiographically by any of the following: a significant increase or decrease in the rate of the pacemaker artifact (a 10 percent or greater change from the original rate, or a 5 percent change if confirmed by electronic analysis of the pacemaker pulse); irregular appearance or absence of pacemaker artifacts; failure of a pacemaker artifact to initiate a QRS complex; a change in the amplitude or vector position of the pacemaker artifact.
2. Malfunction of a ventricular-inhibited or of a ventricular synchronous pacemaker may be manifested electrocardiographically by any of the following: failure of a pacemaker artifact to initiate a QRS complex; change in the amplitude or vector position of the pacemaker artifact; failure of a pacemaker artifact to appear at the preset escape interval of the pulse generator; appearance of a pacemaker artifact before the escape interval has elapsed; significant increase or decrease in the rate of the artifact when the pulse generator is operating in its fixed rate mode; failure of spontaneous impulses occurring outside the refractory period of the generator to inhibit the pacemaker, so that the time interval between the QRS complex which precedes and the pacemaker artifact which follows the spontaneous impulse equals the escape interval of the generator; continuous function of the generator in the fixed rate mode when the rate of spontaneous impulses exceeds the automatic rate of the pacemaker. Malfunction of a ventricular synchronous pacemaker is also indicated by the absence of a pacemaker artifact superimposed on the QRS complex of spontaneous impulses.

3. Malfunction of atrial synchronous pacemakers may be manifested by: absence of pacemaker artifacts following P waves; failure of pacemaker artifact to initiate a QRS complex; failure of the generator to function in the fixed rate mode when the spontaneous atrial rate is less than the automatic rate of the generator; failure of the pacemaker artifact to follow every second or third P wave when the atrial rate exceeds 125 beats per minute; continuous function of the generator in the fixed rate mode when the spontaneous atrial rate is between 60 and 125 beats per minute.
4. Any electrocardiographic evidence of malfunction of a pacemaker system, together with radiologic evidence of malposition of the electrode tip, unusual angulation, or fracture of the electrode.

3.2 Disturbances in Conduction

3.2.1 SINO-ATRIAL EXIT BLOCK

Sino-atrial exit block (Figs. 21A and 21B) is caused by increased vagal tone, digitalis, quinidine, and intrinsic disease of the sino-atrial node. During sinus rhythm and despite normal impulse formation within the sino-atrial node, there is periodic failure of the sinus impulse to reach the right atrium and initiate atrial excitation. A sinus beat, P and QRS–T, fails to appear at the expected time. The dropped beats may occur sporadically or in regularly recurring patterns after every second, third, or fourth normal beat. The resulting pause is an exact multiple of the P to P cycle length, that is, it has the precise duration of two normal cycles, which identifies it as a 2:1 sinus exit block. Occasionally, more than one sinus impulse in succession fails to reach the atrium, and there is dropping of two or three successive P waves, indicating a 3:1 or 4:1 sinus exit block, resulting in a long pause, which escape beats may interrupt. In the incomplete form of exit block, sino-atrial exit block with the Wenckebach phenomenon, there is gradual slowing of conduction from the sino-atrial

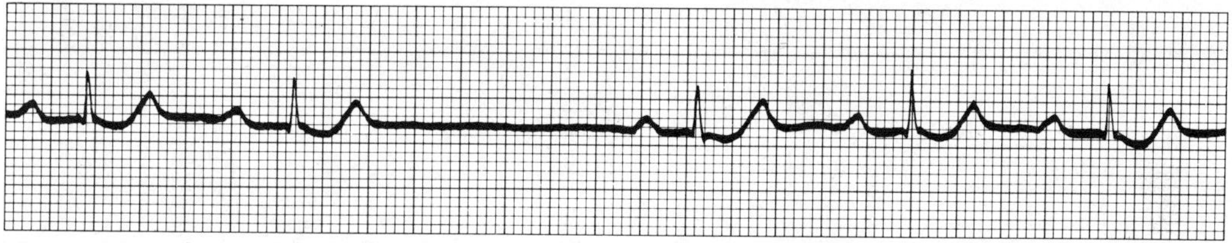

Figure 21A. *Sino-atrial exit block (2:1).* A dropped beat occurs after the second sinus beat, and the pause equals two cycle lengths, identifying this rhythm as 2:1 exit block. The P–R interval is prolonged (0.26 sec). (Figure is recorded on lead II.)

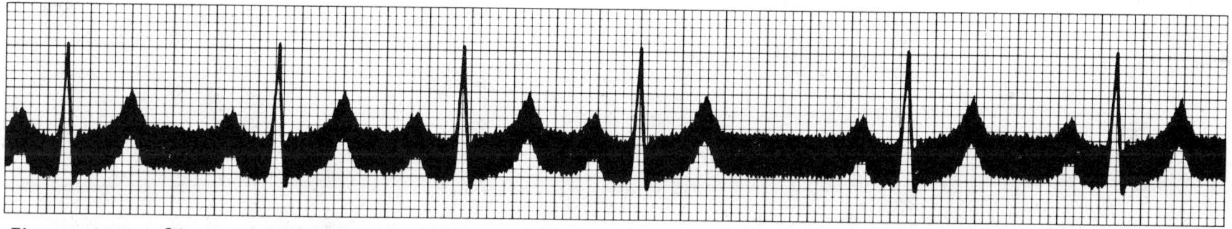

Figure 21B. *Sino-atrial exit block with Wenckebach phenomenon.* The P to P intervals preceding the pause (which occurs after the fourth beat) progressively shorten. The pause is less than a multiple of the basic P to P interval, and the P to P cycle time following the pause is longer than the P to P interval immediately preceding the pause. (Figure is recorded on lead II.)

node to the atrium, until finally one sinus impulse is totally blocked from reaching the atrium, and a P wave drops out. The P to P intervals preceding the pause progressively shorten, the pause is less than a multiple of the basic sinus rate (P to P interval), and the P to P interval following the pause is longer than the preceding P to P interval.

Long pauses will produce the same symptoms that may be encountered with sinus bradycardia.

3.2.2 INTRA-ATRIAL BLOCK

A delay in conduction through the atrial myocardium, or an abnormality of the spread of atrial excitation in the interatrial or internodal tracts, or both is manifested by prolongation of the P wave to 0.12 sec or longer. The widened P wave may be notched and its amplitude increased or decreased. Notching of the P wave alone is not abnormal.

Atrial disease, digitalis, or quinidine can produce this abnormality. Symptoms are not associated with this abnormality.

3.2.3 ATRIOVENTRICULAR CONDUCTION DISTURBANCES

The area involved in atrioventricular conduction disturbances includes the atrioventricular node, the nodal-His bundle junction, and the common bundle of His down to its bifurcation.

These disturbances (Figs. 22A through 22D) are encountered in atherosclerotic, rheumatic, diphtheritic, and syphilitic heart disease. They may be congenital in origin or result from fibrotic or sclerotic lesions limited to the specific tissues. Digitalis, quinidine, procainamide, reserpine, propanolol, and vagal stimuli may induce atrioventricular block. Failure of the atrioventricular conducting mechanisms can be complete or incomplete. The latter defect implies a slowing of conduction velocity within some portion of the atrioventricular junctional tissue.

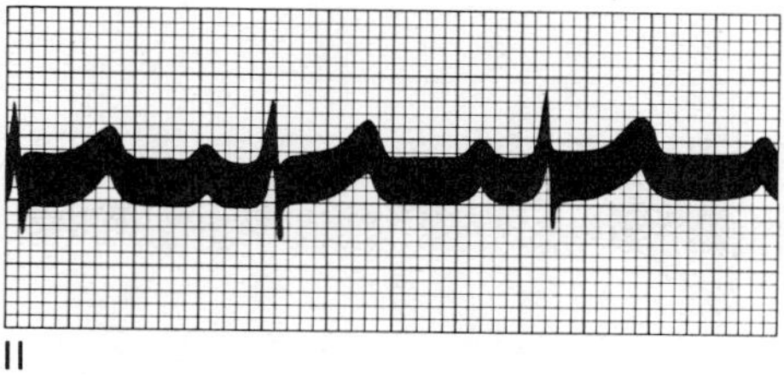

Figure 22A. *Prolonged P–R interval (0.24 sec).*

Figures 22A–D. *Atrioventricular conduction disturbances.* A prolonged P–R interval (0.24 sec) is seen in Figure 22A. A Wenckebach phenomenon with progressive prolongation of the P–R interval with the third P wave completely blocked (no QRS) is seen in Figure 22B. A Mobitz block appears twice in lead II in Figure 22C (the second and seventh P waves are not followed by a QRS). Incomplete atrioventricular block with 2:1 atrioventricular response and a fixed P–R interval occurs in the first line of Figure 22D. Complete atrioventricular block is illustrated in the second line of Figure 22D with atrial and ventricular rates of 88 and 45 per minute, respectively; there is no constant relationship of P to QRS.

3.2.3.1 Incomplete Atrioventricular Block

3.2.3.1.1 PROLONGED P–R INTERVAL (FIRST DEGREE ATRIOVENTRICULAR BLOCK)

In the presence of sinus rhythm and the absence of bundle branch block, prolongation of the P–R interval (Fig. 22A) is due to intra-atrial block or a slowing of conduction of the impulse through the atrioventricular node, or both. The P–H interval of the His bundle electrogram, which describes atrial and atrioventricular nodal conduction time, or time through the upper junctional tissue, is prolonged (normally, the P–H interval is 80–140 msec in duration). The H spike in the His bundle electrogram divides the P–R interval into two parts, separating the upper (P–H) from the lower (H–QRS or H–V) junctional region.

No symptoms result from this form of atrioventricular block.

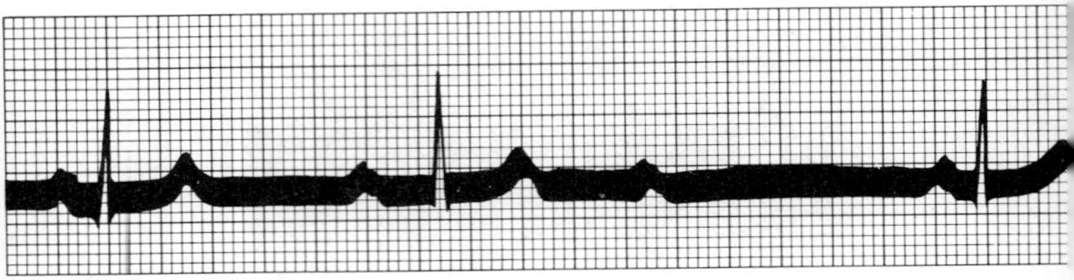

II

Figure 22B. *Incomplete atrioventricular block, type I (Wenckebach periods).*

3.2.3.1.2 INCOMPLETE ATRIOVENTRICULAR BLOCK WITH PERIODICALLY DROPPED BEATS (SECOND DEGREE ATRIOVENTRICULAR BLOCK)

In this type of atrioventricular block, there is periodic complete failure of atrioventricular conduction for one or more beats.

3.2.3.1.2.1 *Type I (Wenckebach periods).* In this conduction disturbance, sinus rhythm is associated with progressive prolongation of the P–R interval until one P wave is completely blocked, and no QRS is generated; hence one ventricular beat is dropped (Fig. 22B). The area of block, as shown by the prolongation in P–H interval in the His bundle electrogram, is usually proximal to the His bundle and probably is in the atrioventricular node itself, but can occur rarely in the bundle branches. In the latter case the H–V and not the P–H interval is prolonged.

Since there are decreasing increments in the P–R intervals, there are progressively shorter and shorter QRS to QRS cycles before the dropped beat. The first cycle following the pause is longer than the preceding cycle, the duration of the pause is shorter than any two consecutive short cycles, and the P–R interval of the first conducted beat in the sequence has the shortest P–R interval. The maximum increment in P–R interval occurs between the first and second conducted beats of the Wenckebach period. The dropped beats may not always occur after the same

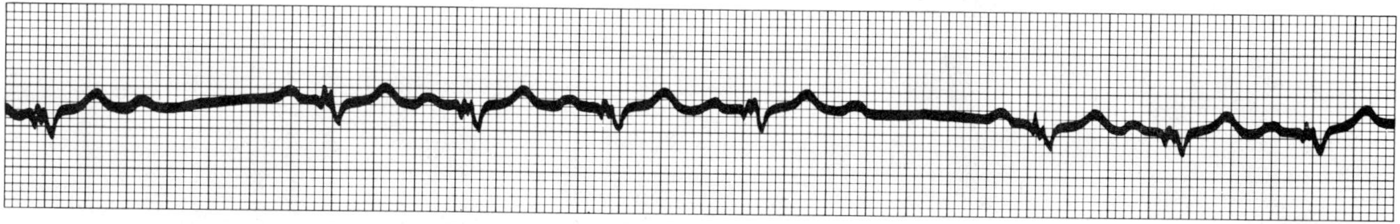

Figure 22C. *Incomplete atrioventricular block, type II (Mobitz block).*

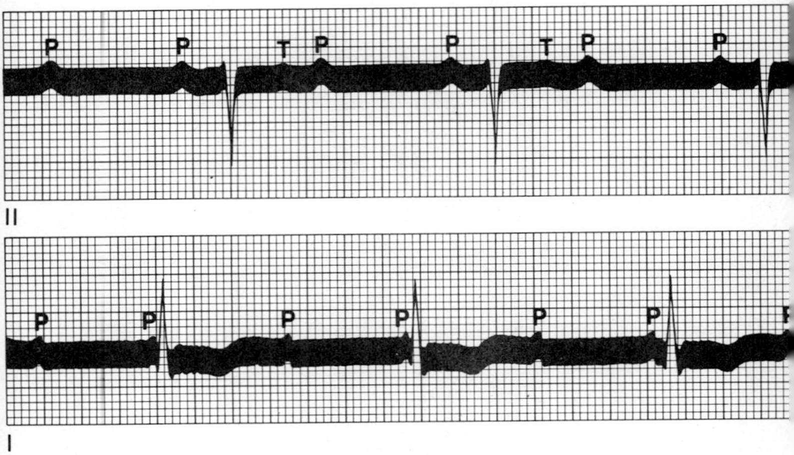

Figure 22D. *Incomplete atrioventricular block with 2:1 atrioventricular response (top) and complete atrioventricular block (bottom).*

number of conducted beats, and hence there may be 3:2, 4:3, 5:4 atrioventricular ratios in succession. Thus the ventricular rate in this form of atrioventricular block may be totally irregular or regular with pauses (if the periods are stable as to atrioventricular ratio). Palpitations are therefore often noted.

3.2.3.1.2.2 *Type II (Mobitz block).* In this uncommon form of incomplete atrioventricular block, one or two ventricular beats are suddenly dropped during sinus rhythm, without any change in P–R interval (Fig. 22C). This interval may be normal or prolonged. Following the dropped beats, atrioventricular conduction occurs normally in subsequent beats. The area of atrioventricular block is usually in the lower junctional tissue, that is, in the His bundle or its branching parts. The His bundle electrogram shows a normal P–H interval and prolongation of the H–V interval, normally 35 to 55 msec in duration. Type II atrioventricular block often progresses to complete atrioventricular block.

Other than occasional palpitation, there are no symptoms during this form of incomplete atrioventricular block, unless the basic atrial rate is quite slow and the pauses long, then dizziness or mild failure may occur.

3.2.3.1.2.3 *Incomplete atrioventricular block with 2:1 atrioventricular response (2:1 atrioventricular block).* Here, there is a constant P–R interval, which may be of normal duration or may be prolonged, and a constant degree of atrioventricular block such that every other P wave is completely blocked; there is no following QRS complex. The atrioventricular ratio is stable at 2:1 (Fig. 22D). This form of incomplete atrioventricular block may become advanced, so that more than every other P is blocked; for example, two or three successive P waves without QRS complexes are seen, and the stable atrioventricular ratio in this high grade block reaches 3:1 or 4:1. The area of block can occur in any portion of the junctional tissue, and this form of incomplete atrioventricular block can alternate with type I or type II. Palpitations may be noted.

3.2.3.2 Complete Atrioventricular Block (Third Degree Atrioventricular Block)

In complete atrioventricular block (Fig. 22D), no supraventricular impulses reach the ventricles, and independent pacemakers control the atria and ventricles. There is complete atrioventricular dissociation. The atrial pacemaker may be the sinus node or other atrial foci. The atrial rhythm is faster than the ventricular. The P waves are unrelated to the QRS complexes.

In complete atrioventricular block, His bundle electrograms demonstrate that the most common site of block is distal to the His bundle; there is a normal P–H interval after such P waves, but no H–V interval or H spike preceding the QRS complexes. The block is probably due to complete bilateral bundle branch block. However, in congenital forms of complete atrioventricular block, the block is generally proximal to the His bundle. The His bundle electrogram reveals no H spike after the P waves (absence of P–H interval); the junctional rhythm controlling the ventricles is characterized by a narrow QRS complex preceded by an H spike and a normal H–V interval.

In acute myocardial infarction with complete atrioventricular block, His electrograms place the site of block in two locations. In inferior wall myocardial infarction, the site of block is usually proximal to the His bundle and is in the atrioventricular node; there is no H spike after the P wave. In anterior wall myocardial infarction the block is usually distal to the His bundle and reflects bilateral bundle branch block.

Usually, the pacemaker which controls the ventricles arises in the junctional tissue below the site of the block and fires at a rate of 40 to 55 per minute in adults and around 70 to 80 in children. The regularly occurring QRS complexes have a normal contour and duration. However, when the ventricular pacemaker lies below the bifurcation of the His bundle, the QRS complexes may be abnormally wide. If the pacemaker arises in the ventricular myocardium, the QRS is wider than 0.12 sec, the rate is between 25 and 40 per minute, and the QRS–T complexes resemble ventricular premature contractions.

3.2.3.3 Adams–Stokes Syndrome

Patients with high degrees of atrioventricular block may experience episodes of giddiness, unexplained falls, syncope, and convulsions. If the block is long-standing, marked fatigue and ventricular failure may occur. In children, especially infants, the symptoms may include poor feeding, crying spells after eating, sudden opisthotonic periods, or frank seizures. The decreased cerebral blood flow responsible for these episodes is produced (1) by cardiac asystole when complete atrioventricular block begins and no ventricular pacemaker arises; (2) when the idioventricular rhythm is too slow—25 to 35 beats per minute; (3) when the change from conducted sinus rates to the slow idioventricular rates during heart block reduces the cardiac output; or (4) when there are periodic runs of ventricular tachycardia or ventricular fibrillation, which complicate complete atrioventricular heart block, usually because the idioventricular rates are very slow, and the myocardium is underperfused. This syndrome of lowered cerebral blood flow can be caused by other conditions, such as severe sinus bradycardia, sinus arrest, or sinus exit block, runs of ventricular tachycardia or ventricular fibrillation, and severe vagotonia with peripheral vascular dilatation and bradycardia.

3.2.4 ATRIOVENTRICULAR DISSOCIATION

Atrioventricular dissociation occurs in certain specific situations, and its recognition can thus add considerably to the specificity of cardiac diagnosis. Excess digitalis and quinidine, mild hypoxia, myocarditis of rheumatic, viral, or unknown etiology, and open heart surgery may be responsible.

The disturbance (Fig. 23) is characterized by two independent rhythms, one in the atria and the other in the junctional tissue or ventricle. One of two mechanisms may be responsible for its production:

1. A junctional tissue center suddenly fires at a rate, usually 90 to 120 per minute, which is faster than the atrial (sinus node) rate. The junctional impulses are blocked from entering the atria and hence do not disturb the atrial rhythm, usually a sinus rhythm. This is only a unidirectional (ventriculo-atrial) block because, since there is intact transmission through the atrioventricular node, the sinus beat occasionally falls at a time when the ventricles are no longer refractory (having recovered from the junctional beat excitation), and one sinus beat, called a capture beat, reaches the ventricles in the normal way. In atrioventricular dissociation the P to P interval is longer than the QRS to QRS interval; the ventricular rate, which is quite regular, is faster than the atrial; and there is no fixed relationship between P waves and the QRS complexes. The occasional capture beat momentarily causes the ventricular rate to become irregular. This represents atrioventricular dissociation with occasional ventricular capture; hence the atrioventricular dissociation is incomplete.

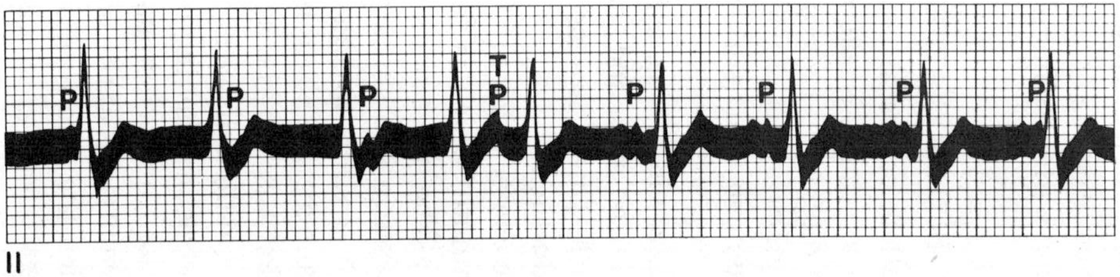

Figure 23. *Atrioventricular dissociation.* The ventricular rate is 107, and the atrial rate (marked with P) is 100 per minute; there is independent beating of atria and ventricles and no fixed P–R interval. The fifth QRS is a capture beat, with the sinus P wave momentarily controlling the ventricles.

2. Atrioventricular dissociation may also appear when there is marked slowing of the rhythmicity of the sinoatrial node. The sinus rate falls below the intrinsic rhythmicity of the junctional tissue, which is usually between 40 and 55 per minute. The junction then escapes and takes control of the ventricular rhythm, but not of the atrial rhythm. The ventricular rate exceeds that of the atria, and there is independence of the two pacemakers, which have rates in the range of 40 to 55 for the junctional tissue and 30 to 50 per minute, as a rule, for the sinus node. If the sinus rate accelerates again, the dissociation ceases, since the junctional escape center is silenced when sinus beats are again conducted to the ventricle in a normal fashion. If a sinus beat does not occasionally capture the ventricles, complete atrioventricular dissociation exists, whether the initiating mechanism is the accelerated junctional rhythm or slowing of the atrial pacemakers with escape junctional rhythm.

3.2.5 INTRAVENTRICULAR CONDUCTION DEFECTS

A complete intraventricular conduction defect may be either a permanent one due to a structural lesion or a functional one related to complete refractoriness of conducting tissue. Incomplete intraventricular conduction implies a more or less uniform slowing of conduction velocity within the tissue. A prolonged P–R interval can be a sign of intraventricular conduction delay, that is, decreased conduction through a part of the His bundle system, as well as a sign of delay in the atrioventricular nodal tissue.

Bilateral bundle branch block implies a combination of defects involving both branches of the His bundle (Fig. 24). Incomplete bilateral bundle branch block exists when one branch, such as the right bundle, is completely blocked while one or the other of the two left fascicles is also blocked. This may be a fixed state, or one or the other of the components may be blocked and then unblocked in an intermittent fashion. Complete bilateral bundle branch

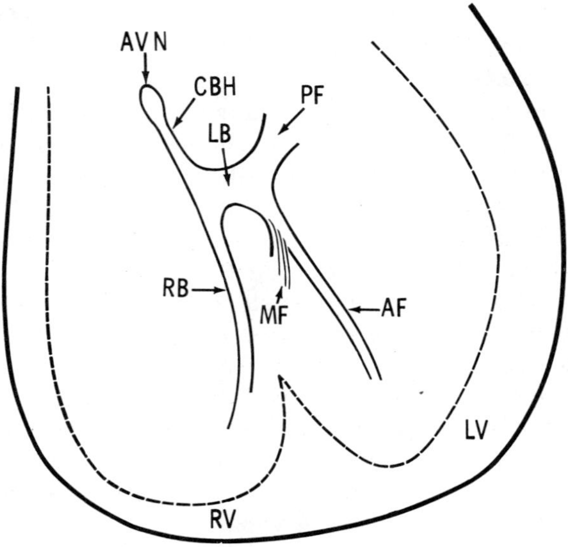

Figure 24. *Diagram of the intraventricular conduction system.* A posteroanterior view of the ventricles illustrates the atrioventricular node (AVN); common bundle of His (CBH); left main stem of the left bundle branch (LB) and its two fascicles, posterior (PF) and anterior (AF), and the right bundle branch (RB). A small medial branch (MF)) of the AF is also shown. The broken line marks the subendocardial terminal network of Purkinje cells.

block implies that all pathways to the ventricles over both bundle branches and their fascicles are blocked, with resultant complete atrioventricular block.

Intraventricular conduction defects can be classified as monofascicular, bifascicular, and trifascicular (multifascicular). With trifascicular block, the right bundle and both left fascicles are involved. Functional block occurs in the main bundle branches and fascicular areas and is usually a rate-dependent phenomenon. It accounts for the aberrant form of the QRS complex which appears when a long QRS to QRS interval is followed shortly by a ventricular complex induced either by an atrial premature contraction or by atrial fibrillation. Each of the major fascicles probably has a different degree of vulnerability, with the right bundle branch most vulnerable, the left anterior fascicle next most vulnerable, and the left posterior fascicle much less vulnerable.

The major anatomic sites of the intraventricular conduction defects appear in Figure 24. The electrocardiographic criteria for their diagnosis are given in Table 1.

3.2.5.1 MONOFASCICULAR BLOCK

3.2.5.1.1 RIGHT BUNDLE BRANCH BLOCK

In this conduction disturbance there is complete block of, or delay in conduction over, the main right bundle.

The diagnostic criteria (Table 1) consist of a prolongation of the QRS complex (0.12 sec or more for right bundle branch block and 0.11 or 0.10 sec for incomplete right bundle branch block), an S wave in leads I, V5, and V6, and two R waves (rR′) in V1 and V2 (Fig. 25). The only difference between right bundle branch block and incomplete right bundle branch block is the duration of the QRS complex. However, if a QRS measures only 0.09 sec or less, and there is an rR′ in V1 and V2, this is considered only a normal variant and not an intraventricular conduction defect. The axis may change little or may be rightward in right bundle branch block.

Both forms of right bundle branch block may occur in normal healthy persons; hence their presence does not necessarily imply a cardiac abnormality. This is in contrast to left bundle branch block, which almost always arises from a cardiac lesion. Right bundle branch block is seen in congenital heart disease, particularly in an atrial septal defect of the ostium secundum type; in Ebstein's anomaly; in rheumatic, atherosclerotic, or pulmonary heart disease; in myocarditis and myocardial infiltrative or fibrotic lesions; with right ventricular hypertrophy; and iatrogenically after cardiac surgery.

Right bundle branch block does not disturb cardiac dynamics significantly. Its importance depends upon the underlying cardiac disease, if any, and whether there are any other conduction abnormalities.

Table 1. *EKG Criteria for Diagnosis of Common Forms of*

	AQRS (degrees)	QRS Dur. (sec)	Axis Dev.
MONOFASCICULAR BLOCK			
RBBB (Right bundle branch block)	+90° to +120°	0.12 or >	NAD or RAD
IRBBB (Incomplete RBBB)	+90° to +120°	0.10–0.11	NAD or RAD
LBBB (Left bundle branch block)	+75° to −75°	0.12 or >	NAD or LAD
ILBBB (Incomplete LBBB)	+75° to −75°	0.10–0.11	NAD or LAD
AFB (Anterior fascicular block)	−45° to −90°	0.09–0.10	MLAD
PFB (Posterior fascicular block)	+90° to +120°	0.09–0.10	RAD
BIFASCICULAR BLOCK			
RBBB + LBBB (complete bilat. BBB→ complete AV block)	—	0.13–0.15	—
RBBB + ILBBB	+90° to +120°	0.12 or >	NAD or RAD
RBBB + AFB	−45° to −120°	0.12 or >	MLAD
RBBB + PFB	+100° to +120°	0.12 or >	RAD
AFB + PFB (LBBB)	+75° to −75°	0.12 or >	NAD or LAD
TRIFASCICULAR BLOCK			
RBBB + AFB + PFB (complete bilat. BBB→ complete AV block)	—	0.13–0.15	—
RBBB + AFB + IPFB	−45° to −120°	0.12 or >	MLAD
RBBB + PFB + IAFB	+100° to +120°	0.12 or >	RAD
RBBB + IAFB + IPFB	+90° to +120°	0.12 or >	NAD or RAD
RBBB + AFB + ILBBB	−45° to −120°	0.12 or >	MLAD
RBBB + PFB + ILBBB	+100° to +120°	0.12 or >	RAD
AFB + PFB(LBBB) + IRBBB	+75° to −75°	0.12 or >	NAD or LAD
DIFFUSE INTRAVENTRICULAR BLOCK	Unchanged	>0.10	Normal

AQRS = Frontal plane axis of QRS
AV = Atrioventricular
Axis Dev. = Axis deviation
H-LB = From the H wave in the His bundle electrogram to the wave from the left main stem
H-RB = From the H wave in the His bundle electrogram to the main right bundle potential
H-V Int. = Interval from H wave (main His bundle) of His bundle electrogram to onset of QRS (or ventricular complex)
IAFB = Incomplete AFB
Incr. = Increased, indicating conduction delay in portion of bundle branch system
IPFB = Incomplete PFB
LAD = Left axis deviation
LB-V = Left main stem potential (or wave) in the His bundle electrogram to the QRS complex

Leads								Intervals		
I	II	III	aVL	aVF	V1	V2	V5, V6	P-R	P-H*	H-V*
qrS†	qRs, Rs	Rs, R qR	rS	R, qR	rR′	rR′	RS	N	N	N
qrS	qRs, Rs	Rs, R, qR	rS	R, qR	rR′, rr′	rR′, rr′	RS	N	N	N
R (no q)	R, RS	R, RS	R (no q)	R, RS	rS, QS	rS, QS	RR′ (no q)	N	N	N
R (no q)	R, RS	R, RS	R (no q)	R, RS	rS, QS	rS, QS	RR′ (no q)	N	N	N
qR	rS	rS	qR	rS	rS	rS	qR	N	N	N
rS	qR	qR	rS	qR	QS	rS	Rs	N	N	N
—	—	—	—	—	—	—	—	—	N	Not seen (H wave only)
qrS	qRS, Rs	Rs, R, qR	rS	R, qR	rR′	rR′	RS	Incr.	N	Incr. (H-LB Incr.)
qRS	rS	rS	qRS	rS	rR′	rR′	RS	N	N	N
rS	qR	qR	rS	qR	rR′	rR′	RS	N	N	N
R (no q)	R, RS	R, RS	R (no q)	R, RS	rS, QS	rS, QS	RR′ (no q)	N	N	N
—	—	—	—	—	—	—	—	—	N	H-LB seen, but No LB-V
qRs	rS	rS	qRs	rS	rR′	rR′	RS	Incr.	N	Incr. (LB-V Incr.)
rS	qR	qR	rS	qR	rR′	rR′	RS	Incr.	N	Incr. (LB-V Incr.)
qrS	qRs, Rs	Rs, R, qR	rS	R, qR	rR′	rR′	RS	Incr.	N	Incr. (LB-V Incr.)
qRs	rS	rS	qRs	rS	rR′	rR′	RS	Incr.	N	Incr. (H-LB Incr.)
rS	qR	qR	rS	qR	rR′	rR′	RS	Incr.	N	Incr. (H-LB Incr.)
R (no q)	R, RS	R, RS	R (no q)	R, RS	rS, QS	rS, QS	RR′ (no q)	Incr.	N	Incr. (H-RB Incr.)

MLAD = Marked LAD
N = Normal
NAD = No axis deviation
P-H Int. = Interval from P wave to the H wave of the His bundle electrogram
P-R Int. = P-R interval (and includes P-H interval plus H-V interval)
QRS Dur. = QRS duration
RAD = Right axis deviation

*Determined from His bundle electrograms.
†The small letters indicate small waves in the electrocardiogram; the large letters indicate the dominant or large-sized waves.

Adapted by permission from Ferrer, M I., Intraventricular conduction defects: New facts, new concepts, new problems. *Med. Times* 99:45, 1972.

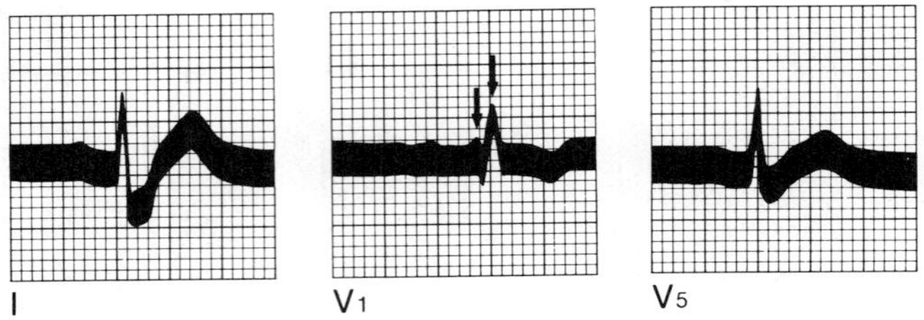

Figure 25. *Right bundle branch block.* A wide S wave is present in leads I and V5; rR′ is present in V1 (at arrows). The QRS is prolonged (0.12 sec).

3.2.5.1.2 LEFT BUNDLE BRANCH BLOCK

In this conduction disturbance there is complete block of, or delay in conduction at, the main stem of the left bundle (LB in Fig. 24).

The diagnostic criteria (Table 1) consist of a prolongation of the QRS complex (0.12 sec or more for left bundle branch block and 0.11 or 0.10 sec for incomplete left bundle branch block), with neither a Q nor an S in leads I, aVL, V5, and V6, and with an RR′ in V5 and V6 (Fig. 26). The only difference between left bundle branch block and incomplete left bundle branch block is the duration of the QRS complex.

Both forms of left bundle branch block are found in rheumatic and atherosclerotic heart disease, left ventricular hypertrophy, myocarditis, and diffuse infiltrative or fibrotic myocardial lesions. It is very rare in congenital heart disease and, if present, is associated with congenital aortic stenosis, coarctation of the aorta, or tricuspid atresia. It is seldom a postoperative complication of cardiac surgery.

The functional consequences of left bundle branch block are negligible. Its importance depends on the underlying disease and whether there are any other conduction abnormalities.

3.2.5.1.3 ANTERIOR FASCICULAR BLOCK

This form of intraventricular conduction defect consists of complete block in the anterior fascicle of the left bundle

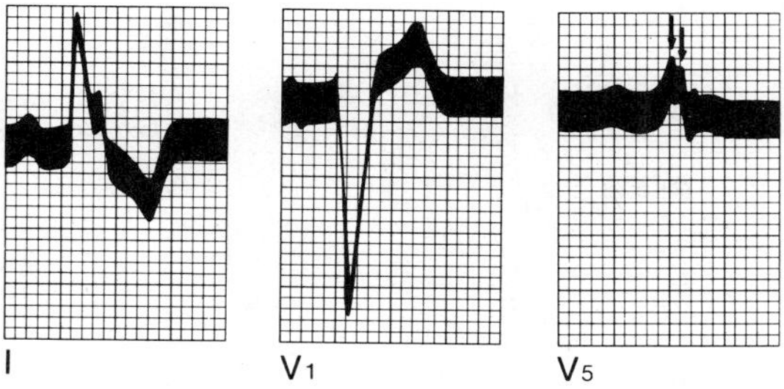

Figure 26. *Left bundle branch block.* A wide R wave is present, without a Q or S in lead I; RR′ is present in V5 (at arrows), and the QRS is prolonged (0.14 sec).

(Fig. 24), with normal conduction through the posterior fascicle and right bundle branch.

The diagnostic criteria (Table 1) depend largely upon the presence of marked left axis deviation. In terms of the frontal plane projection of this QRS vector, marked left axis deviation lies between −30° and −90° (Figs. 6, 9, and 27). Since there is little or no increase in the QRS duration with anterior fascicular block—an increase of 0.01 to 0.02 sec over the original QRS duration is all that occurs—the diagnosis of anterior fascicular block rests upon the presence of this particular axis orientation. It is best to require an axis of −45° to −90° in order to be certain that anterior fascicular block is present, because other causes of left axis deviation may occasionally rotate the QRS vector beyond −30°, but do not usually shift it beyond −45°.

The left ventricular excitation in anterior fascicular block occurs over the posterior fascicle (thus the initial forces are directed inferiorly and to the right), then travels through the Purkinje network, and later spreads superiorly, anteriorly, and to the left over the area normally supplied by the anterior fascicle. The terminal forces are directed superiorly and to the left. This results in the mean QRS axis being markedly to the left, with qR in I, aVL, V6 and S in II, III, and aVF.

The commonest cause of this conduction defect is fibrosis of unknown etiology or myocardial infarction (Fig. 6) due to atherosclerotic heart disease. However, it is also

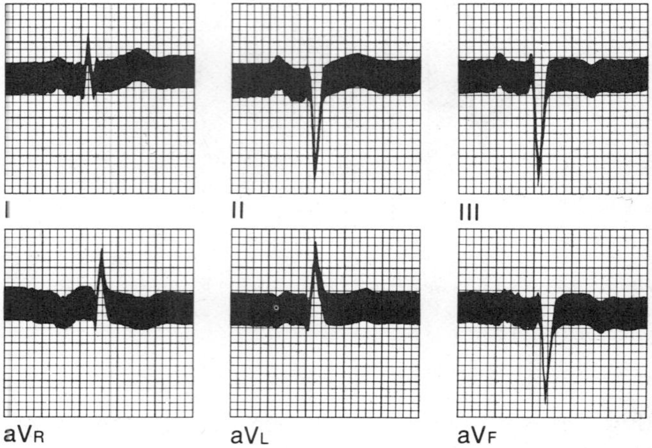

Figure 27. *Left anterior fascicular block.* The mean electrical axis of the QRS is −69°, markedly to the left.

seen in hypertensive heart disease; in disease of the aortic valve that produces fibrosis or calcification at the valve base in the area of the interventricular septum; in diabetes, obesity, and cardiomyopathies; in myocarditis, especially in chronic Chagas' disease; in sclerosis of the left side of the cardiac skeleton in the elderly; and in some types of congenital heart disease, particularly endocardial cushion defects and tricuspid atresia. Surgical injury during operation for left ventricular outflow tract obstruction also is a cause of anterior fascicular block.

The consequences of anterior fascicular block are negligible from a functional point of view. However, it is now known that disease of the ventricular fascicular system can be a slowly progressive one, with one fascicle after another being damaged, or being damaged and recovering, only to be blocked once again. This is true of both the acquired form and a newly described congenital hereditary form. Hence prospective sequential observation of a patient with anterior fascicular block is essential. Monofascicular block which becomes bifascicular or trifascicular has serious consequences. On the other hand, many patients with anterior fascicular block may go a decade or more without complications.

3.2.5.1.4 POSTERIOR FASCICULAR BLOCK

In this form of intraventricular conduction defect there is complete block in the posterior fascicle of the left bundle, with normal conduction through the anterior fascicle and right bundle branch.

Isolated posterior fascicular block is rare and the diagnosis difficult (Table 1). Of the three pathways to the ventricles (right bundle, anterior fascicle, posterior fascicle), the posterior fascicle is least vulnerable to block which probably accounts for the rarity of isolated posterior fascicular block. It usually is seen in association with right bundle branch block. The axis in pure posterior fascicular block lies between +90° and +100° and occasionally as far to the right as +120°. There is minimal change in the QRS duration, which is usually 0.09 to 0.10 sec. Such subtle alterations—slight right axis deviation with a normal QRS duration—make a definitive diagnosis from the electrocardiogram alone almost an impossibility. A normal vertical heart, right ventricular enlargement, emphysema, and extensive lateral wall myocardial infarction must be excluded. A rightward shift in axis which has appeared sequentially, together with large R waves in leads II, III, and aVF, suggests the diagnosis of posterior fascicular block. In posterior fascicular block, left ventricular activation occurs over the healthy anterior fascicle, and initial forces are directed anteriorly, superiorly, and to the left. They later travel over the Purkinje network to invade the area normally served by the posterior fascicle. Thus terminal activation spreads posteriorly, inferiorly, and to the right. The mean QRS thus has a right axis deviation with qR in II, III, and aVF. The R waves in II, III, and aVF are large.

The causes of this block are probably the same as for anterior fascicular block, but it is uncommon as a consequence of cardiac surgical injury and has not been seen in congenital heart disease.

3.2.5.2 Bifascicular Block

3.2.5.2.1 RIGHT BUNDLE BRANCH BLOCK AND LEFT MAIN STEM BUNDLE BRANCH BLOCK

This form of bifascicular block consists of complete block of the right bundle branch and the main stem of the left bundle (Fig. 24).

The diagnostic criteria (Table 1) depend upon evidence of right and left bundle branch block. Such complete bilateral bundle branch block produces complete atrioventricular block; indeed, complete bilateral bundle branch block, rather than damage to the atrioventricular node, is the commonest cause of complete atrioventricular block. In this type of bifascicular block, P waves are not consistently associated with QRS complexes, and the ventricles are under the control of a ventricular pacemaker; this usually arises below the common bundle of His, so that no H–V interval is seen in the His bundle electrogram. An H wave is seen following each sinus beat or P wave, but does not reach the ventricles; there is no H–V interval. The contour of the QRS depends upon its site of origin in either a bundle branch or the ventricular myocardium.

The commonest causes are atherosclerotic heart disease, aortic valvular lesions, cardiomyopathies, and fibrotic or sclerotic lesions of the interventricular septum.

The consequences are similar to those of complete atrioventricular block.

3.2.5.2.2 RIGHT BUNDLE BRANCH BLOCK AND INCOMPLETE LEFT BUNDLE BRANCH BLOCK

In this form of bifascicular block, there is complete block of the right bundle and delayed conduction in the main stem of the left bundle (Fig. 24).

The diagnostic criteria (Table 1) are relatively simple, since the frontal plane axis, the form of the QRS complex, and its prolongation are determined by the right bundle branch block. There is also an increase in the P–R interval. This is occasioned by an increase in the H–V interval of the His bundle electrogram because of the delay through the left bundle. The H–LB interval is prolonged, but the H wave does eventually reach the left ventricle. Right bundle branch block with a prolonged P–R interval can, of course, occur due to a combined disorder of the atrioventricular node and the right bundle branch. The differential diagnosis can be made by the His bundle electrogram, which in the latter disorder would show a prolonged P–H interval with a normal H–V interval. It is of note that the presence of Mobitz type II atrioventricular block associated either with left bundle branch block or right bundle branch block probably implies a form of bifascicular block, since Mobitz type II block almost always occurs in the His bundle system.

The serious consequence of this type of intraventricular conduction defect is progression to complete bilateral bundle branch block and complete atrioventricular block.

3.2.5.2.3 RIGHT BUNDLE BRANCH BLOCK AND ANTERIOR FASCICULAR BLOCK

In this defect there is complete block of these two fascicles (Fig. 24).

The diagnostic criteria (Table 1) are essentially those of right bundle branch block and marked left axis deviation (Figs. 9 and 28); the axis may be quite far to the left (–120°) in such combined lesions.

This conduction defect is seen in atherosclerotic heart disease, calcific aortic stenosis, cariomyopathies, fibrotic or sclerotic diseases of the interventricular septum, and endocardial cushion defects.

The consequences of acquired bifascicular block have recently been intensively surveyed. Five to 15 percent of these patients may progress to complete bilateral bundle branch block and complete atrioventricular block. With acute myocardial infarction, 25 to 50 percent may go on to complete atrioventricular block. This implies that the sole remaining pathway to the ventricle, the posterior fascicle, eventually will also fail to conduct. Thus in these patients

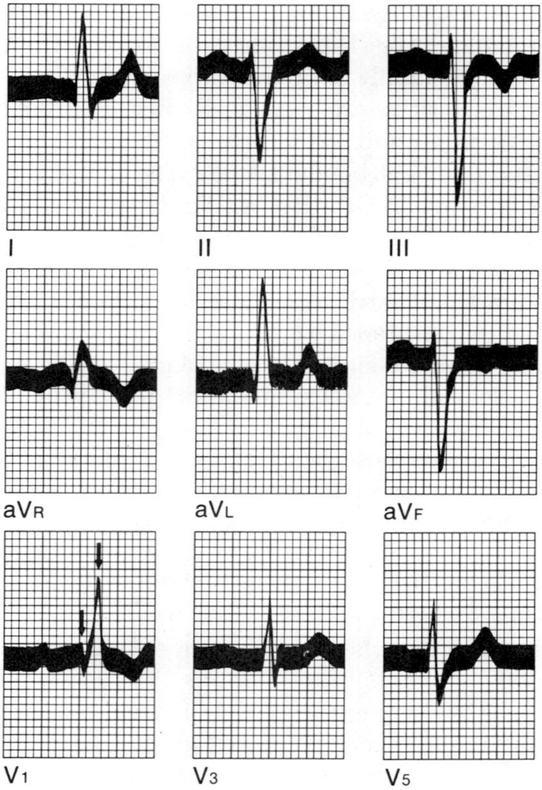

Figure 28. *Right bundle branch block and left anterior fascicular block.* There is a wide S wave in leads I and V5; rR′ is present in V1 (at arrows), and there is prolongation of the QRS (0.14 sec), identifying the right bundle branch block. The marked left axis deviation (–62°) identifies the left anterior fascicular block.

there is a risk that Adams–Stokes episodes, bradycardia, and ventricular failure or cardiac arrest may develop, often suddenly.

3.2.5.2.4 RIGHT BUNDLE BRANCH BLOCK AND POSTERIOR FASCICULAR BLOCK

In this defect there is complete block of these two fascicles (Fig. 24).

The diagnostic criteria (Table 1) essentially require the presence of right bundle branch block with a moderate to marked right axis deviation. If the axis of the QRS is around +120°, or S is seen in I and qR in II, III, and aVF, with the R rather large in these leads, and if one can rule out clinically the same conditions that must be excluded under posterior fascicular block alone, the diagnosis can be made.

This defect occurs in the same pathological conditions as does right bundle branch block with anterior fascicular block.

The consequences are more serious than they are in right bundle branch block with anterior fascicular block. As many as 63 percent of patients may progress to complete atrioventricular block because of the development of permanent damage to the remaining functional pathway, the anterior fascicle. It is likely that coexistence of right bundle branch block and posterior fascicular block indicates some cryptic damage to the more vulnerable anterior fascicle; provocative testing by atrial pacing may reveal this damage.

3.2.5.2.5 ANTERIOR FASCICULAR BLOCK AND POSTERIOR FASCICULAR BLOCK

Complete block of these two fascicles (Fig. 24) results in complete left bundle branch block.

The diagnostic criteria (Table 1) are the same as those due to block in the main stem of the left bundle if both fascicles are blocked simultaneously. If, at first, they are separately blocked, as is usually the case, then serial electrocardiograms will show first one (anterior fascicular block) and then the other (posterior fascicular block), or every other beat may demonstrate a change in block (intermittent alternating fascicular block). When finally a left bundle branch block pattern appears, a diagnosis of bifascicular block due to anterior and posterior fascicular block can be made.

This type of block occurs in the same disease states as

does left bundle branch block, and its consequences are similarly dependent on the underlying disease.

3.2.5.3 Trifascicular (Multifascicular) Block

All forms of trifascicular block arise from the same causes as bifascicular block due to combined right and left bundle branch block. Furthermore, the consequences are dependent upon the development of complete atrioventricular block in all these multifascicular blocks. An increased P–R interval (due to an increased H–V interval) is seen in all the forms of these blocks where atrioventricular conduction occurs.

3.2.5.3.1 RIGHT BUNDLE BRANCH BLOCK, ANTERIOR FASCICULAR BLOCK, AND POSTERIOR FASCICULAR BLOCK

In this defect there is complete bilateral bundle branch block, producing complete atrioventricular block.

The ventricles are under the control of an idioventricular rhythm. Each P wave is followed by an H wave, and a normal H–LB interval is recorded in contrast to right bundle branch block and left main stem bundle branch block (Table 1). However, there is no LB–V interval, since the excitation is blocked in the fascicles of the left branch (Fig. 24), that is, beyond its main stem.

3.2.5.3.2 RIGHT BUNDLE BRANCH BLOCK, ANTERIOR FASCICULAR BLOCK, AND INCOMPLETE POSTERIOR FASCICULAR BLOCK

In this defect there is complete block in the right bundle and anterior fascicle, with delayed conduction in the posterior fascicle (Fig. 24).

The diagnostic criteria (Table 1) consist of right bundle branch block, marked left axis deviation, and an increased P–R interval. The latter occurs because of an increased H–V interval, with a slowing of the LB–V conduction.

3.2.5.3.3 RIGHT BUNDLE BRANCH BLOCK, POSTERIOR FASCICULAR BLOCK, AND INCOMPLETE ANTERIOR FASCICULAR BLOCK

In this defect there is complete block in the right bundle and posterior fascicle, with delayed conduction in the anterior fascicle (Fig. 24).

The diagnostic criteria (Table 1) consist of right bundle branch block, right axis deviation, and a prolonged P–R interval. The H–V and LB–V intervals also are prolonged.

3.2.5.3.4 RIGHT BUNDLE BRANCH BLOCK, INCOMPLETE ANTERIOR FASCICULAR BLOCK, AND INCOMPLETE POSTERIOR FASCICULAR BLOCK

In this defect there is complete block in the right bundle and delayed conduction in both anterior and posterior fascicles of the left branch (Fig. 24).

The diagnostic criteria (Table 1) consist of right bundle branch block and a prolonged P–R interval. The pattern is similar to the bifascicular combination of right bundle branch block and incomplete left bundle branch block. However, in bifascicular block, the H–V interval is increased by a lengthened H–LB interval due to delay at the main stem of the left bundle. In the trifascicular block, the H–V interval is prolonged by a lengthened LB–V interval due to delay in both left fascicles; the H–LB interval is normal.

3.2.5.3.5 RIGHT BUNDLE BRANCH BLOCK, ANTERIOR FASCICULAR BLOCK, AND INCOMPLETE LEFT BUNDLE BRANCH BLOCK

In this defect there is complete block in the right bundle branch and anterior fascicle and delayed conduction in the main stem of the left bundle (Fig. 24).

The diagnostic criteria (Table 1) are those of right bundle branch block, marked left axis deviation, and a prolonged P–R interval. The latter is due to an increase in H–V interval and not a prolonged P–H interval. A prolonged H–LB interval accounts for the increased H–V period.

3.2.5.3.6 RIGHT BUNDLE BRANCH BLOCK, POSTERIOR FASCICULAR BLOCK, AND INCOMPLETE LEFT BUNDLE BRANCH BLOCK

In this defect there is complete block in the right bundle and posterior fascicle and delayed conduction in the main stem of the left bundle (Fig. 24).

The diagnostic criteria (Table 1) are those of right bundle branch block with posterior fascicular block and a prolonged P–R interval. The latter is due to an increase in the H–V and H–LB intervals and not to a long P–H interval.

3.2.5.3.7 ANTERIOR FASCICULAR BLOCK, POSTERIOR FASCICULAR BLOCK, AND INCOMPLETE RIGHT BUNDLE BRANCH BLOCK

In this defect there is complete block in the two fascicles and delay in conduction over the right bundle branch (Fig. 24).

The diagnostic criteria (Table 1) are essentially those of left bundle branch block and a prolonged P–R interval. The latter results from an increase in the H–V interval by virtue of a lengthened H–RB interval.

3.2.5.4 Diffuse Intraventricular (Myofibrillar) Block

In this conduction defect (Table 1), delay occurs in the myofibrillar structures, the impulse having traveled normally over the specialized atrioventricular tissues.

The diagnostic criterion is an abnormally wide QRS complex whose contour is the same as during normal intraventricular conduction. No evidence of bundle branch block or fascicular block is seen.

The defect occurs in severe myocarditis, extensive infiltrative myocardial disease, and chronic diffuse myocardial diseases such as rheumatic heart disease or atherosclerotic heart disease, particularly in the presence of ventricular aneurysms. It may be seen with severe hypoxia, hypothermia, hyperkalemia, and excessive doses of quinidine or procainamide.

3.2.5.5 Rarer Forms of Intraventricular Conduction Defects

The common forms of intraventricular conduction defects are permanent forms of block. It is now well known that transitory blocks of all these types may occur, some even on a purely functional basis in normal hearts. For example, if supraventricular premature contractions fall during the period of relative refractoriness which follows the preceding beat, one can see QRS complexes of the fascicular block type. Right bundle branch block alone is the commonest, but may coexist with anterior fascicular block or posterior fascicular block.

Similarly, changing intraventricular conduction can be seen when abnormalities of impulse transmission vary from one fascicle to another, or the degree of delay varies in the same fascicle from time to time or beat to beat. Hence there can be a Wenckebach (type I) type of block in a single fascicle when decremental conduction exists there, such that the impulse takes longer and longer to get through and finally is blocked. A Mobitz (type II) type of block also can occur, such that in any one fascicle there is intermittent (2:1, 3:1) complete fascicular block. Every second or third beat will then show complete fascicular block. These are rare phenomena however.

In early trifascicular blocks, each one of the three fascicles—right bundle, anterior fascicle, and posterior fascicle (Fig. 24)—can be blocked at different times, but only one may be blocked at any one time. Thus only serial electrocardiograms showing right bundle branch block, anterior fascicular block, and posterior fascicular block, each at different times, permit the diagnosis of trifascicular, not just monofascicular, disease.

Two fascicles blocked at once, but with variation in the pairing, have also been seen. For example, right bundle branch block with anterior fascicular block may be seen at first; then, at a later date, right bundle branch block with posterior fascicular block may appear. This type of block is likely to progress, even suddenly, to trifascicular block of the bilateral bundle branch block variety.

The relationship of abnormal atrioventricular conduction, as indicated by prolongation of the P–R interval or type I (Wenckebach) or type II (Mobitz) forms of second degree atrioventricular block, assumes new importance in intraventricular conduction disturbances. As seen in Table 1, the presence of such abnormalities, which formerly were ascribed to atrioventricular nodal disease and not to disease of the bundle branches, can indicate a bifascicular block (right bundle branch block with prolonged P–R interval) or a trifascicular block (the six forms noted in Table 1) when the QRS abnormalities alone would suggest lower degrees of fascicular block.

3.2.6 ANOMALOUS ATRIOVENTRICULAR CONDUCTION (VENTRICULAR PREEXCITATION)

A bypass tract at the atrioventricular margin acts as a bridge to permit early excitation of some basal portion of the ventricular mass (Fig. 29). These short-circuit paths circumvent the atrioventricular node and its delaying action, and excitation over the bypass can thus precede the normal sequence to some part, at least, of the ventricle. It is characterized electrocardiographically by a short P–R interval (<0.12 sec in adults and <0.09 sec in children), a prolonged QRS (>0.10 sec in adults and >0.09 sec in children) and a delta wave, or slow slurring, in the initial part of the QRS complex (Fig. 30). This slow component occurs at the initial inscription of the widened QRS, in contrast to any form of intraventricular conduction defects where the slow component is later. This can be demonstrated by vectorcardiography when the slow initial component may be seen to last for 0.02 to 0.06 sec. The wide QRS may be followed by abnormal T waves. The point of entry of the preexcitation into the ventricle determines the form of QRS complex. If the atrioventricular bridge terminates in the posterior basal portion of either ventricle, it is termed type A. The major deflection in all of the six V leads of the electrocardiogram is an R wave, and there is often a right axis deviation.

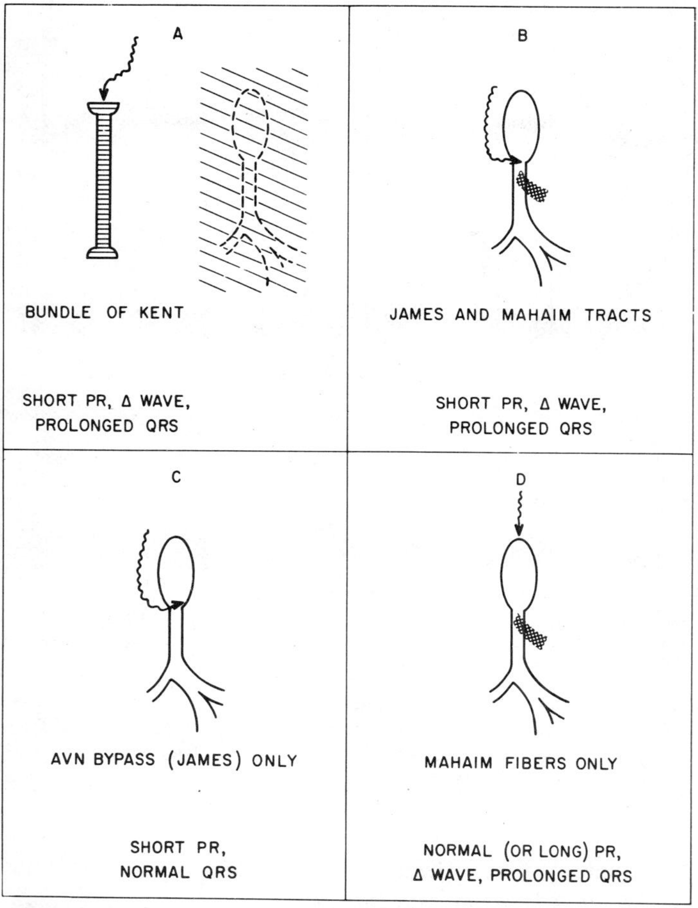

Figure 29. *Various anatomic bypass tracts capable of producing anomalous atrioventricular conduction (ventricular preexcitation).* The expected electrocardiographic features are noted beneath each of the four pathways (A–D). (Reproduced by permission from Ferrer, M. I., *Electrocardiographic Notebook* [4th ed.]. Futura Publishing Company, Mt. Kisco, N.Y., 1973.)

If the preexcitation begins anteriorly and laterally at the base of the right ventricle, it is a type B, with negative QRS complexes (QS) in V1, R waves in V6, and often a left axis deviation. If the bypass ends at the anterior lateral margin of the left ventricle, it is a type C: excitation moves

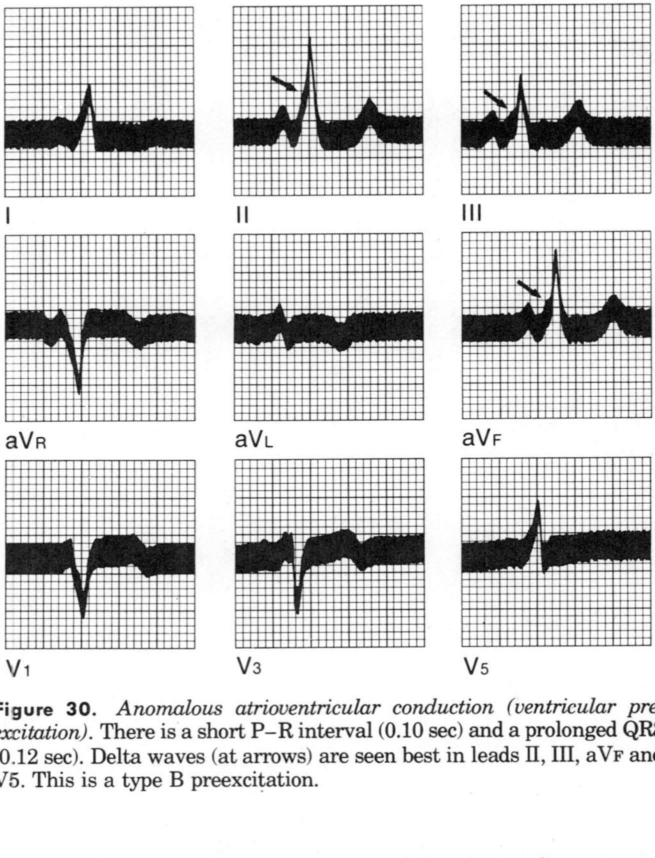

Figure 30. *Anomalous atrioventricular conduction (ventricular preexcitation).* There is a short P–R interval (0.10 sec) and a prolonged QRS (0.12 sec). Delta waves (at arrows) are seen best in leads II, III, aVF and V5. This is a type B preexcitation.

from left to right, V6 has a large and dominant S wave and V1 a large R wave, and right axis deviation is present.

The bypass tracts (Fig. 29) may be a single bundle of Kent or the combined James (periatrioventricular nodal) and Mahaim (His bundle to ventricle) fibers. The ventricles may be totally excited via the bypass, or there may be a double conduction to the ventricles, one by the bypass, the other over normal atrioventricular pathways. The amount of ventricle captured by the bypass may vary, depending upon the degree of preexcitaton and the normal atrioventricular nodal delay. Thus there may be variation in the QRS complex in the same subject.

These atrioventricular bridges are capable of bidirectional conduction, and the arrhythmias seen in these patients are produced by re-entrant mechanisms using the bypass and the normal atrioventricular sequence in series. Over half the patients with preexcitation of the short P–R—long QRS type have paroxysmal tachycardias. Atrial tachycardia and atrial fibrillation or flutter are the most common. This combination of preexcitation and attacks of arrhythmia is called the Wolff-Parkinson-White (WPW) syndrome.

There are two other variants of preexcitation (Fig. 29), one in which there is only a short P–R (no delta wave and no prolongation of QRS), where only the perinodal fibers of James are operative. These patients also may have paroxysmal tachycardia, and when they have tachycardia are said to have the Lown-Ganong-Levine (LGL) syndrome. The other variant has a normal P–R interval, but a long QRS and delta wave, resulting from bypass over Mahaim fibers only. The utilization of any of these atrioventricular bridges need not be constant, and the electrocardiographic evidence for it may therefore be intermittent.

Anomalous atrioventricular conduction usually exists in otherwise normal hearts, but it also occurs in association with certain congenital lesions, notably Ebstein's anomaly and transposition of the great vessels. The only symptoms which are ascribed to this preexcitation are those which are due to the episodes of arrhythmia.

3.3 Disturbances in Supravalvular, Valvular, or Subvalvular Function

3.3.1 AORTIC OBSTRUCTION

3.3.1.1 Supravalvular Obstruction

3.3.1.2 Valvular Obstruction

3.3.1.3 Subvalvular Obstruction

Obstruction to blood flow from the left ventricle can occur as the result of congenital anomalies or acquired disease and can involve the valve or regions above or below the valve. Stenosis of the valve can result from congenital abnormalities, from changes induced by rheumatic fever, and from calcific changes of unknown cause affecting a previously normal, unicuspid, or bicuspid valve. Supravalvular obstruction to blood flow can be caused by narrowing of the aorta induced by a fibromuscular membrane or hypoplasia of the aorta. Subaortic obstruction may result from a discrete fibrous diaphragm below a normal valve or from diffuse hypertrophy of the ventricular septum, which abuts the anterior leaflet of the mitral valve during systole.

When the area involved is considerably reduced, an increase in left ventricular systolic pressure ensues. A systolic pressure gradient is present between points proximal and distal to the obstruction. The left ventricle can hypertrophy, dilate, or fail as a consequence of the increased work induced by the obstruction.

A paucity of symptoms characterizes lesser degrees of obstruction. Severe obstruction may be manifested by dizziness, syncope, anginal syndrome, left ventricular failure, or sudden death.

With obstruction due to valvular deformity or to a subvalvular discrete fibrous membrane, the aortic component of the second sound can be reduced in intensity and delayed sufficiently to produce paradoxical splitting of the second sound. In the more severe degrees of obstruction, when hypertrophy of the left ventricle is marked, a fourth heart sound is audible. A harsh crescendo-decrescendo ejection systolic murmur of variable intensity is usually heard best to the right of the upper sternum and is also audible in the carotid arteries. The murmur is less well transmitted to the apical area, although sometimes this is the only site where it can be heard. A systolic thrill to the right of the sternum or over the carotid areas can accompany louder murmurs. Ejection clicks may occur. The pulse pressure in the systemic arteries may be small, and the pulse may rise slowly and have an anacrotic notch. Echocardiographic findings are discussed in Sections 2.15.3, 2.15.4, and 2.15.5.

Supravalvular obstruction is almost always accompanied by other extracardiac anomalies. The aortic component of the second sound may be normal in intensity; the other physical findings resemble those encountered in valvular obstruction, except that ejection clicks are rare.

In patients with diffuse subvalvular hypertrophy of the septum, the aortic component of the second sound may be faint and delayed, with paradoxical splitting of the second sound. The systolic ejection murmur and thrill may be maximal along the left sternal border. The degree of obstruction and the intensity of the murmur are often increased by the Valsalva maneuver, inotropic agents, amyl nitrite, and premature beats. Echocardiographic evidence of dynamic obstruction may likewise be brought out by these procedures. (See Section 2.5.2.12.) Systolic clicks are common. The systemic arterial pulse rises and falls rapidly, with a secondary rise before the dicrotic notch. Characteristically, there are variations in the systolic pressure gradient between the left ventricular cavity and the subvalvular area. These variations result from changes in the force of left ventricular contraction, the size of the left ventricular cavity, and the transmural pressure that distends the outflow tract during systole. In addition, a systolic pressure gradient may exist across the right ventricular outflow tract caused by protrusion of the hypertrophied septum to the right. Mitral regurgitation is frequently present.

ONE OF THE FOLLOWING CRITERIA IS REQUIRED FOR THE DIAGNOSIS OF AORTIC OBSTRUCTION.

1. Demonstration of a pressure gradient during systole between points proximal and distal to the obstruction.
2. Angiocardiographic evidence of the stenotic area and evidence of left ventricular enlargement.
3. The presence of a harsh, crescendo-decrescendo systolic murmur at the right base of the heart which radiates to the neck, with an absent or faint aortic component of the second sound and a small systemic arterial pulse pressure.
4. The presence of a harsh, crescendo-decrescendo

systolic murmur at the right base of the heart which radiates to the neck, and evidence of calcification of the aortic valve cusps.

5. The presence of a harsh crescendo-decrescendo murmur along the left sternal border; paradoxical splitting of the second heart sound; a bifid systemic arterial pulse; and increase in the intensity of the murmur or of echocardiographic signs of outflow obstruction by the Valsalva maneuver, inotropic agents, or nitrites.

3.3.2 AORTIC REGURGITATION

A wide variety of lesions can induce aortic regurgitation. The valve cusps can be deformed by rheumatic fever, infective endocarditis, calcification, or myxomatous degeneration. Lesions of the aorta induced by syphilis, cystic medial necrosis, ankylosing spondylitis, or dissecting hematoma can also result in aortic regurgitation, as may severe systemic hypertension. Downward displacement of an aortic cusp as a result of a congenital malformation may also produce regurgitation.

Regurgitation causes an increase in left ventricular diastolic volume and work; consequently, the left ventricle may dilate and hypertrophy. Dilatation of the ascending aorta is frequently present. Although regurgitation may be tolerated for long periods without symptoms, ultimately it may lead to left ventricular failure or anginal syndrome.

A blowing, decrescendo diastolic murmur starting with the aortic component of the second sound is characteristic of aortic regurgitation. The murmur is best heard in the third and fourth intercostal spaces to the left of the sternum with the patient leaning forward and with the breath expelled. It occasionally radiates to the cardiac apex. Because of the large stroke volume, there may be a systolic murmur heard over or cephalad to the aortic area. The pulse can be bounding, with an elevated systolic and a decreased diastolic pressure.

Secondary echocardiographic manifestations of aortic regurgitation include a fine fluttering motion of the anterior leaflet of the mitral valve and signs of left ventricular volume overload such as chamber dilatation and exaggerated wall motion.

ONE OF THE FOLLOWING CRITERIA IS REQUIRED FOR THE DIAGNOSIS OF AORTIC REGURGITATION.

1. Evidence of regurgitation into the left ventricle of angiocardiographic contrast medium or other suitable indicators following an aortic injection.
2. A blowing, decrescendo diastolic murmur starting with the second heart sound, heard best in the third and fourth intercostal spaces close to the sternum, in the absence of causes for pulmonic regurgitation.

3.3.3 MITRAL OBSTRUCTION

Obstruction to the flow across the mitral valve most often results from valvular deformities following rheumatic fever. Rarely, congenital deformation of the valve or obstruction of the valve orifice by tumors can be encountered. Obstruction due to left atrial tumors may be intermittent and related to change in position as the tumor prolapses into the mitral orifice.

When the area of the valve orifice is reduced considerably, the mean pressure in the left atrium exceeds that in the left ventricle during diastole. The increased pressure in the left atrium is reflected throughout the pulmonary vasculature. Left atrial, pulmonary arterial, and right ventricular enlargement ensue. Vascular changes may appear in the pulmonary arteries, further elevating pulmonary arterial pressures.

Patients usually present with symptoms of pulmonary congestion with or without concomitant evidence of right ventricular failure. The first heart sound and the pulmonic component of the second heart sound may be accentuated. Closely following the second heart sound, a short, high-pitched sound, the *opening snap*, is often audible in patients with valvular deformity. An early diastolic low-pitched, rumbling murmur which is localized to the apex, or a presystolic crescendo murmur, or both are characteristic of mitral obstruction. Frequently, these murmurs can only be heard when the patient is placed in the left lateral decubitus position after exercise.

In patients with intermittent obstruction due to left atrial tumors, the abrupt fall in cardiac output may lead to dizziness or syncope with changes in position. The murmurs described above may be present. However, the first heart sound is often not accentuated and an early diastolic sound caused by movement of the tumor occurs later than an opening snap.

M-mode echocardiography is most helpful in evaluating the amplitude of excursion and the closing velocity of the anterior mitral leaflet, posterior leaflet motion, and evidence of leaflet thickening and calcification. Left atrial tumors causing intermittent or fixed obstruction can also be seen by this technique. Cross-sectional imaging has a high degree of correlation with actual mitral valve orifice size.

ONE OF THE FOLLOWING CRITERIA IS REQUIRED FOR THE DIAGNOSIS OF MITRAL OBSTRUCTION.

1. **Demonstration of a pressure gradient across the mitral valve during diastole.**
2. **Angiocardiographic or echocardiographic evidence of mitral stenosis and evidence of left atrial enlargement or pulmonary congestion not otherwise explained.**
3. **The characteristic murmur as previously described, with one of the following: accentuation of the first heart sound, an opening snap, radiologic evidence of enlargement of the left atrium or calcification of the valve leaflets.**

3.3.4 MITRAL REGURGITATION

Inability of mitral valve leaflets to appose precisely or to close completely may be caused by a wide variety of lesions. The valve leaflets may be damaged by rheumatic fever, infective endocarditis, or myxomatous degeneration. Rarely, extensive subanular calcification of the zone of attachment of the mitral valve to the left ventricular myocardium, with extension of the calcification to the mitral leaflets, can produce regurgitation. Regurgitation can also result from congenital clefts in the mitral leaflets, rupture or fibrosis of the papillary muscles, rupture of the chordae tendineae, or prolapse of mitral leaflets. Occasionally, dilatation, aneurysm, or asynergy of the left ventricle can interfere with the function of the papillary muscles and chordae tendineae so that valve closure is incomplete. Hypertrophy of the ventricular septum such as may be encountered in "idiopathic hypertrophic subaortic stenosis" also may interfere with mitral valve closure. Regurgitation can also be produced by a variety of arrhythmias, particularly when atrial systole is absent or misplaced in relation to ventricular systole.

The failure of the valve to achieve complete closure permits flow of blood from the ventricle into the left atrium during systole. This results in an added volume load on the left ventricle during diastole. Consequently, the left ventricle may dilate, hypertrophy, or fail. Left atrial enlargement usually is conspicuous with mitral regurgitation of long duration, especially when the onset is in childhood. Mitral regurgitation arising in adult life, especially in middle age, is often not associated with enlargement of the left atrium.

The presenting symptoms may be those of easy fatigability or of pulmonary congestion. The first heart sound is usually diminished in intensity, and a third heart sound is commonly present. The timing, duration, and site of associated systolic murmurs and thrills vary and are dependent on the severity and the cause of the lesion. With regurgitation due to valvular deformity, a harsh, holosystolic, high-pitched murmur is present at the apex and is transmitted to the axilla. Regurgitation following rupture of the chordae tendineae predominantly involving the posterior mitral leaflet is associated with an holosystolic murmur best heard along the left sternal border, while rupture of the chordae tendineae of the anterior leaflet is often associated with an holosystolic murmur at the apex which radiates to the axilla or head. Fibrosis of a papillary muscle may be associated with an apical systolic murmur which begins after the first heart sound and ends before the second. The finding of mid-systolic clicks and a late apical systolic murmur is frequently associated with a mild degree of regurgitation and is often found with myxomatous degeneration of the valve.

A mid-diastolic murmur secondary to a high rate of flow may be heard at the apex in the absence of mitral obstruction.

Left atrial pressure curves characteristically show a loss of the X descent and a prominent V wave. There are at present no reliable echocardiographic criteria for the qualitative or quantitative assessment of mitral regurgitation per se, although secondary hemodynamic effects of increased left atrial or left ventricular volume load may be appreciated.

ONE OF THE FOLLOWING CRITERIA IS REQUIRED FOR THE DIAGNOSIS OF MITRAL REGURGITATION.

1. Evidence of regurgitation into the left atrium of angiocardiographic contrast material or other suitable indicators following a left ventricular injection.
2. Loss of the X descent in the left atrial pressure curves.
3. An holosystolic murmur at the apex which is transmitted to the axilla, and enlargement of the left ventricle and left atrium.
4. The abrupt appearance of a systolic murmur at the apex or along the lower left sternal border which radiates to the axilla, back, base, or head, and the rapid development of pulmonary congestion.

3.3.5 PULMONIC OBSTRUCTION

3.3.5.1 VALVULAR OBSTRUCTION

3.3.5.2 SUBVALVULAR OBSTRUCTION

Obstruction to blood flow from the right ventricle is almost invariably the consequence of a congenital abnormality, either valvular stenosis or massive hypertrophy of the outflow tract of the right ventricle. Rarely, disseminated carcinoid tumor may affect the valve cusps, thereby producing stenosis. Right ventricular endocardial tumors may produce fixed or intermittent obstruction of the valve orifice.

As a result of the obstruction, the right ventricular systolic pressure becomes elevated and exceeds that distal to the lesion, and right ventricular hypertrophy develops. Lesser degrees of obstruction may not produce symptoms. However, with severe obstruction, syncope is not unusual.

The pulmonic component of the second sound may be delayed and diminished in intensity. A characteristic loud, harsh, medium-pitched ejection systolic murmur, accompanied by a thrill, is best heard in the first and second left intercostal spaces, but may be heard down the left sternal border, in the back, or in the neck. Ejection clicks are commonly present with valvular stenosis. Post-stenotic dilatation of the pulmonary artery, frequently restricted to the left main pulmonary artery, may be revealed by radiologic studies.

Echocardiography of the pulmonic valve may demonstrate an exaggerated "a" wave with moderate or severe stenosis, as well as premature opening of the pulmonic valve. These findings, however, are more dependent on diastolic than on systolic pressure relationships, and may not be present.

ONE OF THE FOLLOWING CRITERIA IS REQUIRED FOR THE DIAGNOSIS OF PULMONIC OBSTRUCTION.

1. Demonstration of a systolic pressure gradient between the inflow tract of the right ventricle and some point distal to it.
2. Angiocardiographic evidence of the stenotic area and evidence of right ventricular enlargement.
3. The characteristic systolic murmur previously described, with evidence of right ventricular enlargement.

3.3.6 PULMONIC REGURGITATION

Pulmonic regurgitation is an uncommon physiologic abnormality that may result from congenital malformations of the cusps, infective endocarditis, surgical correction of pulmonary valvular stenosis, severe pulmonary hypertension of unknown cause or that following mitral obstruction, or the rarer forms of pulmonary heart disease. The pulmonary arterial diastolic pressure sometimes is reduced to the level of the elevated end-diastolic pressure of the enlarged right ventricle.

A high-pitched, blowing decrescendo murmur heard in the second, third, or fourth interspaces to the left of the sternum is characteristic of regurgitation through the pulmonic valve.

ONE OF THE FOLLOWING CRITERIA IS REQUIRED FOR THE DIAGNOSIS OF PULMONIC REGURGITATION.

1. Evidence of regurgitation into the right ventricle of angiocardiographic contrast medium or other suitable indicators following a pulmonary arterial injection.
2. Close approximation of the pressure at the end of diastole in the pulmonary artery and right ventricle in the presence of the murmur as previously described.
3. Demonstration of the murmur in the right ventricular outflow tract by intracardiac phonocardiography.
4. The murmur as described previously, occurring in the presence of severe pulmonary hypertension of unknown cause or in patients with pulmonary heart disease secondary to multiple pulmonary emboli, granulomatous lesions, or extensive pulmonary fibrosis.

3.3.7 TRICUSPID OBSTRUCTION

Tricuspid obstruction can result from scarring of the valve due to rheumatic fever, carcinoid tumor, occlusion of the valve orifice by tumors or thrombi, and, rarely, congenital anomalies.

As a result of the obstruction, blood flow from the

right atrium to the right ventricle is impeded during ventricular diastole, with a consequent rise in pressure in the right atrium and the appearance of a diastolic pressure gradient across the valve. Right atrial enlargement and systemic venous congestion ensue.

The diastolic or presystolic murmur associated with tricuspid obstruction is relatively low-pitched, blowing, and heard best to the right or left of the lower sternum. It frequently is accentuated during inspiration.

ONE OF THE FOLLOWING CRITERIA IS REQUIRED FOR THE DIAGNOSIS OF TRICUSPID OBSTRUCTION.

1. Demonstration of a pressure gradient across the valve during diastole.
2. Angiocardiographic evidence of tricuspid stenosis and evidence of right atrial enlargement or systemic congestion not otherwise explained.
3. Presence of the murmur previously described and evidence of right atrial enlargement or systemic venous congestion.

3.3.8 TRICUSPID REGURGITATION

Regurgitation of blood from the right ventricle into the right atrium during ventricular systole may arise as a result of damage to the valves induced by rheumatic fever, carcinoid tumor, trauma, or infective endocarditis. Rupture of the chordae tendineae may also produce regurgitation. Marked dilatation of the right ventricle can interfere with the function of the papillary muscle and chordae tendineae, so that valve closure is incomplete. Loss of atrial contraction, as in atrial fibrillation, may contribute to the poor closure of the valve.

Regurgitation induces a rise in pressure during ventricular systole in the right atrium and consequently in the systemic veins. Right atrial enlargement and systemic venous congestion result, with loss of the X descent in the right atrial pressure curve and a prominent V wave.

The murmur associated with tricuspid regurgitation

is pansystolic, blowing, of medium pitch, and best heard in the fourth or fifth intercostal spaces close to or over the sternum. The murmur is accentuated by inspiration.

ONE OF THE FOLLOWING CRITERIA IS REQUIRED FOR THE DIAGNOSIS OF TRICUSPID REGURGITATION.

1. **Evidence of significant regurgitation into the right atrium of angiocardiographic contrast medium or other suitable indicators following a right ventricular injection.**
2. **Loss of the X descent in the right atrial pressure curve.**
3. **Presence of a murmur as previously described and enlargement of the right atrium.**

3.3.9 MALFUNCTION OF PROSTHESES AND HOMOGRAFTS

Malfunction of intracardiac prostheses may be due to a paravalvular leak, deterioration in the poppet portion of the prosthesis, formation of a thrombus in and about the prosthesis, ingrowth of fibrous tissue, or vegetations following infection. Malfunction soon after implantation of the prosthesis suggests paravalvular leak rather than the other causes.

The manifestations of malfunction are those of valvular obstruction or regurgitation at the site of the prosthesis. Palpitations, syncope, ventricular failure, venous congestion, or new murmurs may suddenly appear. Hemolytic anemia may occur when trauma to the erythrocytes increases in the malfunctioning prosthesis. Rarely, the poppet is dislodged from the cage and may embolize. Ball variance is less frequent with metallic than with plastic poppets.

Prosthetic malfunction may be accompanied by diminution or absence of the prosthetic opening sound or variation in its intensity from beat to beat. Serial changes in the phonocardiogram may be useful in early detection. Echocardiography or fluoroscopy may show restricted ball movement.

Malfunction of an aortic homograft or porcine zenograft in the aortic or mitral area is suggested by the onset of ventricular failure or progressive widening of the pulse pressure. A diastolic murmur is often associated with homograft implantation and does not necessarily mean graft malfunction.

ONE OF THE FOLLOWING CRITERIA IS REQUIRED FOR THE DIAGNOSIS OF MALFUNCTION OF PROSTHESES OR HOMOGRAFTS.

1. **New appearance of valvular obstruction or regurgitation at the site of the implanted prosthesis.**
2. **Appearance of changes in sounds generated by the prosthetic valve.**
3. **Radiographic or echocardiographic evidence of abnormal motion or altered dimensions of the prosthesis.**

3.3.10 PROLAPSE OF VALVES

3.3.10.1 Prolapse of the Aortic Valve

Prolapse of one or more cusps of the aortic valve may result from Marfan's syndrome, myxomatous degeneration, or dissecting hematoma. It may also develop in association with ventricular septal defects.

Aortic regurgitation may result. Aortography may demonstrate the abnormal displacement of a cusp.

THE FOLLOWING CRITERION IS REQUIRED FOR THE DIAGNOSIS OF PROLAPSE OF THE AORTIC VALVE.

Aortographic demonstration of a cusp displaced downward toward the left ventricle.

3.3.10.2 Prolapse of the Mitral Valve

Marfan's syndrome or myxomatous degeneration of valve leaflets or the chordae tendineae may cause displacement of one or both mitral leaflets into the left atrium during ventricular systole. Barlow's syndrome, a common but relatively benign form of mitral prolapse, may long be asymptomatic.

Prolapse is frequently associated with an apical mid-systolic click and a late systolic murmur. Associated mitral regurgitation is common, and abnormalities in left ventricular contraction are sometimes seen. Although left ventriculography has been considered necessary for a definitive diagnosis, echocardiographic evaluation has gained increasing importance. There may be characteristic late or pansystolic posterior displacement of one or both of the mitral leaflets, often most prominent for the posterior leaflet.

THE FOLLOWING CRITERION IS REQUIRED FOR THE DIAGNOSIS OF PROLAPSE OF THE MITRAL VALVE.

Angiocardiographic or echocardiographic demonstration of prolapse of one or more leaflets of the mitral valve.

3.4 Disturbances in Myocardial Function

3.4.1 VENTRICULAR FAILURE

Ventricular failure occurs when myocardial function renders the heart unable to perform normally as a pump. Abnormal myocardial function can result from loss or malfunction of contractile elements or from changes in the anatomic arrangements of the muscle fiber. Ventricular failure is present when the ratio of forward stroke volume to the end-diastolic volume (ejection fraction) of the involved ventricle is diminished. At present, direct measurements of end-diastolic volume by ventriculography or indicator dilution techniques are not sufficiently standardized for reliable clinical application. Accordingly, the hemodynamic consequences of a reduction in this ratio are utilized to indicate the presence of ventricular failure. Although M-mode echocardiography does not directly measure left ventricular volume, clinically useful calculations of ventricular dimensions, ejection fraction, and mean rate of circumferential shortening can be derived from echocardiographic measurements when the shape of the ventricle is not grossly distorted. Serial measurements in a patient over an extended period of time may be useful.

Failure of the left ventricle may be accompanied by manifestations of pulmonary hypertension and pulmonary circulatory congestion; failure of the right ventricle may lead to elevation of systemic venous pressure and to systemic circulatory congestion. Combined ventricular failure can occur; indeed, right ventricular failure often results from the pulmonary hypertension induced by left ventricular failure.

The diagnosis of ventricular failure in infants is often difficult, but may be manifested by poor feeding, occasionally accompanied by sweating, irritability, a rapid respiratory rate, and failure to gain weight. An enlarged liver is difficult to evaluate unless it increases rapidly in size. Often it is necessary to give an infant digitalis and observe changes in symptoms and heart or liver size before reaching a diagnosis.

The diagnosis of ventricular failure cannot be made with certainty in the presence of pericardial disease severe enough to impair the filling of the heart.

Severe anemia, thyrotoxicosis, hypoxia, fever, and systemic arteriovenous fistula may be accompanied by normal or high levels of blood flow even in the presence of ventricular failure. This fact must be considered when using some of the diagnostic criteria enumerated below.

3.4.1.1 Left Ventricular Failure

ONE OF THE FOLLOWING CRITERIA IS REQUIRED FOR THE DIAGNOSIS OF LEFT VENTRICULAR FAILURE.

1. Radiologic evidence of a sudden increase in left ventricular size.
2. An S_3 or a summation gallop located over the left ventricle in adults in the absence of mitral regurgitation.
3. In the absence of aortic or mitral valvular disease, angiocardiographic evidence of a dilated left ventri-

cle and a cardiac output below 2.7 L/min/m² BSA, the latter value measured at rest in the supine position and in a basal state.

4. In the absence of aortic or mitral valvular disease or massive hypertrophy of the left ventricle:
   a. Elevation at rest of the left ventricular end-diastolic pressure above 10 mm Hg, or mean left atrial or pulmonary arterial wedge pressure above 12 mm Hg (zero reference is 5 cm below the second costochondral junction with the patient supine) and a resting level of systemic blood flow below 2.7 L/min/m² BSA; *or*
   b. Elevation of left ventricular end-diastolic pressure (or mean left atrial or pulmonary arterial wedge pressure) above 14 mm Hg on moderate supine leg exercise, and an inability either to increase cardiac output more than 800 ml for every 100 ml increase in oxygen consumption or to increase stroke volume; *or*
   c. Manifestations of pulmonary congestion or pulmonary edema in the presence of a large left ventricle.
5. In the presence of aortic obstruction or regurgitation, radiologic evidence of a sudden change in left ventricular size. This criterion reflects the fact that the valvular lesions themselves may reduce the level of systemic blood flow, both at rest and during exercise, and cause elevation of the end-diastolic pressure as a result of ventricular hypertrophy. However, reversal of these physiologic abnormalities by digitalis glycosides does constitute evidence of left ventricular failure.
6. In the presence of mitral obstruction or regurgitation, evidence of an elevated left ventricular end-diastolic pressure. This criterion reflects the fact that elevation of the left atrial or pulmonary arterial wedge pressure and a reduced level of systemic blood flow both at rest and during exercise can result from the valvular lesions themselves. Similarly, in the presence of mi-

tral obstruction, pulmonary congestion cannot be utilized as a criterion of left ventricular failure, even in the presence of a large left ventricle.

3.4.1.2 Right Ventricular Failure

ONE OF THE FOLLOWING CRITERIA IS REQUIRED FOR THE DIAGNOSIS OF RIGHT VENTRICULAR FAILURE.

1. Radiologic evidence of a sudden change in right ventricular size.
2. An S_3 or a summation gallop located over the right ventricle in adults which increases in intensity with inspiration.
3. Pulsus alternans in the pulmonary artery or right ventricle.
4. In the absence of pulmonic or tricuspid valvular disease, angiocardiographic evidence of a dilated right ventricle and a cardiac output below 2.7 L/min/m^2 BSA, the latter value measured at rest in the supine position and in the basal state.
5. In the absence of pulmonary or tricuspid valvular lesions or massive right ventricular hypertrophy:
   a. Elevation of right ventricular end-diastolic (or right atrial mean) pressure above 5 mm Hg and a cardiac output below 2.7 L/min/m^2 BSA. These criteria apply when the patient is supine, at rest in a basal state, and with the zero reference level for measurement of pressure 5 cm below the second costochondral junction; *or*
   b. Elevation of right ventricular end-diastolic (or right atrial mean) pressure above 5 mm Hg on moderate supine leg exercise and an inability either to increase cardiac output more than 800 ml for every 100 ml increase in oxygen consumption or to increase stroke volume; *or*
   c. Evidence of systemic circulatory congestion in the presence of a large right ventricle.
6. In the presence of tricuspid obstruction or regurgitation, demonstration of an elevated right ventricular

end-diastolic pressure. This criterion reflects the fact that elevation of right atrial pressure and a reduced level of blood flow at rest or during exercise may result from the valvular disturbances themselves.

7. In the presence of pulmonic obstruction or regurgitation, angiocardiographic evidence of a dilated right ventricle or radiologic evidence of a sudden change in right ventricular size. This criterion reflects the fact that elevation of right ventricular end-diastolic pressure and a reduced level of pulmonary blood flow, both at rest and during exercise, may result solely from the valvular lesion and the ensuing myocardial hypertrophy and not from ventricular failure alone.

3.4.2 VENTRICULAR ASYNERGY

Localized areas of the ventricular wall may deviate from the coordinated pattern of contraction of the myocardium during systole. Such asynergic regions may show dyskinesis, or paradoxical expansion during systole; akinesis, or absence of motion; hypokinesis, or decreased motion; and asynchrony, or altered sequence of contraction. The type of asynergy reflects the number and contractility of the surviving myocardial fibers in a damaged or ischemic area, the elastic characteristics of inert scar tissue, and alterations in excitation or excitation-contraction coupling. Several patterns of regional asynergy can be present in the same heart.

Asynergic areas can decrease cardiac performance by several mechanisms. The contribution of the asynergic region to force development is lost or decreased, and the surviving muscle must perform more work; blood may be displaced into a large dyskinetic or aneurysmal area; and the performance of adjacent myocardium may be affected by a change in the series elastic component contributed by the asynergic area. Cardiac output and the rate of force development will decrease, especially if the asynergic areas occupy more than 20 percent of the ventricular surface. Asynergy is usually a consequence of myocardial infarction, but can occur in cardiomyopathy. It is usually permanent, but can be transient, as during anginal syndrome or ectopic beats.

Clinical findings usually include evidence of ventricular failure, an enlarged heart, and a double apical impulse. Ventriculography, particularly with cineangiography, is essential to demonstrate the presence, size, and motion of asynergic areas, although changes may be demonstrated by chest roentgenogram, fluoroscopy, echocardiography, or apexcardiography.

THE FOLLOWING CRITERION IS REQUIRED FOR THE DIAGNOSIS OF VENTRICULAR ASYNERGY.

Radiologic demonstration of asynergy, usually by ventriculography or direct observation at the time of surgery.

3.4.3 PERICARDIAL RESTRICTION

A decrease in the compliance of the pericardium as a consequence of widespread fibrosis, calcification, neoplasia, and/or the accumulation of fluid in the pericardial sac may restrict filling of the heart during diastole. In these situations, the dissimilar compliance characteristics of the two ventricles are replaced by those of the effusion or the thickened pericardium. The end-diastolic pressures in the ventricles no longer reflect their individual compliances, but that of the limiting fluid or pericardium. Hence the diastolic pressure in the two ventricles, their atria, and venous beds becomes elevated and virtually the same. The pulmonary arterial and right ventricular systolic pressures are only modestly elevated. The atrial curves show an accentuation of the Y descent, the X descent or both. The ventricular pressure contours show an early diastolic dip at the time of rapid ventricular filling that is more prominent in the presence of pericardial thickening than with fluid accumulation. Evidence of pulmonary and systemic congestion appears, although the manifestations of the latter are dominant. Low voltage of the QRS complexes is often seen.

When the accumulation of fluid is abrupt (pericardial

tamponade), not only is there a rise in ventricular, atrial, and venous pressures, but the stroke volume and cardiac output fall, and ultimately so does the systemic arterial pressure. Dyspnea, orthopnea, engorged neck veins, and a picture resembling cardiogenic shock may ensue.

When restriction is due to a more gradual accumulation of fluid or to pericardial thickening, cardiac output and systemic blood pressure can be well preserved, and manifestations of circulatory congestion predominate.

Both excessive pericardial fluid and scar tissue can cause accentuation of the normal inspiratory fall in systolic pressure in the systemic arteries (pulsus paradoxus). The magnitude of this fall may be 10 to 20 mm Hg. Abnormal filling of the neck veins during inspiration can also be observed. Pericardial restriction due to thickening is usually associated with a heart sound early in diastole (pericardial knock). Removal of fluid and fall to normal of pericardial pressure with persistent elevation of right atrial pressure indicates that thickening rather than effusion is the cause of the restrictive phenomenon. In the presence of cardiac tamponade the electrocardiogram can show electrical alternans, which is a regular alternation in the amplitude of either the P wave, or the QRS complex, or both during normal sinus rhythm. If restriction is due to pericardial thickening, the right lateral border of the cardiac silhouette on x-ray remains straight; it is usually concave with significant pericardial effusion. Chest roentgenograms can show calcification of the pericardium.

Pericardial effusion or thickening can also be demonstrated by radiologic examination following the injection of gas (usually 100 percent carbon dioxide) or contrast material into the right atrium. Scanning of the chest with an automatic scintillation counter following the intravenous injection of radioisotopes can indicate pericardial fluid and thickening if there is a discrepancy between the heart as outlined by the radioisotope scanning and the cardiac silhouette as visualized by a supine 6-foot roentgenogram of the chest. Pericardial fluid, and, in some instances, evidence of restriction, can also be revealed by ultrasound recording (echocardiography), which has become the primary diagnostic tool in this condition. In certain cases computerized tomography may be helpful diagnostically.

ONE OF THE FOLLOWING CRITERIA IS REQUIRED FOR THE DIAGNOSIS OF PERICARDIAL RESTRICTION.

1. Evidence of pericardial effusion, calcification, or thickening confirmed by direct aspiration of fluid or by radiographic studies, radioisotope studies, or echocardiography, and evidence of peripheral and pulmonary congestion.
2. Evidence of peripheral and pulmonary congestion and the characteristic equalization of left and right heart diastolic pressures, small pulmonary arterial pulse pressure, accentuation of the Y or X descent or both in the atrial pressure curves, and an early diastolic dip in the ventricular pressure curves.

3.4.4 MYOCARDIAL RESTRICTION

Decreased compliance of the ventricles may produce disturbances in ventricular filling. The underlying abnormality may be diffuse, severe myocardial hypertrophy, extensive fibrosis, endocardial fibroelastosis, or diffuse infiltrative processes such as amyloidosis, progressive systemic sclerosis, hemochromatosis, or sarcoidosis.

As a consequence of the reduced compliance of the ventricular chamber, its diastolic pressure rises. This is accompanied by elevation of pressure in the corresponding atrium and venous beds. The ventricular pressure curves show an early diastolic dip, while the atrial pressure curves show an accentuation of the Y descent and a large A wave. A fourth heart sound is usually heard. Manifestations of pulmonary and peripheral congestion result from the elevated ventricular diastolic pressure.

ONE OF THE FOLLOWING CRITERIA IS REQUIRED FOR THE DIAGNOSIS OF MYOCARDIAL RESTRICTION.

1. Radiologic evidence of a hypertrophied ventricle, without dilatation, and either an elevated ventricular

end-diastolic pressure or evidence of congestion in the proximal venous bed.

2. **The presence of some infiltrative disease known to be associated with myocardial restriction and evidence of an elevated end-diastolic pressure in the affected ventricle, with an early ventricular diastolic dip.**

3.4.5 CARDIOGENIC SHOCK

The syndrome of cardiogenic shock is characterized by apprehension, cold wet skin, sustained systemic arterial hypotension, tachycardia, and decreased urine flow, all occurring as a consequence of a marked decrease in effective peripheral blood flow secondary to heart disease.

Cardiogenic shock most often follows acute myocardial infarction, but can also be produced by tachycardias with rapid ventricular rates or acute left ventricular failure; it sometimes follows cardiac surgery. The cardiac output is severely reduced, and the systolic blood pressure in the systemic arteries in previously normotensive individuals is below 80 mm Hg.

THE FOLLOWING CRITERIA ARE REQUIRED FOR THE DIAGNOSIS OF CARDIOGENIC SHOCK.

Evidence of the syndrome of shock occurring as a result of acute myocardial infarction, sustained tachycardia, or cardiac surgery.

3.5 Disturbances in Intravascular Pressures

3.5.1 PULMONARY ARTERIAL HYPERTENSION

At the moment of birth, pulmonary arterial pressure is approximately the same as systemic arterial pressure. Soon thereafter, pulmonary arterial pressure falls and continues to do so until, after the first two weeks of life, it lies at levels encountered in the normal adult.

After two weeks of age, pulmonary arterial hypertension exists when the pulmonary arterial pressure exceeds 30 mm Hg systolic, 10 mm Hg diastolic, and 15 mm Hg mean (zero reference is 5 cm below the second costochondral junction) at rest. Under the stress of moderate leg exercise, pulmonary arterial pressures do not normally exceed 30 mm Hg systolic, 14 mm Hg diastolic, and 20 mm Hg mean. Levels of pressure in excess of these limits indicate the presence of pulmonary hypertension, although strenuous exercise may normally be accompanied by higher levels of pressure.

Pulmonary arterial hypertension may develop solely as a consequence of pulmonary venous hypertension. It may also stem from an abnormal resistance to blood flow in the pulmonary arterial tree due to a variety of causes. Disturbances in respiratory gas exchange which lead to hypoxia and acidosis may produce pulmonary arterial vasoconstriction and hypertension. An anatomic curtailment of the pulmonary vascular bed as a result of disease processes either intrinsic or extrinsic to the vessels may also cause pulmonary hypertension. In certain patients the cause of pulmonary hypertension has not been identified, but has been attributed to vasoconstriction. Although pulmonary vascular lesions are associated with this form of hypertension, it is not known whether these lesions result from or cause the elevation in blood pressure.

Right ventricular hypertrophy, dilatation, and failure may ultimately result from pulmonary arterial hypertension.

Echocardiography of the pulmonic valve in patients with pulmonary hypertension has shown absence of the normal "a" wave, a flattening of the diastolic e-f slope, prolongation of the preejection period, and mid-systolic notching; however, these findings are relatively recently described and their exact reliability remains to be determined.

ONE OF THE FOLLOWING CRITERIA IS REQUIRED FOR THE DIAGNOSIS OF PULMONARY ARTERIAL HYPERTENSION.

1. **Elevation of pulmonary arterial pressures above 30 mm Hg systolic, 10 mm diastolic, and 15 mm mean at rest.**
2. **Elevation of pulmonary arterial pressures above 30 mm Hg systolic, 14 mm diastolic, and 20 mean during moderate leg exercise.**

3. Radiologic evidence of enlargement of the main pulmonary artery and its major branches, with narrowing of the more distal segmental and subsegmental branches, which may be irregular and tortuous, especially in the lower lobes.
4. Evidence of right ventricular enlargement in the absence of pulmonary stenosis or left-to-right shunt at the atrial level.
5. Evidence of pulmonary venous hypertension.

3.5.2 PULMONARY VENOUS HYPERTENSION

Pulmonary venous hypertension exists when the mean pressure in the left veno-atrial system exceeds 12 mm Hg at rest (zero reference level is 5 cm below the second costochondral junction) or 14 mm Hg on moderate supine leg exercise.

Pulmonary venous hypertension results from any lesion which causes elevation of the left ventricular end-diastolic or mean left atrial pressure: left ventricular failure, massive hypertrophy of the left ventricle, mitral obstruction or regurgitation, or tumors or thrombi which obstruct the flow of blood from either the pulmonary veins or left atrium. Pericardial or myocardial lesions which affect filling of the left ventricle may also cause pulmonary venous hypertension.

Pulmonary congestion and pulmonary arterial hypertension frequently result from pulmonary venous hypertension.

ONE OF THE FOLLOWING CRITERIA IS REQUIRED FOR THE DIAGNOSIS OF PULMONARY VENOUS HYPERTENSION.

1. Elevation of mean left atrial or pulmonary arterial wedge pressure above 12 mm Hg or of the left ventricular end-diastolic pressure above 12 mm Hg at rest or 14 mm Hg on moderate leg exercise.
2. Evidence of pulmonary congestion or pulmonary arterial hypertension in the presence of left ventricular failure, left ventricular enlargement, or mitral valvular or pericardial disease.

3.5.3 SYSTEMIC ARTERIAL HYPERTENSION

Persistent elevations of the systemic arterial blood pressure greater than 10–15 mm Hg above the appropriate mean for the age, sex, and race of the patient indicate the presence of hypertension. Systemic arterial pressure measurements obtained in a representative sample of the normal adult population are shown in Table 2. Tables 3 and 4 provide mean blood pressures for sample populations of children and adolescents differing in geographic and racial characteristics.

Combined systolic and diastolic hypertension is the common and significant abnormality. Isolated systolic hypertension (decreased aortic compliance) and diastolic hypertension (increased arterial resistance) each produce characteristic changes in left ventricular performance. Peak ventricular pressure is more sensitive to increased arterial resistance than to decreased compliance (according to in vitro comparisons of the two changes in afterload). Sustained arterial hypertension can lead to left ventricular hypertrophy and failure. Isolated systolic hypertension occurs most frequently in the aged and in the developing phase of hypertension in the young.

Primary or essential hypertension connotes hypertension without any identifiable cause. Its estimated prevalence in adults is 15 percent in white and 30 percent in black populations. It occurs in adolescents less frequently and in children apparently rarely. Three subgroups have been defined according to plasma renin activity. Low renin essential hypertension is observed in 20–30 percent, normal renin in 50–60 percent and high renin in the remainder. The etiologic implications of renin heterogeneity in primary hypertension remains to be defined. Anti-hypertensive therapy reduces the incidence of cerebral and renal disease and of left ventricular hypertrophy and failure at diastolic pressures of 103 mm Hg or greater according to studies in adult males. The incidence of coronary artery disease is unaffected.

Secondary hypertension is related to identifiable disorders. It may be associated with bilateral intrinsic renal

Table 2. *Mean Blood Pressures (mm Hg) of Adults*
Health and Nutrition Examination Survey, U.S.A. 1971–1974†*

Blood Pressure and Age (Years)	Female						Male					
	White			Black			White			Black		
	Mean‡	+10	+15	Mean	+10	+15	Mean	+10	+15	Mean	+10	+15
Systolic												
18–24	115.1	**125**	**130**	113.2	**123**	**128**	123.7	**134**	**139**	122.9	**133**	**138**
25–34	116.2	**126**	**131**	121.5	**132**	**137**	125.2	**135**	**140**	129.3	**139**	**144**
35–44	122.6	**133**	**138**	130.5	**141**	**146**	127.0	**137**	**142**	136.7	**147**	**152**
45–54	131.1	**141**	**146**	150.8	**161**	**166**	134.7	**145**	**150**	147.7	**158**	**163**
55–64	143.0	**153**	**158**	153.4	**163**	**168**	139.6	**150**	**155**	144.2	**154**	**159**
65–74	151.6	**162**	**167**	161.3	**171**	**176**	146.0	**156**	**161**	156.6	**167**	**172**
Diastolic												
18–24	71.3	**81**	**86**	72.7	**83**	**88**	76.4	**86**	**91**	76.2	**86**	**91**
25–34	74.6	**85**	**90**	78.0	**88**	**93**	80.8	**91**	**96**	84.3	**94**	**99**
35–44	79.3	**89**	**94**	86.9	**97**	**102**	84.2	**94**	**99**	91.2	**101**	**106**
45–54	82.6	**93**	**98**	93.5	**104**	**109**	87.5	**98**	**103**	91.9	**102**	**107**
55–64	86.2	**96**	**101**	90.6	**101**	**106**	86.4	**96**	**101**	93.4	**103**	**108**
65–74	85.4	**95**	**100**	90.4	**100**	**105**	84.9	**95**	**100**	90.9	**101**	**106**

*These data provide an estimate of mean blood pressures in individuals of specific age, race, and sex. They may be used in comparing an individual blood pressure against group values. Values in boldface represent 10 and 15 mm Hg increments above the mean systolic and diastolic pressures. Serial observations remain the appropriate method of determining arterial pressure pattern and indications of abnormal regulation in the individual patient.

†Total n (6–74 years) = 17,796 ‡Values in bold face represent 10 and 15 mm Hg increments above the mean.

Table 3. *Mean Blood Pressures of Female Children and Adolescents (Data from Samples Differing in Geographic and Racial Characteristics)*

Age (Years)	Health and Nutrition Examination Survey Total $n = 17,796$ male and female				Iowa–Mayo Pool Predominantly white Total $n = 10,988$ male and female		New York, New York Predominantly black and Latin Total $n = 3,537$ male and female	
	Systolic		*Diastolic*					
	White	Black	White	Black	*Systolic*	*Diastolic*	*Systolic*	*Diastolic*
					Females (6–11 years) $n = 3,243$			
6	96.5	95.1	62.1	59.2	97.5	64.7	—	—
7	97.2	102.3	61.3	65.7	101.8	67.5	—	—
8	102.6	101.4	63.3	60.0	105.4	69.5	—	—
9	104.1	106.7	65.3	65.8	108.0	71.2	—	—
10	103.4	106.4	63.9	66.5	110.6	72.1	—	—
11	107.7	104.5	66.8	65.4	115.2	73.8	—	—
					Females (12–18 years) $n = 2,267$		*Females* (14–19 years) $n = 2,022$	
12	109.9	109.5	67.3	68.2	117.3	73.6	—	—
13	111.2	113.1	68.0	71.2	119.1	75.4	—	—
14	113.1	112.5	68.7	67.6	119.4	77.2	110	71
15	112.4	108.3	70.1	67.7	117.9	76.4	110	71
16	113.2	117.9	69.0	72.5	119.6	76.4	112	72
17	112.0	111.6	71.1	70.7	119.5	75.9	113	73
18	—	—	—	—	121.4	77.1	113	72
19	—	—	—	—	—	—	114	75

Table 4. *Mean Blood Pressures of Male Children and Adolescents (Data from Samples Differing in Geographic and Racial Characteristics)*

Age (Years)	Health and Nutrition Examination Survey Total $n = 17{,}796$ male and female				Iowa–Mayo Pool Predominantly white Total $n = 10{,}988$ male and female		New York, New York Predominantly black and Latin Total $n = 3{,}537$ male and female	
	Systolic		*Diastolic*					
	White	Black	White	Black	*Systolic*	*Diastolic*	*Systolic*	*Diastolic*
					Males (6–11) $n = 3{,}288$			
6	94.2	98.6	59.4	63.9	99.1	65.6	—	—
7	101.7	100.6	63.9	63.0	103.5	67.7	—	—
8	100.7	100.7	63.0	63.0	106.5	70.0	—	—
9	104.4	99.7	66.5	61.8	108.6	71.7	—	—
10	105.6	104.4	66.2	65.4	110.8	72.5	—	—
11	105.0	105.6	66.8	66.2	113.8	74.6	—	—
					Males (12–18 years), $n = 2{,}190$		*Males* (14–19 years), $n = 1{,}515$	
12	109.7	104.6	67.7	66.9	115.4	73.6	—	—
13	111.4	111.0	69.9	67.0	118.6	73.4	—	—
14	114.8	110.1	67.8	72.4	121.7	75.6	113	69
15	115.8	117.6	70.8	73.1	123.4	76.2	116	71
16	119.3	117.6	72.3	76.0	127.1	76.6	117	74
17	120.1	115.6	73.9	72.5	129.2	78.8	118	75
18	—	—	—	—	132.2	80.7	120	78
19	—	—	—	—	—	—	121	78

disease such as acute and chronic glomerulonephritis, polycystic disease, amyloidosis, and acute and chronic pyelonephritis. Diseases of the renal vasculature that may give rise to hypertension include the fibromuscular dysplasia usually observed in young persons, primarily female, and atherosclerotic disorders in older populations. Polyarteritis nodosa may also cause persistent hypertension, possibly due to the high frequency of renal involvement. Disorders of the adrenal gland such as primary aldosteronism, Cushing's disease, and pheochromocytoma may lead to persistent secondary hypertension. Disorders of the central nervous system occasionally give rise to systemic arterial hypertension. Secondary hypertension may be produced by contraceptive drugs, and by licorice excess which promotes renal sodium retention.

Malignant (accelerated) hypertension may appear during the course of essential or secondary forms of hypertension. It is characterized clinically as a form of severe and often suddenly and rapidly advancing hypertension which is attended by evidences of renal, cardiac, and cerebral damage, and usually neuroretinopathy (papilledema). Pathologically, necrotizing or fibrinoid arteriolitis is present, particularly involving the kidneys. Elevated renin levels are usually observed in this syndrome.

Prolonged hypertension can lead to left ventricular hypertrophy and, more rarely, to left ventricular failure.

THE FOLLOWING CRITERION IS REQUIRED FOR THE DIAGNOSIS OF SYSTEMIC ARTERIAL HYPERTENSION.

Persistent elevation of the systolic and diastolic blood pressure to the levels previously indicated.

3.5.4 PULMONARY CIRCULATORY CONGESTION

3.5.5 SYSTEMIC CIRCULATORY CONGESTION

Circulatory congestion is defined as distention of systemic or pulmonary veins or capillaries by an abnormally large volume of blood. Pressures in these vessels may become elevated, and fluid can then shift from the vascular compartment to the adjacent interstitial spaces. The magnitude of such fluid shifts depends upon the interplay of such factors as the level of intravascular pressures, tissue pressure, the vascularity of the organ or tissue involved, the presence and competence of venous valves, gravitational forces, oncotic pressures, and lymphatic drainage.

Congestion can result from reduced venous outflow, as in ventricular failure, pericardial or myocardial restriction, lesions of the mitral or tricuspid valves, and venous or lymphatic occlusive disease. When hypervolemia develops in such conditions as cirrhosis of the liver and acute glomerulonephritis, congestion can arise. Furthermore, redistribution of the circulating blood volume, as in severe anemia, can cause regional congestion. It follows that congestion can involve single organs, regional circulations, or the greater part of the circulation.

ONE OF THE FOLLOWING CRITERIA IS REQUIRED FOR THE DIAGNOSIS OF CONGESTION OF THE PULMONARY CIRCULATION.

1. Radiologic evidence of enlargement of the hilar shadows (particularly in their upper portions), with dilatation of upper lung vessels and the occurrence of interstitial edema in the lower lung fields, particularly as manifested by horizontal, parallel septal lines (B lines of Kerley), best seen in the costophrenic sinuses.
2. Dyspnea, orthopnea, frothy pink sputum, or rales over the more dependent regions of the lungs in the presence of lesions which result in pulmonary venous hypertension.

ONE OF THE FOLLOWING CRITERIA IS REQUIRED FOR THE DIAGNOSIS OF CONGESTION OF THE SYSTEMIC CIRCULATION.

1. Edema, pleural effusion, ascites, or hepatomegaly constitute acceptable evidences of congestion in the presence of either hypervolemia or elevation of right atrial or vena caval pressures (central venous pressure) above 5 mm Hg or 70 mm H_2O with the subject

at rest (zero reference level is 5 cm below the second costochondral junction).

2. **Elevation of the circulating blood volume above 2.9 L/m² BSA in men and above 2.6 L/m² BSA in women.**
3. **The vertical height of the jugular venous pulse is above the level of the second costochondral junction.**

3.6 Abnormal Communications in the Heart or Great Vessels

Abnormal connections between the heart chambers, between the great vessels and the heart, or between the large arteries and veins permit direct transfer of blood from one vascular system to another without traversing capillaries. Such lesions are most often congenital in origin; rarely, they may be acquired.

Pressures in the left heart chambers and systemic arteries are normally greater than the pressures in the corresponding chambers or vessels of the right side of the circulation. Hence the flow of blood through such abnormal communications usually is from left to right. Only in the instance of abnormal connections between pulmonary arteries and veins is flow from right to left. The magnitude of blood flow depends both on the size of the defect and on the difference in pressures between the chambers or vessels it connects.

3.6.1 INTRACARDIAC SHUNTS

3.6.1.1 LEFT-TO-RIGHT SHUNTS

Left-to-right intracardiac flow of blood occurs in atrial septal defect, ventricular septal defects, and left ventricular–right atrial communications.

The physiologic consequences of a left-to-right intracardiac shunt are enlargement of the cardiac chambers traversed by the augmented blood flow and engorgement of the pulmonary circulation. With prolonged pulmonary overperfusion, secondary changes in the media and intima of the small pulmonary arteries may occur, resulting in the development of increased resistance to pulmonary blood flow and in pulmonary hypertension. As pressures in the right ventricle, or atrium, or both approach or exceed pressures in the corresponding left heart chamber, the magnitude of left-to-right shunt flow is reduced, and blood flow across the shunt may be reversed.

3.6.1.2 Right-to-left Shunts

In the presence of pulmonary hypertension and the consequent rise in right ventricular and atrial pressures secondary to hypertrophy or ventricular failure, there may be right-to-left shunting of blood through an atrial defect, a foramen ovale, or large ventricular septal defect (Eisenmenger's syndrome).

Right-to-left shunting may also occur in the absence of pulmonary hypertension if anatomic obstruction to blood flow through the right heart or lungs accompanies defects in the partitions between the right and left hearts. Valvular or infundibular pulmonary stenosis or atresia, downward displacement of the tricuspid valve (Ebstein's malformation), and tricuspid stenosis or atresia may accompany a ventricular septal defect, an atrial septal defect, or a patent foramen ovale. In such instances, shunt flow may be from right to left.

The physiologic consequences of such a shunt are a reduction in pulmonary blood flow and in systemic arterial oxyhemoglobin saturation, at rest or at varying levels of exercise. Cyanosis, polycythemia, digital clubbing, exertional dyspnea, and fatigue may ensue.

3.6.2 EXTRACARDIAC SHUNTS

3.6.2.1 Left-to-right Shunts

Abnormal communications may exist between the great vessels themselves or between the right heart and great vessels. Because of the usual differences between systemic and pulmonary (or right heart) pressures, the flow of blood is from left to right. Examples of such lesions are a congenital or acquired fistula between the aorta and right heart chambers, a fistula between a coronary artery and a right heart chamber, direct communication of one or more pulmonary veins to the right atrium, patent ductus arteriosus, aorticopulmonary window, truncus arteriosus, and systemic arteriovenous fistula.

The physiologic consequences of these lesions are increased pulmonary blood flow and possible enlargement of the involved right-sided chambers or vessels. The various atriovenous communications may produce enlargement of the left ventricle as well.

3.6.2.2 Right-to-left Shunts

Venous blood may flow directly into the systemic circulation in the presence of complete or incomplete transposition of the great arteries. In the presence of total anomalous pulmonary venous drainage, the systemic circulation is perfused through a patent foramen ovale or atrial septal defect. With the development of sufficiently severe pulmonary hypertension, the direction of flow through a patent ductus arteriosus or an aorticopulmonary window may reverse. The physiologic consequences of such right-to-left shunts are the same as are encountered in intracardiac right-to-left shunts.

The diagnosis of shunts involving the heart and great vessels may be entertained on clinical grounds. The location of such abnormal communications may be demonstrated by a number of indicator dilution techniques that utilize oxygen, optically active or radiopaque dyes, and inert gases in conjunction with a wide variety of sensing devices.

ONE OF THE FOLLOWING CRITERIA IS REQUIRED FOR THE DIAGNOSIS OF A LEFT-TO-RIGHT SHUNT.

1. The demonstration of an increase in blood oxygen content at the point of entry of the shunt and distal to it.
2. The early arrival of hydrogen or other indicator at the point of entry of the shunt.
3. Demonstration of a left-to-right shunt by angiocardiography.

ONE OF THE FOLLOWING CRITERIA IS REQUIRED FOR THE DIAGNOSIS OF A RIGHT-TO-LEFT SHUNT.

1. **Demonstration of a right-to-left shunt by angiocardiography.**
2. **Demonstration of a right-to-left shunt by hydrogen or other indicator.**

3.7 Anginal Syndrome

The anginal syndrome consists of pain in the chest which is precipitated in patients with organic heart disease by effort, excitement, ingestion of a heavy meal, or exposure to cold. The pain is typically in the upper retrosternal area and most often radiates down the medial aspect of the left arm, but it may occur in other areas such as the anterior neck, the jaw, both shoulders, or the interscapular region. The quality of the pain is typically squeezing, but it may be pressing, burning, or choking and may vary in intensity from mild to severe. The pain is usually relieved by rest or use of nitrites. The duration of the sensation rarely exceeds fifteen minutes. In some patients, pain may begin at rest or during sleep.

Although the actual mechanism which produces anginal pain is unknown, the discomfort is characteristically associated with episodic disproportions between the need of the myocardium for oxygen and the delivery of oxygen by the coronary arterial blood. The syndrome is most often caused by coronary atherosclerosis, and severe narrowing or occlusion of the coronary arteries can usually be demonstrated by arteriography. During episodes of anginal pain, there is often evidence of transient abnormalities in left ventricular function. Coronary venous blood obtained during an anginal attack often shows biochemical evidence of anaerobic metabolism in the involved segments of myocardium. Electrocardiographic changes—typically, depression of the S–T segment and inversion of the T waves—may be present at rest and can often, but not always, be elicited by carefully supervised exercise if they are not present at rest. In atypical or variant forms of angina, S–T segments may be elevated.

Anginal syndrome can appear abruptly or slowly, can precede or follow acute myocardial infarction, and can disappear following infarction. The pain of acute myocardial infarction may be qualitatively identical with the pain of the anginal syndrome, but is usually of greater intensity and duration.

Anginal syndrome is not limited to patients with coronary atherosclerosis, but may also be present with coronary arteritis, coronary ostial stenosis, or severe ventricular hypertrophy due to aortic stenosis or regurgitation. It can also be precipitated or aggravated by anemia in patients with those diseases.

THE FOLLOWING CRITERIA ARE REQUIRED FOR THE DIAGNOSIS OF ANGINAL SYNDROME.

Pain in the chest (usually localized to the retrosternal area), neck, shoulder, or left arm in patients with organic heart disease which is usually produced by effort and relieved by rest or nitrites.

Cardiac Status and Prognosis

4

The purpose of this classification, "Cardiac Status and Prognosis," is to assess the present cardiac status of the patient and to make a prognosis of the future status as modified by optimal therapy. *Cardiac status* represents a total assessment of the etiologic, anatomic, and physiologic diagnoses. *Prognosis* is based on an assessment of the potential effects of optimal current medical and surgical therapies. The classification should be reviewed frequently and revised when indicated. This appraisal should communicate to others the physician's opinion of the patient's status and prognosis without consideration of details of management.

Recommendations for further diagnostic procedures, medical and surgical therapies, and limitation of physical activity should be detailed at the end of this classification.

Cardiac Status	*Prognosis*
1. Uncompromised	1. Good
2. Slightly compromised	2. Good with therapy
3. Moderately compromised	3. Fair with therapy
4. Severely compromised	4. Guarded despite therapy

Specific Recommendations: (Further diagnostic procedures; medical or surgical correction of the underlying defect; limitation of physical activity; use of antibiotics, digitalis glycosides, diuretics; dietary restrictions; and so forth).

Uncertain Diagnosis

5

NO HEART DISEASE: PREDISPOSING ETIOLOGIC FACTOR

The diagnostic category No Heart Disease: Predisposing Etiologic Factor includes patients in whom no cardiac disease is discovered, but whose course should be followed by periodic examinations because of the presence of a history of an etiologic factor which might cause heart disease. These should be recorded as No Heart Disease: History of (stating the etiologic factor).

NO HEART DISEASE: UNEXPLAINED MANIFESTATION

The diagnostic category No Heart Disease: Unexplained Manifestation includes patients with symptoms or signs referable to the heart, but in whom a diagnosis of cardiac disease is uncertain at the time of examination. These cases should be recorded as No Heart Disease: Unexplained Manifestation, with a further recommendation that reexamination be performed after a stated interval.

When there is a reasonable certainty that the symptoms or signs are not of cardiac origin, the diagnosis should be: No Heart Disease.

Appendix

Analysis of the Plain Chest Roentgenograms in Heart Disease

Chest roentgenographic examination has become essential to the proper diagnosis and management of cardiac disease. The heart configuration and size, the contours of the great vessels in the mediastinum, and the state of the lungs and pleural spaces are to be considered when examining the chest roentgenograms of patients with cardiovascular disease. While few roentgenographic features are pathognomonic, they are always guides in the evaluation of the patient. A discrepancy between the roentgenographic findings and the clinical diagnosis warns that the patient's status is not correctly or fully understood.

After full examination of the chest roentgenograms, a useful approach is to consider heart disease from three aspects: (1) heart size, (2) heart shape, and (3) the great vessels and lungs.

HEART SIZE

The overall heart size can be determined accurately by plain film examination. It has been found, however, that the normal range in heart sizes greatly overlaps the abnormal, so that elaborate efforts to define the normal limits of the heart size are unrewarding.

Some of the factors affecting the normal heart size on chest roentgenograms are: the roentgen-ray geometry of the image; body build; body weight; variations in the bony thorax (pectus excavatum, scoliosis, "straight spine," and so forth); size of lungs; abdominal organs (position of diaphragm); the physiologic state (pregnancy, age, training, nutrition, metabolic rate, and so forth); and the phase of heart cycle, heart rate, and phase of respiration at the time of roentgenogram exposure.

Since it is not practicable to control all of these variables, only a rough estimate of heart size on chest roentgenograms is feasible. It should be remembered that heart disease often does not affect overall heart size appreciably: for example, heart disease due to atherosclerosis, pulmonary disease and pericardial restriction.

The examiner must therefore decide whether the heart size is (1) normal, (2) significantly enlarged, implying that heart disease is present, or (3) borderline enlarged.

Estimates of heart size based on comparative measurements of the heart and bony thorax are of limited value, but may be helpful to the beginner in accumulating experience. Relative changes in heart size on serial films of the same patient are much more likely to be significant.

HEART SHAPE

Analysis of the size of individual cardiac chambers on plain film examination has many inherent difficulties. Conventional signs of individual chamber enlargement are frequently difficult or impossible to apply. The cardiac chambers are intimately clustered together and, in addition, they are cloaked externally, not only by pericardium but also by mediastinal fat, pleura, and diaphragm.

The cardio-mediastinal silhouette is conveniently analyzed in the frontal projection (Fig. 31) by considering the four segments of the left heart border: (1) The distal aortic arch, or aortic knob, which continues caudally as the descending aorta; (2) the main pulmonary arterial segment; (3) the left atrial appendage segment; and (4) the ventricular segment (usually the left ventricle). On the right side, two segments are considered: the upper one, in which the superior vena cava (or in older persons, the ascending aorta) forms the border, and the lower segment, in which the right atrium normally forms the border.

In the left lateral view (Fig. 32) the posterior wall of

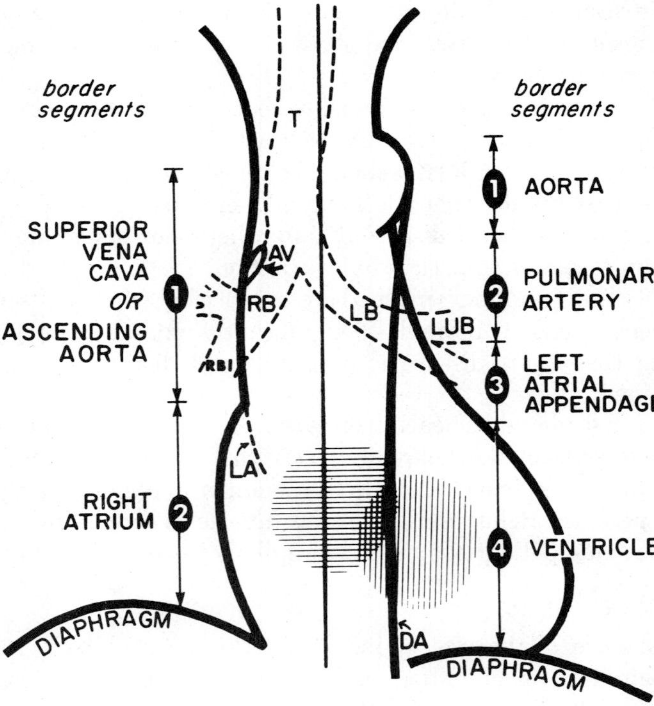

Figure 31. *Diagram of normal adult heart as shown on the frontal chest roentgenogram.* The left border of the mediastinum is divided into four segments: (1) distal aortic arch segment; (2) main pulmonary artery segment; (3) left atrial appendage segment; (4) ventricular segment. The right border is divided into two segments: (1) the superior vena cava or ascending aortic segment; (2) right atrial segment. LA indicates the right margin of the left atrium, often seen in this region in the normal person. T: trachea. AV: azygous vein. RB: right main bronchus. RBI: right intermediate bronchus. LB: left main bronchus. LUB: left upper lobe bronchus. DA: left margin of descending aorta. The horizontally-lined area represents usual position of the aortic valve, while vertically-lined area represents usual position of the mitral valve. The dashed lines represent the tracheal and main bronchial outlines.

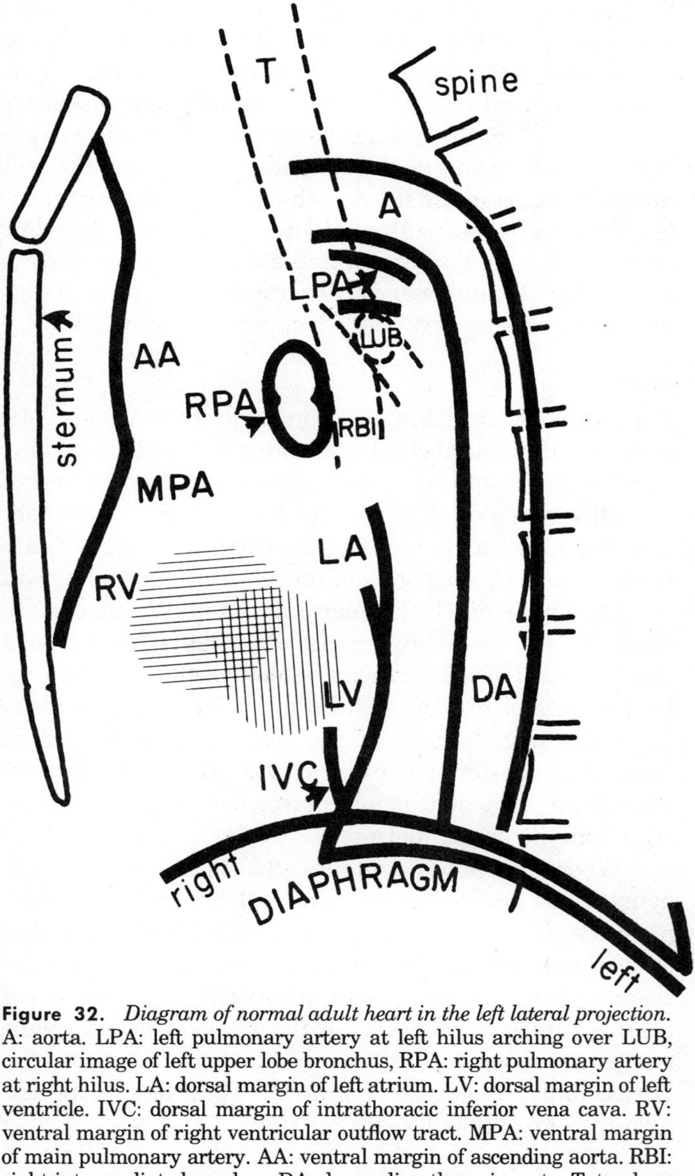

Figure 32. *Diagram of normal adult heart in the left lateral projection.* A: aorta. LPA: left pulmonary artery at left hilus arching over LUB, circular image of left upper lobe bronchus, RPA: right pulmonary artery at right hilus. LA: dorsal margin of left atrium. LV: dorsal margin of left ventricle. IVC: dorsal margin of intrathoracic inferior vena cava. RV: ventral margin of right ventricular outflow tract. MPA: ventral margin of main pulmonary artery. AA: ventral margin of ascending aorta. RBI: right intermediate bronchus. DA: descending thoracic aorta. T: trachea. The horizontally-lined area represents usual position of the aortic valve while vertically-lined area represents usual position of the mitral valve.

the left ventricle is often seen contrasted against the lung. Opacification of the esophagus with barium can improve the outline of the dorsal margin of the left atrium. Commonly, a curved margin (concave dorsally), representing the back wall of the inferior vena cava, is seen intersecting the right dome of the diaphragm. The ventral and cephalad aspect of the heart is the usually indistinct margin of the right ventricular outflow tract, often obscured in older persons because of a prominent elongated ascending aorta. The left pulmonary artery can sometimes be recognized as it crosses over the left upper lobe bronchus.

Left Atrium

The outline of the left atrium can be quite accurately estimated on the frontal chest film using: the medial margins of the right main and right intermediate bronchi and of the left main and left lower lobe bronchi; the second contour due to left atrium often seen close to the right heart border (Fig. 31); the region of the left atrial appendage on the left. There may be a general increase in heart density caused by the dorsal prominence of the left atrium. Mitral and aortic valve calcifications, when present, are also useful markers of the left atrial margins. The lateral view, especially with barium in the esophagus, is helpful in locating the posterior margins of the left atrium, particularly since slight left atrial enlargement is most impressive along its dorsal margin.

When left atrial contours deform the cardiac silhouette (by producing, e.g., unusual bronchial displacement, straightening or convexity of the left heart border, or a prominent double contour on the right), disproportionate left atrial enlargement is present. In most cases of chronic left ventricular disease, the left atrial size parallels and is not disproportionate to that of the left ventricle. Occasionally, as is typical of atrial septal defect, the left atrium is exceptionally small.

Left Ventricle

In the frontal view, the ventricular region of the cardiac shadow can be considered to be that part inferior and to the left of a line connecting the right cardiophrenic angle with the pulmonary artery segment, or, more simply, that part to the left of the midline not accounted for by the left atrium. Enlargement of this region in adults is due to left ventricular enlargement in more than 90 percent of cases, but precisely the same appearance can be caused by right ventricular dilatation or pericardial effusion. Lengthening of the axis of the ventricular region toward the left costophrenic angle and increased prominence of the lower lateral ventricular border suggest left ventricular enlargement. Increased thickness of the heart on the lateral view at the level of the diaphragm, especially when the posterior left ventricular border overlaps the inferior vena caval margin, also suggests left ventricular enlargement. Again, calcifications in both aortic and mitral valves may help identify the margins of the left ventricle.

Right Ventricle

Since the right ventricle seldom contributes to the cardiac border in the frontal projection, its dilatation per se produces mainly nonspecific enlargement of the ventricular region. Enlargement of the right ventricle does, however, tend to displace the outflow tract and main pulmonary artery upward and to the left. The pulmonary artery segment becomes more prominent in the frontal projection, and in the lateral view, encroachment from below on the retrosternal clear space may be seen. This latter feature has limited value because of frequent obscuration by a large ascending aorta, thymus, or a narrow anteroposterior mediastinal dimension. With extreme dilatation of the right ventricle, this chamber often forms the left border of the cardiac silhouette and may produce a long convexity on the left heart border which can be confused with prominence of the left atrial appendage.

Right Atrium

The length and prominence of the right heart border (lower segment) in the frontal projection is a rough indicator of right atrial size. The right atrium is most likely to be large when the right ventricle is large. Persistent prominence of the caval margins or of the azygos vein suggests elevation of right atrial pressure.

GREAT VESSELS AND THE LUNGS

Prominence of the right ventricular outflow tract and dilatation of the central pulmonary arteries are the most important, though indirect, indicators of right ventricular enlargement. Dilatation of the main pulmonary arteries indicates pulmonary hypertension (or post-stenotic dilatation) and therefore right ventricular hypertension, suggesting that right ventricular hypertrophy is likely to be present. The central pulmonary vessels (after discounting the effects of aging and normal variations) provide an extremely valuable index of pulmonary arterial pressure, or of turbulence, in the case of post-stenotic dilatation.

The appearance of the peripheral lung vessels also has great importance in diagnosis. The lungs are the only organs in which the macroscopic vasculature is seen on plain roentgenograms. The sizes of the more peripheral pulmonary vessels reflect pulmonary blood volume and flow (as well as acute pressure changes). Pulmonary edema (interstitial or alveolar) in heart disease usually implies pulmonary capillary and venous hypertension.

Characteristic patterns in the appearance of the pulmonary vasculature reflect different hemodynamic states. In Figure 33A the normal appearance of the lung vessels of the right lung on the normal erect chest roentgenogram is diagramed. Note the relatively more distended pulmonary vessels at the lung bases, sharply contrasted against the surrounding aerated lung. Figure 33B shows the generally distended pulmonary vasculature that can be produced by increased pulmonary blood volume and flow at modestly elevated pressures secondary to a left-to-right shunt in congenital heart disease, severe anemia, or pregnancy. Figure 33C diagrams the state of the lung vessels in the presence of pulmonary arterial hypertension induced by the pulmonary capillary and venous hypertension of left ventricular failure or mitral obstruction. Note the relatively small caliber of both the arteries and the

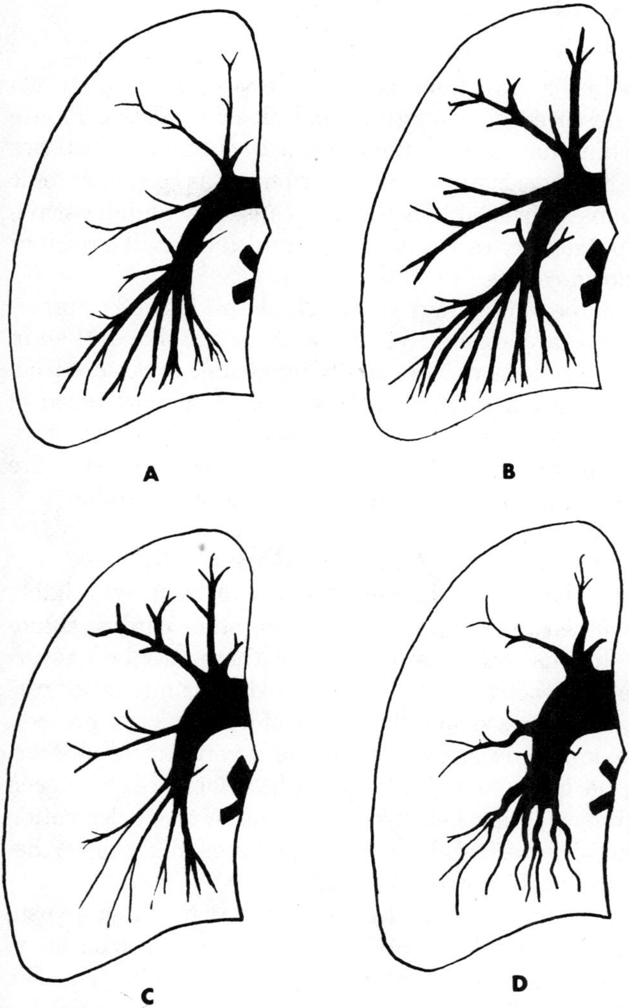

Figure 33. *Schematic representations in the right lung of some characteristic pulmonary vascular patterns as shown on chest roentgenograms in the frontal view.* A. Normal lung, showing the relatively larger vessels in the lower lung fields. B. Generally distended pulmonary vasculature that may be found in large left-to-right shunts. C. Relatively distended central and upper lung field vessels and small lower lung vessels, which may arise secondary to pulmonary capillary and venous hypertension. D. Disproportionately enlarged central pulmonary arteries abruptly tapering to normal or small peripheral pulmonary vessels, which may be encountered in acquired chronic pulmonary arterial hypertension.

veins in the lower lung fields; these vessels are often further obscured by interstitial and alveolar edema. Figure 33D diagrams the tortuous central pulmonary arteries abruptly tapering toward the periphery, as seen in chronic pulmonary arterial hypertension caused by a high peripheral pulmonary resistance due to multiple small emboli or unknown causes.

In the infant and young child the heart is proportionately larger compared to the size of the thorax than in adults. In addition, it is usually impossible to be sure from plain chest roentgenographic examination how much of the mediastinum is heart and how much is thymus. Standards for normal heart size and heart configuration are thus even more broad and uncertain than in adults.

Three diagnostic features need special emphasis:

1. The size of the left atrium can be more reliably determined than can the size of the other cardiac chambers. It must be remembered that there is only a rough correlation between the left atrial size (or any other cardiac chamber size) and the degree of heart disease present. For example, in some instances of severe mitral obstruction, no impressive left atrial enlargement may be seen despite very high left atrial pressures. Valve calcification or chronic interstitial edema in the lungs might nevertheless lead to the correct diagnosis.

2. Enlargement of the ventricular region, though usually the result of left ventricular disease, can also be due to right ventricular dilatation or pericardial effusion. The appearance of the pulmonary arteries and the lungs, as well as the clinical data, helps to differentiate between these possibilities.

3. The great vessel configurations and vascular changes in the lungs are extremely important in indicating cardiac function. The appearance of the lung fields is often more helpful in the diagnosis of heart disease than is the appearance of the heart itself.

Table A. *Normal Deflections in Standard Leads I, II, and III in Adults.**

Normal P is a curved or pointed upward deflection 0.5–2.5 mm in height.

Normal Q is any initial downward ventricular deflection which is neither slurred nor splintered, and has a maximum absolute and relative size in the three leads as follows:

Lead	Absolute Size (mm)	% of Largest QRS Deflection in Any Standard Lead
I	2.0	15
II	2.5	20
III	3.0	25

These criteria are not applicable to curves showing high voltage or RAD.

Normal R is an upward deflection, neither slurred nor splintered, varying in size from 1.5 to 20 mm.

Normal S is a downward deflection preceded by an upstroke. It is neither slurred nor splintered, and does not exceed 6 mm in depth.

Normal T is a rounded or pointed upward deflection 1.0–7.0 mm in height. A small deflection known as the *U wave* may follow the T wave and is normally upright in standard leads.

Normal S–T is one which is not displaced at its origin by more than 0.9 mm in either direction from the isoelectric level. It is not fused with the T and is not convex to, or from, the baseline, but is relatively horizontal in its extent.

The reference level for measurement of P wave, T_p wave, S–T segment, T wave, and U wave is the T–P line. Q, R, S, and J are measured from P–R segment.

The normal QRS interval in adults is 0.06–0.10 sec; 0.06–0.09 sec in children from 5–14 years of age; and 0.04–0.08 sec in children under 5 years.

Low voltage of QRS is present whenever the amplitude of the whole QRS complex is 5 mm or less in all six limb leads (I, II, III, aVR, aVL, aVF).

* Standardization: 1 mv = 10 mm. *N.B.* 1 mm = 1 small box.

Reprinted by permission from Ferrer, M. I., *Electrocardiographic Notebook* (4th ed.). Futura Publishing Company, Mt. Kisco, N.Y., 1973.

Table B. *Normal Values for ECG Waves in aV and V Leads in Adults.*

Criteria for Normal Deflections (in mm) in Adults in Augmented Extremity Leads aVR, aVL, aVF. (With normal instrument sensitivity)

	P		Q		R*		S		S–T†		T‡	
	Min.	Max.	Min.	Max.	Min.	Max.	Min.	Max.	Min.	Max.	Min.	Max.
aVR	−1.5	−0.8	0	12.0	0	4.5	0	16.0	0	0	−6.0	−1.0
aVL	−1.0	1.0	0	2.0	0	8.0	0	10.0	0	0	−1.5	2.0
aVF	0	3.0	0	2.5	1.5	20.0	0	7.0	0	0	0.2	5.0

Criteria for Normal Deflections (in mm) in Adults in Precordial Leads V1 to V6. (With instrument sensitivity at half normal [1 mv = 0.5 cm]. Values must be doubled if records are made at normal sensitivity [1 mv = 1 cm].)

	P		Q		R*		S		S–T†		T‡	
	Min.	Max.	Min.	Max.	Min.	Max.	Min.	Max.	Min.	Max.	Min.	Max.
V1	0	1.0	0	0	0.5	5.0	2.0	12.5	0	0.5	−1.5	2.5
V2	−0.3	1.0	0	0	1.5	10.0	2.0	20.0	0	0.5	1.0	6.0
V3	0.3	1.0	0	0.5	3.0	20.0	0	12.0	0	1.0	1.0	8.0
V4	0	1.0	0	2.0	4.0	22.0	0	8.0	0	0.5	0.8	7.0
V5	0	0.5	0	1.5	4.0	17.0	0	4.0	0	0	0.5	5.0
V6	0	0.5	0	1.5	3.5	11.0	0	1.5	0	0	0.5	3.0

* Includes value of R′ if present.
† S–T junction with reference to P–R segment.
‡ T with reference to isoelectric line.
Reprinted by permission from Ferrer, M. I., *Electrocardiographic Notebook* (4th ed.). Futura Publishing Company, Mt. Kisco, N.Y., 1973.

Table C. *Normal Values for P–R Intervals.*

Upper Limits of the Normal P–R Interval (Corrected for rate).*

Rate	Below 70	71–90	91–110	111–130	Above 130
Large adults	0.21	0.20	0.19	0.18	0.17
Small adults	0.20	0.19	0.18	0.17	0.16
Children, ages 14 to 17	0.19	0.18	0.17	0.16	0.15
Children, ages 7 to 13	0.18	0.17	0.16	0.15	0.14
Children, ages 1½ to 6	0.17	0.165	0.155	0.145	0.135
Children, ages 0 to 1½	0.16	0.15	0.145	0.135	0.125

Range of the Normal P–R Interval and P Wave Duration (Uncorrected for rate).†

Age	P–R Interval (sec) Range	P Wave Duration (sec) Range
0–1 week	0.08–0.15	0.04–0.08
1 week–1 month	0.08–0.14	0.03–0.08
1 month–3 months	0.08–0.14	0.04–0.08
3 months–6 months	0.08–0.14	0.04–0.08
6 months–1 year	0.08–0.15	0.04–0.08
1 year–3 years	0.08–0.15	0.06–0.09
3 years–5 years	0.10–0.17	0.05–0.11
5 years–16 years	0.10–0.20	0.05–0.12
16 years–20 years	0.12–0.20	0.08–0.12

* Reprinted by permission from Ferrer, M. I., *Electrocardiographic Notebook* (4th ed.). Futura Publishing Company, Mt. Kisco, N.Y., 1973.
† Adapted by permission from Burch, G. E., and DePasquale, N. P., *Electrocardiography in the Diagnosis of Congenital Heart Disease*. Lea & Febiger, Philadelphia, 1967.

Table D. *Data for Computation of Heart Rate and Values for the Maximum Normal Q–T Intervals at Various Rates in Adults.**†

Cycle Time (0.04-sec intervals)	Rate	Max. Q–T (sec) Male	Max. Q–T (sec) Female	Cycle Time (0.04-sec intervals)	Rate	Max. Q–T (sec) Male	Max. Q–T (sec) Female
5	300	.19	.20	28	52	.42	.47
6	250	.20	.22	29	51	.43	.47
7	214	.21	.23	30	50	.44	.48
8	187	.23	.25	31	48	.45	.49
9	166	.24	.26	32	46	.45	.50
10	150	.25	.28	33	45	.46	.51
11	136	.26	.29	34	43	.47	.51
12	125	.28	.30	35	42	.47	.52
13	115	.29	.32	36	41	.48	.53
14	107	.30	.33	37	40	.49	.54
15	100	.31	.34	38	39	.49	.54
16	93	.32	.35	39	38	.50	.55
17	88	.33	.36	40	37	.51	.56
18	83	.34	.37	41	36	.51	.56
19	78	.35	.38	42	35	.52	.57
20	75	.36	.39	43	35	.52	.58
21	71	.37	.40	44	34	.53	.58
22	68	.38	.41	45	33	.54	.59
23	65	.38	.42	46	32	.54	.60
24	62	.39	.43	47	32	.55	.60
25	60	.40	.44	48	31	.56	.61
26	57	.41	.45	49	30	.56	.62
27	55	.42	.46	50	30	.57	.62

* Rate computation for regular rhythms only.
† For children, see Table H.
Reprinted by permission from Ferrer, M. I., *Electrocardiographic Notebook* (4th ed.). Futura Publishing Company, Mt. Kisco, N.Y., 1973.

Table E. *Normal Values for ECG Waves in Standard aV and V Leads in Infants, Children and Adolescents.*

Part I. Normal Infants, Newborn to 1 Year Old, Supine. Size of the Electrocardiographic Deflections in the Bipolar Extremity, Augmented Unipolar Extremity, and Precordial Leads Is Given in Tenths of a Millivolt.*

	P				Q				R				S				RS				S–T				T			
Lead	No. Cases	Min.	Max.	Mean	No. Cases	Min.	Max.	Mean	No. Cases	Min.	Max.	Mean	No. Cases	Min.	Max.	Mean	No. Cases	Min.	Max.	Mean	No. Cases	Min.	Max.	Mean	No. Cases	Min.	Max.	Mean
I	158	−1.0	2.5	0.94	164	0	3.0	1.15	165	0	17.0	5.58	165	0	15.0	4.34	—	—	—	—	195	−0.1	0.1	—	143	−2.0	6.0	2.23
II	158	0	2.5	1.63	165	0	5.5	1.95	165	1.0	25.0	10.04	165	0	8.5	2.99	—	—	—	—	197	−0.1	0.2	—	143	0	7.0	2.84
III	158	−1.0	2.0	0.80	165	0	9.0	3.26	164	1.0	24.0	8.91	164	0	6.5	2.18	—	—	—	—	197	−0.2	0.2	—	143	−3.0	5.0	0.73
aVR	158	−2.5	1.5	−1.09	165	0	13.0	5.92	165	0	9.0	2.32	165	0	18.0	7.45	—	—	—	—	197	−0.1	0.1	—	143	−5.0	2.0	−2.39
aVL	158	−1.5	1.5	0.22	164	0	5.5	1.34	165	0	10.0	3.33	165	0	16.0	5.23	—	—	—	—	197	−0.1	0.1	—	143	−1.5	3.5	0.97
aVF	158	−1.0	3.0	1.17	165	0	6.0	2.36	165	1.5	21.5	8.15	165	0	7.5	2.29	—	—	—	—	197	−0.05	0.2	—	143	−2.0	5.0	1.68
V_1	155	−1.0	2.5	0.69	186	0	0	0	137	3.0	29.0	13.61	123	0	28.0	8.57	142	3.0	50.0	22.73	161	−0.2	0.1	—	126	−8.0	6.0	−2.65
V_2	139	0	2.5	1.13	186	0	0	0	137	3.0	43.0	19.98	121	1.0	42.0	18.35	162	3.0	66.0	40.14	159	−0.2	0.2	—	126	−9.0	9.0	−2.84
V_3	115	0	3.0	1.44	117	0	3.0	1.09	114	5.5	40.0	20.49	112	1.0	39.0	17.72	116	(18.0)†	73.0	38.71	116	−0.2	0.25	—	116	−7.0	6.0	−1.37
V_4	142	0	2.0	1.05	161	0	3.0	1.32	139	3.0	37.0	21.21	123	0	42.0	12.88	146	4.0	63.0	31.73	157	−0.1	0.2	—	123	−7.0	6.5	2.46
V_5	122	0	2.0	1.14	122	0	5.5	2.09	118	3.0	34.0	14.49	119	0	30.0	7.00	121	5.0	48.0	21.89	121	—	0.2	—	122	−4.0	7.0	2.93
V_6	141	0	2.0	0.84	142	0	5.0	1.64	119	0	24.0	8.00	138	0	30.0	2.72	161	3.0	34.0	12.17	161	—	0.1	—	125	−3.0	6.0	2.27

* Based on normal series studied by Ziegler.

† 6 months–1 year age group only.

Table E. *(Continued)*

Part II. Normal Children, 1 to 10 Years Old, Supine. Size of the Electrocardiographic Deflections in the Bipolar Extremity, Augmented Unipolar Extremity, and Precordial Leads Is Given in Tenths of a Millivolt.*

	P				Q				R				S				RS				S–T				T			
Lead	No. Cases	Min.	Max.	Mean	No. Cases	Min.	Max.	Mean	No. Cases	Min.	Max.	Mean	No. Cases	Min.	Max.	Mean	No. Cases	Min.	Max.	Mean	No. Cases	Min.	Max.	Mean	No. Cases	Min.	Max.	Mean
I	225	0.5	2.5	1.04	227	0	2.5	1.11	223	1.5	17.0	6.75	225	0	8.0	2.88	—	—	—	—	227	−1.0	1.0	—	223	1.0	6.5	2.53
II	224	0	3.0	1.63	228	0	5.4	1.55	223	2.0	28.0	12.21	223	0	6.5	2.38	—	—	—	—	227	−1.0	2.0	—	223	0	7.0	3.25
III	224	−1.5	2.0	0.62	227	0	8.0	2.50	223	1.0	23.0	7.99	223	0	9.0	1.70	—	—	—	—	228	−1.0	1.0	—	223	−3.0	4.0	0.52
aVR	293	−2.0	0	−1.56	347	0	14.0	5.70	342	0	6.5	1.60	342	0	19.5	7.77	—	—	—	—	227	−1.0	1.0	—	292	−6.0	−0.2	−2.79
aVL	293	−1.0	2.0	0.32	347	0	4.0	0.84	342	0	11.8	3.15	342	0	11.0	3.72	—	—	—	—	227	−1.0	1.0	—	292	−4.0	4.0	1.10
aVF	293	−0.6	2.0	1.03	347	0	5.0	1.33	342	0.5	21.0	9.30	342	0	14.0	1.61	—	—	—	—	227	−1.0	1.0	—	292	−1.0	6.0	1.84
V_1	198	−1.0	2.5	0.72	203	0	0	0	198	0.4	20.0	7.15	197	0	36.5	11.02	103	6.5	46.5	28.85	134	−1.0	2.0	—	197	−6.0	3.0	−2.86
V_2	201	−0.6	2.0	0.92	204	0	0	0	192	2.0	28.0	12.90	196	3.0	44.0	18.31	101	9.0	61.0	37.45	133	−1.0	2.5	—	197	−8.5	6.0	−1.91
V_3	182	0.1	2.0	0.80	185	0	1.0	0.44	181	4.0	42.0	14.00	180	0	36.0	13.66	87	14.0	60.0	32.17	118	0	2.5	—	191	−13.0	12.5	1.30
V_4	200	0	1.5	0.73	203	0	6.0	1.21	199	4.0	50.0	20.16	199	0	26.0	7.53	102	13.0	61.0	32.94	133	0	2.0	—	199	−4.0	14.5	4.54
V_5	188	0	1.5	0.62	190	0	8.0	1.53	186	6.0	40.0	18.97	186	0	15.0	3.62	88	15.0	47.0	23.89	88	−1.0	1.2	—	186	0	12.0	4.51
V_6	197	0	1.5	0.61	201	0	5.0	1.47	196	5.0	23.0	11.94	195	0	13.0	1.23	102	5.0	26.0	14.74	93	−1.0	1.0	—	196	0	8.5	3.41
V_7	28	0	1.0	0.50	28	0	3.0	0.78	28	5.5	20.0	11.13	28	0	5.5	1.29	—	—	—	—	28	0	0.8	—	28	0.7	6.5	3.50
$V_{3}R$	28	−0.8	1.5	0.57	28	0	2.0	0.09	28	1.3	9.9	4.18	28	0	19.5	5.51	—	—	—	—	28	0	0.6	—	28	−4.8	0.9	−1.77
$V_{4}R$	28	−0.4	1.5	0.44	28	0	2.0	0.09	28	1.0	4.8	2.80	28	0	10.5	8.67	—	—	—	—	28	0	0.4	—	28	−4.9	−1.0	−1.59

* This table is based on normal series studied by Ziegler; Switzer and Besoain; Kneese de Melo; and Yu, Joos, and Katsampes.

Part III. Normal Adolescents, 10 to 20 Years, Supine. Size of the Electrocardiographic Deflections in the Bipolar Extremity, Augmented Unipolar Extremity, and Precordial Leads Is Given in Tenths of a Millivolt.*

Lead	No. Cases	P			Q			R			S			T		
		Min.	Max.	Mean	Min.	Max.	Mean	Min.	Max.	Mean	Min.	Max.	Mean	Min.	Max.	Mean
I	124	0.2	1.5	0.74	0	2.5	0.30	1.3	13.0	5.26	0	6.8	1.40	0.2	5.0	2.32
II	124	0	2.1	1.01	0	2.8	0.37	2.9	20.0	9.66	0	6.3	1.59	0.2	6.5	2.89
III	124	−1.0	1.8	0.43	0	4.6	0.50	0.7	15.8	6.05	0	9.0	1.18	−1.19	3.9	0.65
aV_R	214	−1.75	−0.2	−1.03	0	13.7	2.68	0	8.0	1.39	0	17.0	4.94	−5.2	−0.1	−2.36
aV_L	214	−1.0	1.4	0.29	0	4.2	0.34	0	10.1	2.24	0	14.2	2.51	−2.5	3.6	0.87
aV_F	214	−0.8	2.2	0.74	0	3.8	0.42	1.0	21.0	8.22	0	4.9	0.99	−0.5	5.4	1.76
V_1	138	−0.2	2.2	0.77	0	1.5	0.01	0.4	16.7	5.29	0	26.6	11.99	−3.5	7.5	0.22
V_2	139	−0.2	2.0	0.78	0	0	0	0.5	23.5	8.16	2.6	45.5	15.81	−3.8	14.1	2.19
V_3	138	0	1.8	0.73	0	0.7	0.01	1.6	26.0	10.15	0.9	31.1	12.76	−3.7	13.5	3.39
V_4	139	0	1.5	0.62	0	4.4	0.21	3.1	31.6	13.98	0.2	22.2	8.27	−2.8	12.6	4.43
V_5	139	0	1.2	0.55	0	3.1	0.49	4.2	29.0	13.56	0	15.1	3.03	0.1	10.5	3.71
V_6	138	0	1.0	0.50	0	4.2	0.66	3.5	25.0	11.44	0	11.3	1.74	0	7.8	3.04
V_7	24	0.2	0.8	0.4	0	2.5	0.9	5.0	16.0	15.0	0	5.4	0.9	0.7	5.0	2.4
V_3R	24	—	1.2	0.7	0	0	0	1.5	8.0	3.8	0	16.0	7.6	−3.6	1.8	−1.1
V_4R	24	—	1.0	0.4	0	1.5	—	0.7	5.5	2.3	1.0	9.5	5.4	−2.4	1.1	−1.1

* This table is based on normal series studied by Vaquero, Limón, and Limón; Switzer and Besoain; Kneese de Melo; Yu, Joos, and Katsampes.

Table F. *Determination of the Frontal Plane Mean Electrical Axis of QRS Complex or P Wave.*

Table F_1

Lead III Positive	Lead I Positive 0.0	0.5	1.0	1.5	2.0	2.5	3.0	3.5	4.0	4.5	5.0	6.0	7.0	8.0	9.0	10.0	11.0	12.0	13.0	14.0	15.0	20.0
0.0		30	30	30	30	30	30	30	30	30	30	30	30	30	30	30	30	30	30	30	30	30
0.5	90	60	49	44	41	39	38	37	36	35	35	34	33	33	33	32	32	32	32	32	32	31
1.0	90	71	60	53	49	46	44	42	41	40	39	38	37	36	35	35	34	34	34	33	33	32
1.5	90	76	67	60	55	52	49	47	45	44	43	41	39	38	38	37	36	36	36	35	35	33
2.0	90	79	71	65	60	56	53	51	49	47	46	44	42	41	40	39	38	38	37	37	36	35
2.5	90	81	74	68	64	60	57	54	52	51	49	47	45	43	42	41	40	39	39	38	38	36
3.0	90	82	76	71	67	63	60	57	55	53	52	49	47	45	44	43	42	41	40	39	39	37
3.5	90	83	78	73	69	66	63	60	58	56	54	51	49	47	46	44	43	42	42	41	40	38
4.0	90	84	79	75	71	68	65	62	60	58	56	53	51	49	47	46	45	44	43	42	42	39
4.5	90	85	80	76	73	69	67	64	62	60	58	55	53	51	49	48	47	45	44	43	43	40
5.0	90	85	81	77	74	71	68	66	64	62	60	57	55	52	51	49	48	47	46	45	44	41
6.0	90	86	82	79	76	73	71	69	67	65	63	60	57	55	53	52	50	49	48	47	46	43
7.0	90	87	83	81	78	75	73	71	69	67	65	63	60	58	56	54	53	51	50	49	48	44
8.0	90	87	84	82	79	77	75	73	71	69	68	65	62	60	58	56	55	53	52	51	50	46
9.0	90	87	85	82	80	78	76	74	73	71	69	67	64	62	60	58	57	55	54	53	52	48
10.0	90	88	85	83	81	79	77	76	74	72	71	68	66	64	62	60	58	57	56	54	53	49
11.0	90	88	86	84	82	80	78	77	75	73	72	70	67	65	63	62	60	59	57	56	55	50
12.0	90	88	86	84	82	81	79	78	76	75	73	71	69	67	65	63	61	60	59	57	56	52
13.0	90	88	86	84	83	81	80	78	77	76	74	72	70	68	66	64	63	61	60	59	58	53
14.0	90	88	87	85	83	82	80	79	78	77	75	73	71	69	67	66	64	63	61	60	59	55
15.0	90	88	87	85	84	82	81	80	78	77	76	74	72	70	68	67	65	64	62	61	60	55
20.0	90	89	88	87	85	84	83	82	81	80	79	77	76	74	72	71	70	68	67	65	65	60

Lead III Negative	Lead I Negative 0.0	0.5	1.0	1.5	2.0	2.5	3.0	3.5	4.0	4.5	5.0	6.0	7.0	8.0	9.0	10.0	11.0	12.0	13.0	14.0	15.0	20.0
0.0	−150	−150	−150	−150	−150	−150	−150	−150	−150	−150	−150	−150	−150	−150	−150	−150	−150	−150	−150	−150	−150	−150
0.5	−90	−120	−131	−136	−139	−141	−142	−143	−144	−145	−145	−146	−147	−147	−147	−148	−148	−148	−148	−148	−148	−149
1.0	−90	−109	−120	−127	−131	−134	−136	−138	−139	−140	−141	−142	−143	−144	−145	−145	−146	−146	−146	−147	−147	−148
1.5	−90	−104	−113	−120	−125	−128	−131	−133	−135	−136	−137	−139	−141	−142	−142	−143	−144	−144	−144	−145	−145	−147
2.0	−90	−101	−109	−115	−120	−124	−127	−129	−131	−133	−134	−136	−138	−139	−140	−141	−142	−142	−143	−143	−144	−145
2.5	−90	−99	−106	−112	−116	−120	−123	−126	−128	−129	−131	−133	−135	−137	−138	−139	−140	−141	−141	−142	−142	−144
3.0	−90	−98	−104	−109	−113	−117	−120	−123	−125	−127	−128	−131	−133	−135	−136	−137	−138	−139	−140	−141	−141	−143
3.5	−90	−97	−102	−107	−111	−114	−117	−120	−122	−124	−124	−129	−131	−133	−134	−136	−137	−138	−138	−139	−140	−142
4.0	−90	−96	−101	−105	−109	−112	−115	−118	−120	−122	−124	−127	−129	−131	−133	−134	−135	−136	−137	−138	−138	−141
4.5	−90	−95	−100	−104	−107	−111	−113	−116	−118	−120	−122	−125	−127	−129	−131	−132	−133	−135	−136	−137	−137	−140
5.0	−90	−95	−99	−103	−106	−109	−112	−114	−116	−118	−120	−123	−125	−128	−129	−131	−132	−133	−134	−135	−136	−139
6.0	−90	−94	−98	−101	−104	−107	−109	−111	−113	−115	−117	−120	−123	−125	−127	−128	−130	−131	−132	−133	−134	−137
7.0	−90	−93	−97	−99	−102	−105	−107	−109	−111	−113	−115	−117	−120	−122	−124	−126	−127	−129	−130	−131	−132	−136
8.0	−90	−93	−96	−98	−101	−103	−105	−107	−109	−111	−112	−115	−118	−120	−122	−124	−125	−127	−128	−129	−130	−134
9.0	−90	−93	−95	−98	−100	−102	−104	−106	−107	−109	−111	−113	−116	−118	−120	−122	−123	−125	−126	−127	−128	−132
10.0	−90	−92	−95	−97	−99	−101	−103	−104	−106	−108	−109	−112	−114	−116	−118	−120	−122	−123	−124	−126	−127	−131
11.0	−90	−92	−94	−96	−98	−100	−102	−103	−105	−107	−108	−110	−113	−115	−117	−118	−120	−121	−123	−124	−125	−130
12.0	−90	−92	−94	−96	−98	−99	−101	−102	−104	−105	−107	−109	−111	−113	−115	−117	−119	−120	−121	−123	−124	−128
13.0	−90	−92	−94	−96	−97	−99	−100	−102	−103	−104	−106	−108	−110	−112	−114	−116	−117	−119	−120	−121	−122	−127
14.0	−90	−92	−93	−95	−97	−98	−100	−101	−102	−103	−105	−107	−109	−111	−113	−114	−116	−117	−119	−120	−121	−125
15.0	−90	−92	−93	−95	−96	−98	−99	−100	−102	−103	−104	−106	−108	−110	−112	−113	−115	−116	−118	−119	−120	−125
20.0	−90	−91	−92	−93	−95	−96	−97	−98	−99	−100	−101	−103	−104	−106	−108	−109	−110	−112	−113	−115	−115	−102

Table F *(Continued)*

Table F_2

Lead III Negative	Lead I Positive 0.0	0.5	1.0	1.5	2.0	2.5	3.0	3.5	4.0	4.5	5.0	6.0	7.0	8.0	9.0	10.0	11.0	12.0	13.0	14.0	15.0	20.0
0.0		30	30	30	30	30	30	30	30	30	30	30	30	30	30	30	30	30	30	30	30	30
0.5	−90	−30	0	11	16	19	21	22	23	24	25	26	26	27	27	27	28	28	28	28	28	29
1.0	−90	−60	−30	−11	0	7	11	14	16	18	19	21	22	23	24	25	25	26	26	26	27	27
1.5	−90	−71	−49	−30	−16	−7	0	5	7	11	13	16	18	20	21	22	23	23	24	24	25	26
2.0	−90	−76	−60	−44	−30	−19	−11	−5	0	4	7	11	14	16	18	19	20	21	22	22	23	25
2.5	−90	−79	−67	−53	−41	−30	−21	−14	−8	−4	0	6	9	12	14	16	17	19	20	20	21	23
3.0	−90	−81	−71	−60	−49	−39	−30	−22	−16	−11	−7	0	5	8	11	13	15	16	17	18	19	22
3.5	−90	−82	−74	−65	−55	−46	−38	−30	−23	−18	−13	−6	0	4	7	10	12	14	15	16	17	21
4.0	−90	−83	−76	−68	−60	−52	−44	−37	−30	−24	−19	−11	−5	0	4	7	9	11	13	14	15	19
4.5	−90	−84	−78	−71	−64	−56	−49	−42	−36	−30	−25	−16	−9	−4	0	3	6	8	10	12	13	18
5.0	−90	−85	−79	−73	−67	−60	−53	−47	−41	−35	−30	−21	−14	−8	−4	0	3	6	8	9	11	16
6.0	−90	−86	−81	−76	−71	−66	−60	−54	−49	−44	−39	−30	−22	−16	−11	−7	−3	0	3	5	7	13
7.0	−90	−86	−82	−78	−74	−69	−65	−60	−55	−51	−46	−38	−30	−23	−18	−13	−9	−6	−3	0	2	10
8.0	−90	−87	−83	−80	−76	−72	−68	−64	−60	−56	−52	−44	−37	−30	−24	−19	−15	−11	−8	−5	−2	7
9.0	−90	−87	−84	−81	−78	−74	−71	−67	−64	−60	−56	−49	−42	−36	−30	−25	−20	−16	−13	−9	−7	3
10.0	−90	−87	−85	−82	−79	−76	−73	−70	−67	−63	−60	−53	−47	−41	−35	−30	−25	−21	−17	−14	−11	0
11.0	−90	−88	−85	−83	−80	−77	−75	−72	−69	−66	−63	−57	−51	−45	−40	−35	−30	−26	−22	−18	−15	−3
12.0	−90	−88	−86	−83	−81	−79	−76	−74	−71	−68	−66	−60	−54	−49	−44	−39	−34	−30	−26	−22	−19	−7
13.0	−90	−88	−86	−84	−82	−80	−77	−75	−73	−70	−68	−63	−57	−52	−47	−43	−38	−34	−30	−26	−23	−10
14.0	−90	−88	−86	−84	−82	−80	−78	−76	−74	−72	−69	−65	−60	−55	−51	−46	−42	−38	−34	−30	−27	−13
15.0	−90	−88	−87	−85	−83	−81	−79	−77	−75	−73	−71	−67	−62	−58	−53	−49	−45	−41	−37	−33	−30	−16
20.0	−90	−89	−87	−86	−85	−83	−82	−81	−79	−78	−76	−73	−70	−67	−63	−60	−57	−53	−50	−47	−44	−30

Lead III Positive	Lead I Negative 0.0	0.5	1.0	1.5	2.0	2.5	3.0	3.5	4.0	4.5	5.0	6.0	7.0	8.0	9.0	10.0	11.0	12.0	13.0	14.0	15.0	20.0
0.0		−150	−150	−150	−150	−150	−150	−150	−150	−150	−150	−150	−150	−150	−150	−150	−150	−150	−150	−150	−150	−150
0.5	90	150	180	−169	−164	−161	−159	−158	−157	−156	−155	−154	−154	−153	−153	−153	−152	−152	−152	−152	−152	−151
1.0	90	120	150	169	180	−173	−169	−166	−164	−162	−161	−159	−158	−157	−156	−155	−155	−154	−154	−154	−153	−153
1.5	90	109	131	150	164	173	180	−175	−172	−169	−167	−164	−162	−160	−159	−158	−157	−157	−156	−156	−155	−154
2.0	90	104	120	136	150	161	169	175	180	−176	−173	−169	−166	−164	−162	−161	−160	−159	−158	−158	−157	−155
2.5	90	101	113	127	139	150	159	166	172	176	180	−174	−171	−168	−166	−164	−163	−161	−160	−160	−159	−157
3.0	90	99	109	120	131	141	150	158	164	169	173	180	−175	−172	−169	−167	−165	−164	−163	−162	−161	−158
3.5	90	98	106	115	125	134	142	150	157	162	167	174	180	−176	−173	−170	−168	−166	−165	−164	−163	−159
4.0	90	97	104	112	120	128	136	143	150	156	161	169	175	180	−176	−173	−171	−169	−167	−166	−165	−161
4.5	90	96	102	109	116	124	131	138	144	150	155	164	171	176	180	−177	−174	−172	−170	−168	−167	−162
5.0	90	95	101	107	113	120	127	133	139	145	150	159	166	172	176	180	−177	−174	−172	−171	−169	−164
6.0	90	94	99	104	109	114	120	126	131	136	141	150	158	164	169	173	177	180	−177	−175	−173	−167
7.0	90	94	98	102	106	111	115	120	125	129	134	142	150	157	162	167	171	174	177	180	−178	−170
8.0	90	93	97	100	104	108	112	116	120	124	128	136	143	150	156	161	165	169	172	175	178	−173
9.0	90	93	96	99	102	106	109	113	116	120	124	131	138	144	150	155	160	164	167	171	173	−177
10.0	90	93	95	98	101	104	107	110	113	117	120	127	133	139	145	150	155	159	163	166	169	180
11.0	90	92	95	97	100	103	105	108	111	114	117	123	129	135	140	145	150	154	158	162	165	177
12.0	90	92	94	97	99	101	104	106	109	112	114	120	126	131	136	141	146	150	154	158	161	173
13.0	90	92	94	96	98	100	103	105	107	110	112	117	123	128	133	137	142	146	150	154	157	170
14.0	90	92	94	96	98	100	102	104	106	108	111	115	120	125	129	134	138	142	146	150	153	167
15.0	90	92	93	95	97	99	101	103	105	107	109	113	118	122	127	131	135	139	143	147	150	164
20.0	90	91	93	94	95	97	98	99	101	102	104	107	110	113	117	120	123	127	130	133	136	150

Directions for using Tables F_1 and F_2 for determining the electrical axis:

1. Using amplitudes of deflections, calculate algebraic sum of positive and negative waves in lead I. If sum is positive, use Table F_1; if negative, use Table F_2.

2. Determine algebraic sum of positive and negative waves in lead III.

3. Plot values obtained under appropriate headings. Point of intersection of lead I and lead III columns gives electrical axis in degrees. Electrical axis is expressed as angle alpha and represents the angle (in degrees) subtended from the horizontal by QRS or P vector. Angles above horizontal are defined as negative, those below as positive, as seen in Figure 34 of the Appendix.

Definitions:

Normal axis is present when angle alpha lies between +90° and +30°.

Left axis deviation is present when angle alpha lies between +29° and −90°.

Marked left axis deviation is present when angle alpha lies between −30° and −90°.

Right axis deviation is present when angle alpha lies between +91° and −91°.

Marked right axis deviation is present when angle alpha lies beyond +180° (from −179° to −91°).

Superior axis is considered present when angle alpha lies in the region of −75° to −105°, that is, close to and on either side of −90°, or the most superior orientation.

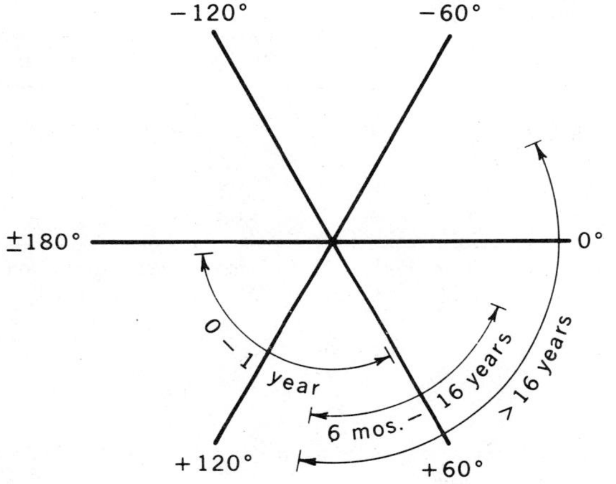

Figure 34. Location of the mean electrical axis of the QRS at different ages. (Reproduced by permission from Ferrer, M. I., *Electrocardiographic Notebook* [4th ed.]. Futura Publishing Company, Mt. Kisco, N.Y., 1973.)

Table G. *Normal Heart Rates in Children.*

Age (yr)	Normal Rate
Birth	110–150
2	85–125
4	75–115
6	65–105
Over 6	60–100

Reprinted by permission from Ferrer, M. I., *Electrocardiographic Notebook* (4th ed.). Futura Publishing Company, Mt. Kisco, N.Y., 1973.

Table H. *Q–T Intervals (Uncorrected for Rate) and QRS Duration in Normal Infants and Children.*

	Q–T (sec)	QRS (sec)
Age	Range	Range
0–1 week	.182–.355	.040–.082
1 week–1 month	.186–.300	.041–.080
1 month–3 months	.180–.346	.048–.080
3 months–6 months	.200–.360	.050–.085
6 months–1 year	.200–.320	.048–.084
1 year–3 years	.200–.340	.042–.086
3 years–5 years	.220–.368	.042–.090
5 years–8 years	.228–.372	.048–.092
8 years–12 years	.260–.400	.051–.098
12 years–16 years	.282–.422	.058–.100
16 years–20 years	.324–.420	.055–.110

Reprinted by permission from Ferrer, M. I., *Electrocardiographic Notebook* (4th ed.). Futura Publishing Company, Mt. Kisco, N.Y., 1973.

Index

Note: Italicized page numbers refer to illustrations.